Look & Cook: A step-by-step guide to healthy meals in family child care homes
by Partners in Nutrition and the Chef Marshall O'Brien Group

First edition

Publisher
Partners in Nutrition and the Chef Marshall O'Brien Group
855 Rice Street, Suite 200
St. Paul, MN 55117

ISBN: 978-0-9966293-1-7

Nutrition regulations, menu planning guidelines and food safety information from USDA Nutrition Standards for CACFP Meals and Snacks, 2016.

Editor & Project Manager - Bonnie McDermid, Wordsmith.Ink

Printed in the United States of America

Ordering Information

RedLeaf Press
10 Yorkton Court
St. Paul, MN 55117-1065

1-800-423-8309
www.RedLeafPress.org

LOOK & COOK

A step-by-step guide to healthy meals in family child care homes

By Partners in Nutrition and
the Chef Marshall O'Brien Group

Partners in Nutrition and the Chef Marshall O'Brien Group
St. Paul, Minnesota

Acknowledgements

This book is dedicated to the hard-working staff at Partners in Nutrition and the Chef Marshall O'Brien Group.

A special thank you to our families. None of this would be possible without you.

Table of Contents

Introduction

The foods children eat and how they eat during their first five years is critical in establishing lifelong eating habits. As Boyd Swinburn of the World Health Organization puts it, "the die is cast by the age of five."

The importance of the formative years in developing taste preferences means that nutrition initiatives should be focused on early care and education programs. For some children, waiting until they are in school to be introduced to fruits, vegetables and whole grains is too late.

We know that early care and education programs are not just miniature schools. We also know that there isn't a nutrition department at most of these programs. One person might be the nutrition department—and also the transportation department, enrollment coordinator, care provider and parent educator!

Look & Cook for Family Child Care Homes has two goals:

1. Make your life as an early care and education provider easy when it comes to meals
2. Get fresh, delicious, colorful foods on kids' plates

Look & Cook meets those goals by:

- Providing you with recipes for over 150 delicious meals that meet all CACFP regulations
- Giving you creative cycle menus for each season to follow or adapt
- Using only simple, affordable, familiar ingredients
- Limiting the number of ingredients
- Providing clear, easy-to-follow preparation instructions
- Sharing photos of recipe assembly instructions and the final product
- Calculating the portions for the USDA Child and Adult Care Food Program for each meal and snack

Children love fresh, delicious, colorful foods

It's time to let go of the myth that there are "kid" foods and "adult" foods. It's all food! And children appreciate fresh, delicious, colorful foods just as much as adults do. It's also important to remember that adults have incredible influence over the eating habits of young children; adults decide what goes on the menu, when meal times occur and are also role models for mealtime habits.

- In feeding young children, we encourage early care and education providers to:
- Plan menus that consider the taste preferences of children, but not at the expense of good nutrition
- Enjoy mealtimes with children whenever possible
- Serve meals and snacks family-style (in large serving bowls or platters that are passed around)
- Empower children to decide what and whether they will eat certain foods.
  Pressure leads to resistance. At mealtimes, your job is to simply provide a balanced meal and establish a pleasant environment.
- Resist the urge to become a short-order cook—the menu for the meal is the menu for the meal. Children may choose from the options available or may choose not to eat.

We hope you enjoy ***Look & Cook for Family Child Care Homes***.

Christine Twait MS, RDN, LDN
Executive Director, Partners in Nutrition

Chef Marshall O'Brien, CEO
Chef Marshall O'Brien Group

How to Use This Book

The two features in ***Look & Cook*** that will guide you to a successful, compliant meal program are the Cycle Menus and the "Grid."

Look & Cook Cycle Menus provide a complete, creditable meal plan that features different recipes every day in every cycle. They offer 16 weeks of lunches (4 weeks per season) and 8 weeks of breakfasts and snacks (2 weeks per season). At the end of each cycle, you simply start again at the beginning.

A few of the advantages of the *Look & Cook* cycle menus include:

- Less time spent planning menus
- Advance planning increases the likelihood that the menu will meet meal pattern requirements
- Repeated exposure to foods, which is important when introducing new foods to young children
- Reduced food cost from bulk purchasing and/or fewer last-minute trips to purchase missing menu items
- Simplified CACFP recordkeeping (for example, the ability to enter the names of food items in food production records ahead of time, or the ability to print a menu for the entire month ahead of time and reduce handwritten notes to menu substitutions)
- The Cycle Menus may be modified, although take extra care to ensure that the meal pattern requirements are being met. The best way to ensure this is to move entire meals and snacks around.

The "Grid" ensures creditable meals and snacks

At the bottom of each recipe, you will see a grid (or table). Under the recipe name is a crediting statement that indicates each meal component(s) that recipe counts toward. The Grid is your guide to a creditable meal; it lists each menu item and the correct portion to be served to each age group.

You may freely substitute fruits and vegetables and the meal will still qualify for CACFP reimbursement. However, be careful in adjusting portions of mixed dishes (those that satisfy multiple meal components) as the calculations for all components must be taken into consideration.

The Cycle Menus, the "Grid," and the recipes in ***Look & Cook*** were all designed to make a delicious, creditable meal program easier. We have done all the measurements, calculations and nutritional analysis—your job is to simply measure the recipe components carefully.

General Tips

Batch cooking - Cook once, eat twice! Several recipes in this book yield enough for two meals so you can freeze half for later. Go ahead and double or triple recipes that refrigerate or freeze well.

Grain/Bread - Serving sizes of grains/breads are given in ounces and, in most cases, by the piece. Weighing is the most accurate way to ensure adequate serving sizes. The USDA divides grain/bread items into different categories. Each category has a different weight that is equivalent to a "serving" of grain/bread. It is critical that programs reference FCS Instruction 783.1 Rev 2: Exhibit A Grains/Breads for the Food-Based Menu Planning in the Child Nutrition Programs when determining grain/bread serving sizes. This chart is in the Food Buying Guide for Grains/Bread.

Luncheon meats - Luncheon meats must be listed in the Food Buying Guide. They must not contain meat or poultry by-products, cereals, binders or extenders. They must have a Child Nutrition "CN" label or have a Product Formulation Statement.

Low-sodium foods - Whenever possible, choose low-sodium meats, sauces and soups.

Pasta - Each type of pasta has a different yield after cooking, so measure carefully to ensure adequate serving sizes. When substituting a different type of pasta, check the Food Buying Guide for the yield. Quantities are given in both ounces and cups, although weight is a more accurate measure.

Yogurt - The maximum amount of sugar allowed per 6 oz. of yogurt is 23 grams.

Cycle Menus - Summer

Breakfast / Snack					
Summer	Monday	Tuesday	Wednesday	Thursday	Friday
Week One Breakfast	Apple-Cinnamon Stuffed French Toast Milk	Sweet Strawberry Oatmeal Milk	Cinnamon Tortilla Chips Diced Berries Milk	Just Peachy Pancakes Peaches Milk	Golden Granola Bars Oranges Milk
Snack	Carrot Swirl Bites	Fresh Fruit Cone Milk	Veggie Kabobs	Sweet Bagel Chips Milk	Apple-Cinnamon Yogurt Granola
Week Two Breakfast	Vanilla French Toast Bananas Milk	Peachy Keen Muffins Pears Milk	Silver Dollar Griddlecakes Applesauce Milk	Strawberry Sunshine Bread Oranges Milk	Good Morning Granola Peaches Milk
Snack	Black Bean Hummus Corn Chips	Mini Bagel Cucumber Sandwiches	Pita Nachos	American Flag Toast	Crackerwiches

Lunch / Supper					
Summer	Monday	Tuesday	Wednesday	Thursday	Friday
Week One	Pizza Sandwich Melon Milk	Apple-Cheddar Ham Salad Cornbread Milk	Mexican Dip Tortilla Chips Pears Milk	Chicken Sandwich Cucumber Watermelon Milk	Pork Lettuce Wraps Breadsticks Grapes Milk
Week Two	California Burger Mixed Berries Milk	Taco Salad Wraps Apple Wedges Milk	Chicken Mozzarella Melt Sandwich Peas Peaches Milk	Honey Mustard Chicken Salad Crackers Mandarin Oranges Milk	Very Veggie Bagel Sandwich String Cheese Grapes Milk
Week Three	Humpty Dumpty Sandwich Celery Sticks Mandarin Oranges Milk	Chicken Pasta Primavera Pineapple Milk	Under the Sea Burgers Green Beans Apples Milk	Southwest Chicken Salad Breadsticks Tropical Fruit Milk	Asian Beef Stir-Fry Brown Rice Melon Milk
Week Four	Summer Veggie Rice Bowl String Cheese Strawberries Milk	Stuffed Zucchini Boats Rolls Oranges Milk	Sesame Chicken Brown Rice Pepper Strips Pineapple Milk	Black Bean Burger Watermelon Milk	Chicken Drumsticks Bread Spinach-Strawberry Salad Milk

Cycle Menus - Autumn

Breakfast / Snack					
Autumn	Monday	Tuesday	Wednesday	Thursday	Friday
Week One Breakfast	Pumpkin Pancakes Cinnamon Apple Chunks Milk	Gingerbread French Toast Bananas Milk	Veggie Omelet Mini Bagels Milk	Apple-Cinnamon Oatmeal Oranges Milk	Pumpkin Muffins Applesauce Milk
Snack	Pretzel Melts	Oatmeal Biscuits Milk	Autumn Apple Squares Milk	Cheesy Baked Broccoli Bites	Potato Nachos
Week Two Breakfast	Cinnamon Granola Pineapple Milk	Ham & Veggie Frittata Toast Grapes. Milk	Cinnamon Swirl Bread Applesauce Milk	Apple Muffins Peaches Milk	Pumpkin Bread Oranges Milk
Snack	Cream Cheese Bagel Butterflies Strawberries	Cheesy Zucchini Sticks Marinara Sauce, Milk	Corn Salsa Tortilla Chips	Lemon Fruit Dip Melon Chunks	Caramel Yogurt Dip Apple Slices

Lunch / Supper					
Autumn	Monday	Tuesday	Wednesday	Thursday	Friday
Week One	Black Bean Burritos Green Pepper Melon Milk	Cheddar-Ham Calzone Broccoli Grapes Milk	Lentil-Beef Meatloaf Rice Mixed Fruit Milk	Sweet & Spicy Glazed Ham Rolls Green Beans Apricots Milk	Quiche Spinach-Strawberry Salad Milk
Week Two	Vegetarian Taco Pizza Apricots Milk	Grilled Ham and Cheese Sandwich Tomato Soup Melon Milk	Chicken Caesar Pita Sandwich Mandarin Oranges Milk	Braised Turkey Wild Rice Peas Apricots Milk	Pork Lo Mein Grapes Milk
Week Three	Two-Bean Veggie Chili Cornbread Tropical Fruit Milk	Ham & Cheese Pasta Bake Peas Peaches Milk	Sweet & Sour Chicken Jicama Milk	Roast Turkey Breast Cranberry Sauce Potatoes, Rolls Pears Milk	Lentil Curry Rice Carrots Apples Milk
Week Four	Chicken Pot Pie Mandarin Oranges Milk	Vegetable Beef Soup Crackers Pears, Milk	Shredded Pork Taco Corn Milk	Club Sandwich Grapes Milk	Chicken-Broccoli Quesadilla Pears, Milk

Cycle Menus - Winter

Breakfast / Snack					
Winter	Monday	Tuesday	Wednesday	Thursday	Friday
Week One Breakfast	Cinnamon Pita Chips Fruit Salsa Milk	Breakfast Tostada Milk	Banana-Chocolate Chip Muffins Bananas Milk	Ham & Veggie Omelet Toast Milk	Banana-Stuffed French Toast Milk
Snack	Taco Cereal Trail Mix Milk	Tuna Stackers	Ham Pinwheels	Orange Bowl Fruit Dip Toast	Creamy Dreamy Whipped Fruit Toast
Week Two Breakfast	Banana Oatmeal Milk	French Toast Sticks Peaches Milk	English Muffin Egg Sandwich Oranges Milk	Gingerbread Muffins Applesauce Milk	Oatmeal Breakfast Treats Pears Milk
Snack	Raisin Energy Snacks Milk	Spinach Ranch Dip Wheat Crackers	Baked Apple Pretzel Boats	Polka Dot Twisters Milk	Fruity Toast Snacks

Lunch / Supper					
Winter	Monday	Tuesday	Wednesday	Thursday	Friday
Week One	Veggie Lasagna Mixed Fruit Milk	Cheese Enchiladas Corn Tropical Fruit Milk	Three-Bean Turkey Chili Breadsticks Pears Milk	Fish Tacos Tropical Fruit Milk	BBQ Chicken Breast Rolls Green Beans Peaches Milk
Week Two	Vegetable Minestrone Crackers Melon Milk	Grilled Tuna Salad Sandwich Baked Beans Mandarin Oranges Milk	Chicken Chow Mein Rice Pineapple Milk	Pork Roast Rolls Peas Apricots Milk	Orange Chicken Rice Pepper Strips Bananas Milk
Week Three	Cheesy Penne with Broccoli Mandarin Oranges Milk	Shredded Beef Sandwich Romaine Salad Peaches Milk	Easy Chicken & Rice Green Beans Oranges Milk	White Chicken Chili Biscuits Melon Milk	Pork Stir-Fry Rice Pineapple Milk
Week Four	Squash Soup Crackerwiches Pears Milk	Beef Burritos Lettuce Grapes Milk	Hot Chicken Pita Sandwich Lettuce & Tomato Pears, Milk	Meatball Subs Marinara Sauce Sweet Potatoes Milk	Pizza Soup Breadsticks Peaches Milk

Cycle Menus - Spring

Breakfast / Snack

Spring	Monday	Tuesday	Wednesday	Thursday	Friday
Week One Breakfast	Jam Muffins Melon Milk	Breakfast Burritos Milk	Strawberry-Stuffed French Toast Milk	Carrot Cake Baked Oatmeal Grapes Milk	Breakfast Quesadillas Milk
Snack	Mini Fruit Pizza	Breadsticks Marinara Sauce Grapes	Broccoli and Cheese Quesadillas	Pretzel Sticks Nectarines	Apple Pie Bites
Week Two Breakfast	Peach Oatmeal Milk	Cinnamon Muffins Applesauce Milk	English Muffin Breakfast Pizza Milk	Banana Pancakes Bananas Milk	Strawberry Muffins Strawberries Milk
Snack	Cinnamon Yogurt Dip Apple Slices	Veggie Pita Pizza	Applesauce-Bran Muffins Milk	Carrot Dip Wheat Crackers	Fruity Dippers Raisin Toast

Lunch / Supper

Spring	Monday	Tuesday	Wednesday	Thursday	Friday
Week One	Broccoli-Cheddar Baked Potatoes Roll Oranges Milk	Pork Fried Rice Pineapple Milk	Chicken-Cheddar Melt Peas Peaches Milk	Beef Stroganoff Green Beans Apple Slices Milk	Quiche Cups Bread Peaches Milk
Week Two	Hummus Wraps Grapes Milk	Chicken Alfredo Mandarin Oranges Milk	On Top of Spaghetti Marinara Sauce Green Beans Milk	Barbeque Sandwich Lettuce Peaches Milk	Parmesan Chicken Noodles Peas Pears Milk
Week Three	Primo Pasta Salad Melon Milk	Hot Ham & Cheese Sandwich Cucumbers Grapes, Milk	Chicken Fajitas Oranges Milk	Tuna Casserole Peaches Milk	Jambalaya Pears Milk
Week Four	Mexican Beans & Rice Celery Mandarin Oranges Milk	Potato & Corn Chowder Roast Beef Sandwich Tropical Fruit Milk	Chinese Beef & Broccoli Rice Peaches Milk	Fiesta Chicken Pasta Corn Oranges Milk	Honey Mustard Turkey Melt Romaine Salad Watermelon Milk

New Meal Patterns

New Nutrition Guidelines for Healthier Children

"Through the Healthy, Hunger-Free Kids Act, championed by the First Lady and signed by President Obama, USDA made the first major changes in the CACFP [Child and Adult Care Food Program] meals and snacks since the Program's inception in 1968, which will help ensure children and adults have access to healthy, balanced meals and snacks throughout the day. The new CACFP nutrition standards will help safeguard the health of children early in their lives and improve the wellness of adults.

Under the new CACFP nutrition standards, meals and snacks served will include a greater variety of vegetables and fruit, more whole grains, and less added sugar and saturated fat. In addition, the standards encourage breast feeding and better align the CACFP with the Special Supplemental Nutrition Program for Women, Infants, and Children (WIC) and with other Child Nutrition Programs.

The new standards for meals and snacks served in the CACFP are based on the Dietary Guidelines for Americans, science-based recommendations made by the National Academy of Medicine, cost and practical considerations, and stakeholder's input. These improvements are expected to enhance the quality of meals served in CACFP to help young children learn healthy eating habits early on in their lives and improve the wellness of adult participants."

CACFP Meal Pattern Requirements for children ages 1 through 12	
Breakfast	Milk, fluid Juice (fruit or vegetable), or fruit(s) or vegetable(s) Grain/Bread
Lunch / Supper	Milk, fluid Meat or meat alternate Vegetable and/or fruit (at least two) Grain/Bread
Snack	*Choose 2 components* Milk, fluid Juice (fruit or vegetable), or fruit(s) or vegetable(s) Grain/Bread Meat or meat alternate *At snack, if serving milk do not serve juice as the second component.*

Acceptable Substitutions & New Requirements

Fruits & Vegetables - The new CACFP meal pattern separates the fruit and vegetable components. That means programs can serve a fruit and a vegetable at snack and it will credit for reimbursement. At lunches and suppers, program operators have the option to serve 1) one fruit and one vegetable or 2) two different vegetables. Lunches and suppers with two fruits and no vegetables do not qualify for reimbursement.

One Whole Grain-Rich Food Per Day: - The new meal pattern requires that programs serve a whole grain-rich food at least once per day. A whole grain-rich food is defined at 51% whole grain by weight. The majority of the recipes in *Look & Cook* qualify as whole grain-rich.

Meeting Grains Requirement at Breakfast - Meat and meat alternates may be used to meet the entire grains requirement a maximum of three times a week. One ounce of meat/meat alternate is equal to one ounce equivalent of grains.

Beans - Beans (legumes) are special foods because they can credit toward the meat/meat alternate component or the vegetable components. Programs can always substitute beans for meat; there is no limit on the number of times per week beans can be served in place of meat. However, be careful because beans (legumes) can be either a meat alternate OR a vegetable in a meal, but never both in the same meal.

Child Meal Pattern - Breakfast

Breakfast Select all three components for a reimbursable meal				
Food Component & Food Items[1]	**Ages 1-2**	**Ages 3-5**	**Ages 6-11**	**Ages 13-18**[2*]
Fluid Milk[3]	4 fluid ounces	6 fluid ounces	8 fluid ounces	8 fluid ounces
Vegetables, fruits, or portions of both[4]	1/4 cup	1/2 cup	1/2 cup	1/2 cup
Grains (oz eq)[5,6,7]				
Whole grain-rich or enriched bread	1/2 slice	1/2 slice	1 slice	1 slice
Whole grain-rich or enriched bread product, such as biscuit, roll or muffin	1/2 serving	1/2 serving	1 serving	1 serving
Whole grain-rich, enriched or fortified cooked breakfast cereal,[8] cereal grain, and/or pasta	1/4 cup	1/4 cup	1/2 cup	1/2 cup
Whole grain-rich, enriched or fortified ready-to-eat breakfast cereal (dry, cold)[8,9]				
Flakes or rounds	1/2 cup	1/2 cup	1 cup	1 cup
Puffed cereal	3/4 cup	3/4 cup	1-1/4 cups	1-1/4 cups
Granola	1/8 cup	1/8 cup	1/4 cup	1/4 cup

*at-risk after school programs and emergency shelters

Breakfast Footnotes

[1] Must serve all three components for a reimbursable meal. Offer versus serve is an option for only adult and at-risk after school participants.

[2] Larger portion sizes than specified may need to be served to children 13 through 18 years old to meet their nutritional needs.

[3] Must be unflavored whole milk for children age one. Must be unflavored low-fat (1 percent) or unflavored fat-free (skim) milk for children two through five years old. Must be unflavored low-fat (1 percent), unflavored fat-free (skim), or flavored fat-free (skim) milk for children six years old and older and adults.

[4] Pasteurized full-strength juice may only be used to meet the vegetable or fruit requirement at one meal, including snack, per day.

[5] At least one serving per day, across all eating occasions, must be whole grain-rich. Grain-based desserts do not count towards meeting the grains requirement.

[6] Meat and meat alternates may be used to meet the entire grains requirement a maximum of three times a week. One ounce of meat and meat alternates is equal to one ounce equivalent of grains.

[7] Beginning October 1, 2019, ounce equivalents are used to determine the quantity of creditable grains.

[8] Breakfast cereals must contain no more than 6 grams of sugar per dry ounce (no more than 21 grams sucrose and other sugars per 100 grams of dry cereal).

[9] Beginning October 1, 2019, the minimum serving size specified in this section for ready-to-eat breakfast cereals must be served. Until October 1, 2019, the minimum serving size for any type of ready-to-eat breakfast cereals is ¼ cup for children ages 1-2; 1/3 cup for children ages 3-5; ¾ cup for children 6-12; and 1½ cups for adults.

Child Meal Pattern - Lunch

Lunch / Supper Select all five components for a reimbursable meal				
Food Component & Food Items[1]	**Ages 1-2**	**Ages 3-5**	**Ages 6-11**	**Ages 13-18**[2*]
Fluid Milk[3]	4 fluid ounces	6 fluid ounces	8 fluid ounces	8 fluid ounces
Meat/meat alternates				
Lean meat, poultry, or fish	1 ounce	1-1/2 ounces	2 ounces	2 ounces
Tofu, soy product, or alternate protein products[4]	1 ounce	1-1/2 ounce	2 ounces	2 ounces
Cheese	1 ounce	1-1/2 ounce	2 ounces	2 ounces
Large egg	1/2	3/4	1	1
Cooked dry beans or peas	1/4 cup	3/8 cup	1/2 cup	1/2 cup
Peanut butter or soy nut butter or other nut or seed butters	2 tablespoons	3 tablespoons	4 tablespoons	4 tablespoons
Yogurt, plain or flavored unsweet-ened or sweetened[5]	4 ounces or 1/2 cup	6 ounces or 3/4 cup	8 ounces or 1 cup	8 ounces or 1 cup
The following may be used to meet no more than 50% of the require-ment: Peanuts, soy nuts, tree nuts, or seeds, as listed in program guidance, or an equivalent quantity of any combination of the above meat/meat alternates (1 oz. of nuts/seeds = 1 ounce of cooked lean meat, poultry, or fish)	½ ounce = 50%	¾ ounce = 50%	1 ounce = 50%	1 ounce = 50%
Vegetables[6]	1/8 cup	1/4 cup	1/2 cup	1/2 cup
Fruits[6,7]	1/8 cup	1/4 cup	1/4 cup	1/4 cup
Grains (oz eq)[8,9]				
Whole grain-rich or enriched bread	1/2 slice	1/2 slice	1 slice	1 slice
Whole grain-rich or enriched bread product, such as biscuit, roll or muffin	1/2 serving	1/2 serving	1 serving	1 serving
Whole grain-rich, enriched or fortified cooked breakfast cereal,[10] cereal grain, and/or pasta	1/4 cup	1/4 cup	1/2 cup	1/2 cup

Lunch/Supper Footnotes

[1] Must serve all five components for a reimbursable meal. Offer versus serve is an option for only adult and at-risk after school participants.

[2] Larger portion sizes than specified may need to be served to children 13 through 18 years old to meet their nutritional needs.

[3] Must be unflavored whole milk for children age one. Must be unflavored low-fat (1 percent) or unflavored fat-free (skim) milk for children two through five years old. Must be unflavored low-fat (1 percent), unflavored fat-free (skim), or flavored fat-free (skim) milk for children six years old and older and adults.

[4] Alternate protein products must meet the requirements in Appendix A to Part 226.

[5] Yogurt must contain no more than 23 grams of total sugars per 6 ounces.

[6] Pasteurized full-strength juice may only be used to meet the vegetable or fruit requirement at one meal, including snack, per day.

[7] A vegetable may be used to meet the entire fruit requirement. When two vegetables are served at lunch or supper, two different kinds of vegetables must be served.

[8] At least one serving per day, across all eating occasions, must be whole grain-rich. Grain-based desserts do not count towards the grains requirement.

[9] Beginning October 1, 2019, ounce equivalents are used to determine the quantity of the creditable grain.

[10] Breakfast cereals must contain no more than 6 grams of sugar per dry ounce (no more than 21 grams sucrose and other sugars per 100 grams of dry cereal).

*at-risk after school programs and emergency shelters

United State Department of Agriculture. Nutrition Standards for CACFP Meals and Snacks. Retrieved from http://www.fns.usda.gov/cacfp/meals-and-snacks

Child Meal Pattern - Snack

Snack Select two of the five components for a reimbursable snack				
Food Component & Food Items[1]	**Ages 1-2**	**Ages 3-5**	**Ages 6-11**	**Ages 13-18**[2*]
Fluid Milk[3]	4 fluid ounces	6 fluid ounces	8 fluid ounces	8 fluid ounces
Meat/meat alternates				
Lean meat, poultry, or fish	1/2 ounce	1/2 ounce	1 ounce	1 ounce
Tofu, soy product, or alternate protein products[4]	1/2 ounce	1/2 ounce	1 ounce	1 ounce
Cheese	1/2 ounce	1 1/2 ounce	1 ounce	1 ounce
Large egg	1/2	1/2	1/2	1/2
Cooked dry beans or peas	1/8 cup	1/8 cup	1/4 cup	1/4 cup
Peanut butter or soy nut butter or other nut or seed butters	1 tablespoon	1 tablespoon	2 tablespoons	2 tablespoons
Yogurt, plain or flavored unsweetened or sweetened[5]	2 ounces or 1/4 cup	2 ounces or 1/4 cup	4 ounces or 1/2 cup	4 ounces or 1/2 cup
Peanuts, soy nuts, tree nuts, or seeds	1/2 ounce	1/2 ounce	1 ounce	1 ounce
Vegetables[6]	1/2 cup	1/2 cup	3/4 cup	3/4 cup
Fruits[6]	1/2 cup	1/2 cup	3/4 cup	3/4 cup
Grains (oz eq)[7,8]				
Whole grain-rich or enriched bread	1/2 slice	1/2 slice	1 slice	1 slice
Whole grain-rich or enriched bread product, such as biscuit, roll or muffin	1/2 serving	1/2 serving	1 serving	1 serving
Whole grain-rich, enriched or fortified cooked breakfast cereal,[9] cereal grain, and/or pasta	1/4 cup	1/4 cup	1/2 cup	1/2 cup
Whole grain-rich, enriched or fortified ready-to-eat breakfast cereal (dry, cold)[9,10]				
Flakes or rounds	1/2 cup	1/2 cup	1 cup	1 cup
Puffed cereal	3/4 cup	3/4 cup	1-1/4 cups	1-1/4 cups
Granola	1/8 cup	1/8 cup	1/4 cup	1/4 cup

Snack Footnotes

[1] Select two of the five components for a reimbursable snack. Only one of the two components may be a beverage.

[2] Larger portion sizes than specified may need to be served to children 13 through 18 years old to meet their nutritional needs.

[3] Must be unflavored whole milk for children age one. Must be unflavored low-fat (1 percent) or unflavored fat-free (skim) milk for children two through five years old. Must be unflavored low-fat (1 percent), unflavored fat-free (skim), or flavored fat-free (skim) milk for children six years old and older and adults.

[4] Alternate protein products must meet the requirements in Appendix A to Part 226.

[5] Yogurt must contain no more than 23 grams of total sugars per 6 ounces.

[6] Pasteurized full-strength juice may only be used to meet the vegetable or fruit requirement at one meal, including snack, per day.

[7] At least one serving per day, across all eating occasions, must be whole grain-rich. Grain-based desserts do not count towards meeting the grains requirement.

[8] Beginning October 1, 2019, ounce equivalents are used to determine the quantity of creditable grains.

[9] Breakfast cereals must contain no more than 6 grams of sugar per dry ounce (no more than 21 grams sucrose and other sugars per 100 grams of dry cereal).

[10] Beginning October 1, 2019, the minimum serving sizes specified in this section for ready-to-eat breakfast cereals must be served. Until October 1, 2019, the minimum serving size for any type of ready-to-eat breakfast cereals is ¼ cup for children ages 1-2; 1/3 cup for children ages 3-5; ¾ cup for children 6-12; and 1½ cups for adults.

*at-risk after school programs and emergency shelters

United State Department of Agriculture. Nutrition Standards for CACFP Meals and Snacks. Retrieved from http://www.fns.usda.gov/cacfp/meals-and-snacks

Food Safety

Safe Minimum Cooking Temperatures			
Category	**Food**	**Temperature** (degrees F)	**Rest Time**
Ground Meat & Meat Mixtures	Beef, Pork, Veal, Lamb	160	None
	Turkey, Chicken	165	None
Fresh Beef, Veal, Lamb	Steaks, Roasts, Chops	145	3 minutes
Poultry	Chicken & Turkey, whole	165	None
	Poultry breasts, roasts	165	None
	Poultry thighs, legs, wings	165	None
	Duck & Goose	165	None
	Stuffing (cooked alone or in bird)	165	None
Pork & Ham	Fresh pork	145	3 minutes
	Fresh ham (raw)	145	3 minutes
	Precooked ham (no reheat)	140	None
Eggs & Egg Dishes	Eggs (cook until yolk and whites are firm)		None
	Egg dishes	160	None
Leftovers & Casseroles	Leftovers	165	None
	Casseroles	165	None
Seafood	Fin Fish (cook to 145 degrees or until flesh is opaque and separates easily with a fork)		None

FoodSafety.gov. Safe Minimum Cooking Temperatures. Retrieved from https://www.foodsafety.gov/keep/charts/mintemp.html

Choking Hazards	
Choking Hazards - The following foods, if served whole or in chunks, are considered choking hazards. Use these simple changes to make them safe options. Be sure all foods are cut into bite-size pieces (no larger than 1/2"), steamed or mashed. Encourage children to chew completely before swallowing to ensure safety. Some foods cannot be safely altered, so it's recommended they not be served at all.	
Food	**Action Step**
Nuts & Seeds†	Chop finely
Hot dogs†	Cut in quarters lengthwise, then cut into smaller pieces
Whole grapes	Cut in half lengthwise, then cut into smaller pieces
Chunks of meat or cheese	Chop finely
Hard chunks of fruit, like apples	Chop finely, cut into thin strips, steam, mash or purée
Raw vegetables	Chop finely, cut into thin strips, steam, mash or purée
Peanut butter†	Spread thinly on crackers or mix with applesauce and cinnamon and spread thinly on bread. Use only creamy style, not chunky.
Dried fruits, vegetables, popcorn*	Do not serve
Note - Tree nuts, peanuts and nut butters are excellent sources of protein for growing children. They are reimbursable meat alternate options and are strongly encouraged if feasible for your center. If your center is nut-free, the nuts listed in this book's recipes are optional.	
*Foods that are not reimbursable. †Foods that are not reimbursable for infants under 1 year old.	

Allergy Warning	
Food Allergies	**Action Steps**
Because food allergies are common in children, it is important to be aware of the ingredients in all foods before serving. The eight most common allergens are milk, eggs, peanuts, tree nuts, fish, shellfish, soy and wheat.	Be sure to speak with all parents/guardians about children's food allergies. If a child has a food allergy, a doctor's note must be kept on file stating the allergy and any appropriate substitutions. If allergies are severe, ask for a list of foods the child is able to eat.

USDA. CACFP Menu Planning Guide, page 5.
Retrieved from http://dpi.wi.gov/fns/cacfpwellness.html

Child Nutrition Labels

Child Nutrition (CN) Labels

A voluntary component of the Federal labeling program for the Child Nutrition Programs. Provides a warranty for CN-labeled products for auditing purposes if the product is used according to manufacturer's directions as printed on the approved CN label. Allows manufacturers to state a product's contribution to the meal pattern requirements on their labels.

What Products are Eligible for CN Labels?

Main dish products that contribute at least ½ ounce to the meat/meat alternate component of the meal pattern requirements. Examples include, but are not limited to, beef patties, cheese or meat pizzas, meat or cheese and bean burritos, egg rolls, breaded fish, and chicken portions. Juice and juice products containing at least 50% full-strength juice by volume. This includes such products as frozen juice drink bars and sherbet. 100% juice products are NOT eligible for a CN label. Since 100% juice credits 1 fluid ounce per 1 fluid ounce, there is no need for a CN label.

How to Identify a CN Label

A CN label will always contain the following information: The CN logo, which is a distinct border. The meal pattern contribution statement. A unique six-digit product identification number (assigned by the USDA Agricultural Marketing Service) appearing in the upper right hand corner of the CN logo. The USDA/FNS authorization statement. The month and year of the original FNS Final Approval appearing at the end of the authorization statement. The remaining required label features: product name, inspection legend, ingredient statement, manufacturer's name, signature/address line and net weight.

For any CN-labeled product to be valid, the purchased product label must have the CN logo on it. A company may have a legitimate CN label approval, but unless the product is produced under inspection following all

CN requirements and the CN logo is part of the printed label on the purchased product, it is not a CN-labeled product and is not warranted by USDA. A valid CN logo will never be a separate sticker. Printing a fact sheet or manufacturer's statement from a website does not document that the CN-labeled product was purchased. In addition, a fact sheet or other manufacturer documentation is never authorized to have the CN logo on it. Proper documentation of a CN-labeled product is an actual label on the purchased product carton.

For a detailed explanation of CN Labeling Regulations for the CACFP, see 7 CFR Part 226, Appendix C or the FBG for CN programs, Appendix C. Program information is also available online at: http://www.fns.usda.gov/cnlabeling/child-nutrition-cn-labeling-program

Product Formulation Statement

(Previously called a Product Analysis Sheet) An information sheet obtained from the manufacturer with a detailed explanation of what the product actually contains and the amount of each ingredient by weight. We strongly recommend that it contain the original signature of an authorized company representative, not that of a sales representative.

A sample Product Formulation Statement for meat/meat alternate products and review checklist has been developed and is provided on pages 73-75 of the *Crediting Handbook of the CACFP*. Additional product formulation templates may be accessed online at: fns.usda.gov/cnd/cnlabeling/ foodmanufacturers.htm.

USDA. Crediting Handbook for the Child and Adult Care Food Program. Food & Nutrition Service. FNS-425. January 2014. Retrieved from http://www.fns.usda.gov/sites/default/files/CACFP_creditinghandbook.pdf

Breakfast

French Toast Master Recipe

Prep time - 10 minutes
Cook time - 15 minutes
Total time - 25 minutes

Bake in oven

Yield - 6 slices

Ingredients

2 eggs
½ cup milk
½ teaspoon vanilla extract
½ teaspoon ground cinnamon
6 slices whole grain bread, at least 1½ ounces each

Directions

1. Position rack at top of oven and preheat to 375 degrees. Line baking sheet with foil or parchment paper, or coat with cooking spray.
2. Whisk eggs, milk, vanilla and cinnamon in a wide, shallow bowl until well-combined.
3. Dip bread in egg mixture, moistening both sides.
4. Lay dipped bread on baking sheet, leaving a small space between slices.
5. Bake until golden brown, about 15 minutes. Rotate pan about halfway through the baking. French toast is done when a toothpick inserted into the center comes out clean.

Variations

Apple-Cinnamon Stuffed French Toast
Banana French Toast
French Toast Sticks
Gingerbread French Toast
Strawberry Stuffed French Toast
Vanilla French Toast

French Toast provides G/B at breakfast			
	Toddler	Pre-School	School Age
French Toast	1/2 oz. or 1/2 slice	1/2 oz. or 1/2 slice	1 oz. or 1 slice
Fruit	1/4 cup	1/2 cup	1/2 cup
Milk	1/2 cup	3/4 cup	1 cup

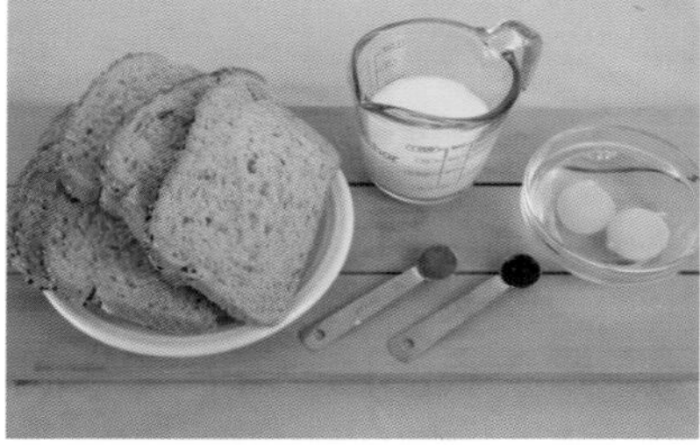

Ingredients

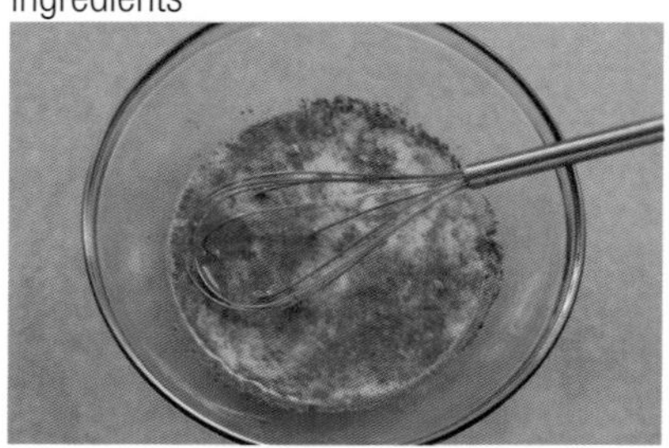

Step 2

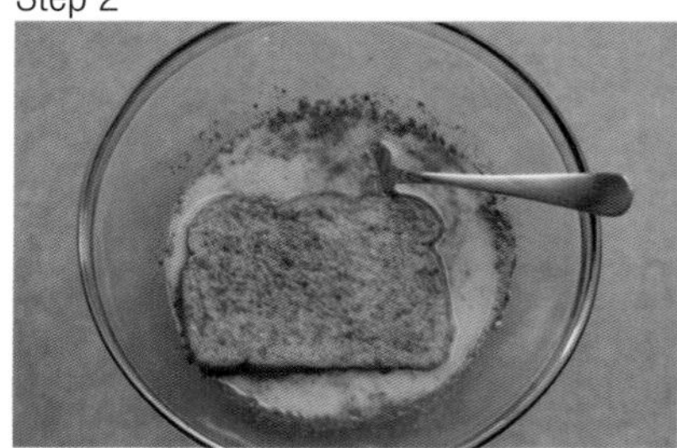

Step 3

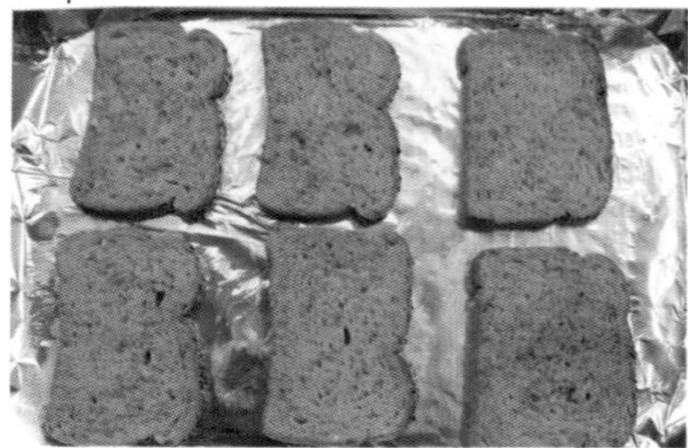

Step 4

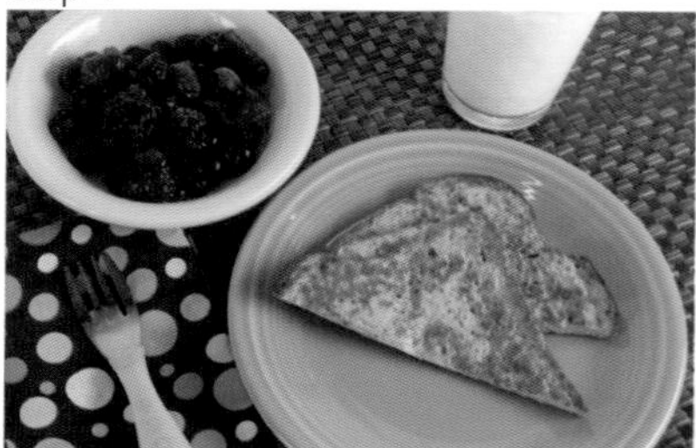

Creditable breakfast

Variations

French Toast Sticks

Use the same Master Recipe ingredients

Follow Master Recipe directions, plus add Step 6:
After baking, cut each slice of French toast into four sticks.

For a creditable breakfast, serve with peaches and milk.

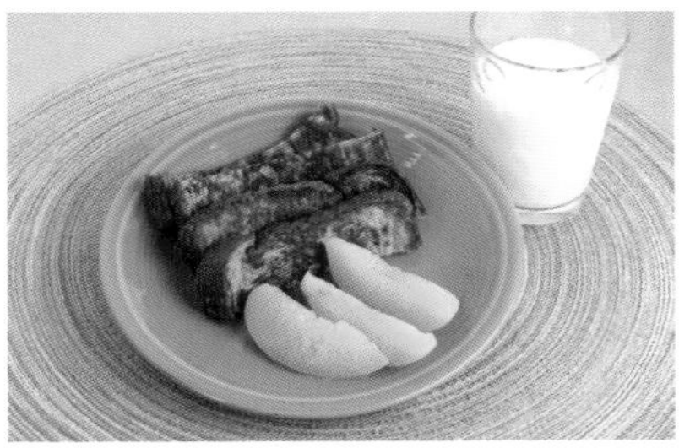
French Toast Sticks

Gingerbread French Toast

Add to the Master Recipe ingredients:
1 teaspoon molasses
½ teaspoon ground ginger

Follow Master Recipe directions, plus:
In Step 2, whisk the molasses and ginger with the eggs.

For a creditable breakfast, serve with bananas and milk.

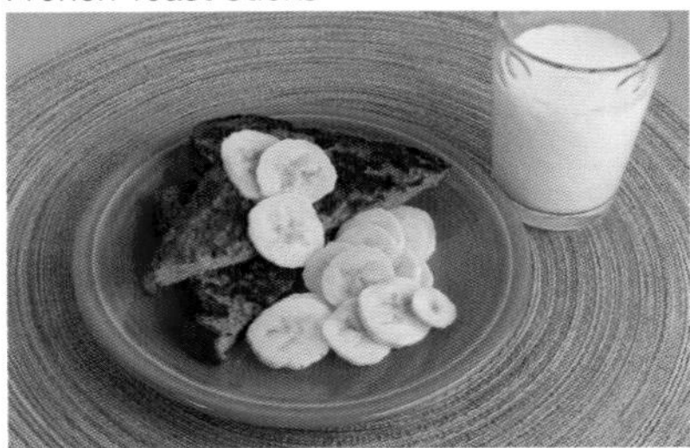
Gingerbread French Toast

Vanilla French Toast

Add to the Master Recipe ingredients:
¼ cup vanilla yogurt

Follow Master Recipe directions, plus:
In Step 2, whisk the yogurt with the eggs.

For a creditable breakfast, serve with bananas and milk.

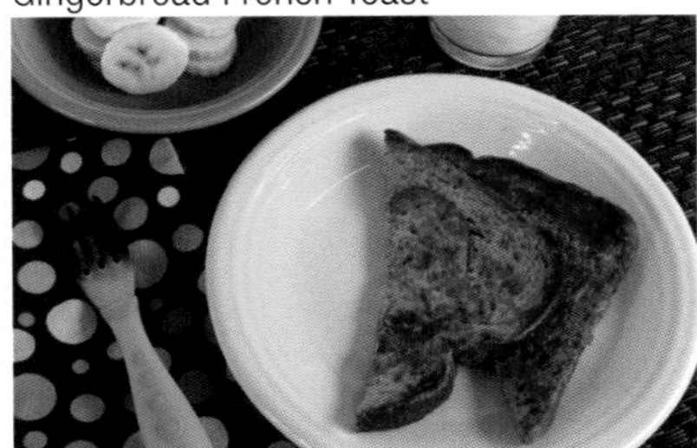
Vanilla French Toast

French Toast Variations
provide G/B at breakfast

	Toddler	Pre-School	School Age
French Toast	1/2 oz. or 1/2 slice	1/2 oz. or 1/2 slice	1 oz. or 1 slice
Fruit	1/4 cup	1/2 cup	1/2 cup
Milk	1/2 cup	3/4 cup	1 cup

Apple-Cinnamon Stuffed French Toast

Prep time - 15 minutes
Cook time - 30 minutes
Total time - 45 minutes

Bake in oven

Yield -
3 French toast sandwiches

Ingredients

2 tablespoons butter
5 cups apples, cored and diced
2 tablespoons brown sugar
¼ cup water
2 eggs
½ cup milk
½ teaspoon vanilla extract
½ teaspoon ground cinnamon
6 slices whole grain bread, at least 1½ ounces each

Directions

1. Preheat oven to 375 degrees. Line baking sheet with foil or parchment paper, or coat with cooking spray.
2. Heat butter in skillet over medium heat. Sauté apples and sugar, stirring frequently, about 5 minutes.
3. Add water, cover and reduce heat to medium-low. Cook apples until tender, 5-10 minutes; set aside.
4. Whisk eggs, milk, vanilla and cinnamon in a wide, shallow bowl until well combined.
5. Dip bread in egg mixture, moistening both sides.
6. Lay 3 slices of the dipped bread on baking sheet, leaving a small space between slices. Top each with one-third of the cooked apples, followed by another slice of dipped bread.
7. Bake until golden brown, 20-25 minutes. Rotate pan about halfway through baking. French toast is done when a toothpick inserted into the center comes out clean.

Apple-Cinnamon Stuffed French Toast
provides G/B and FR at breakfast

	Toddler	Pre-School	School Age
Stuffed French Toast	1/2 sandwich	1/2 sandwich	1 sandwich
Milk	1/2 cup	3/4 cup	1 cup

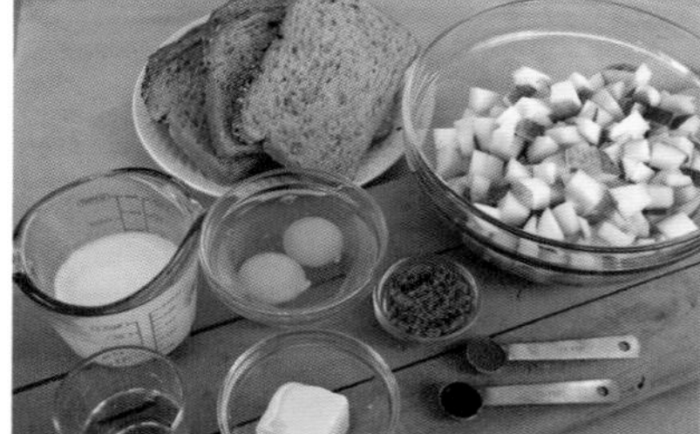

Ingredients

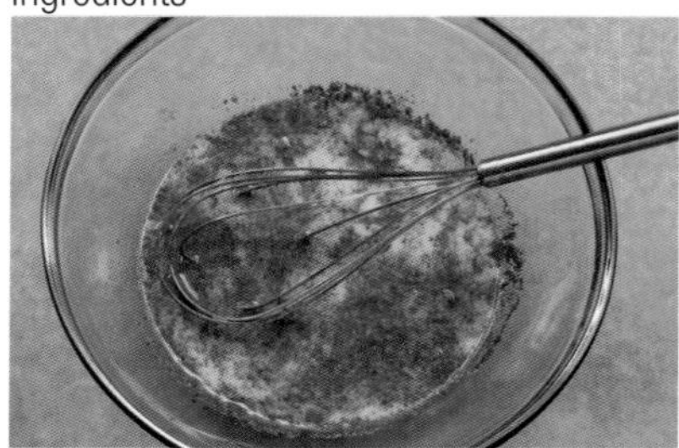

Step 1

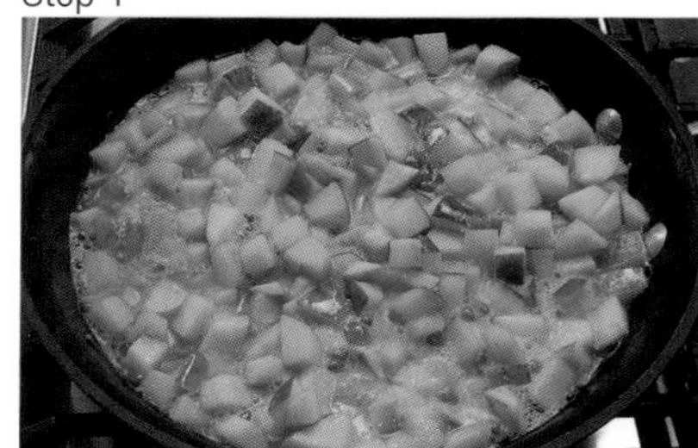

Step 2

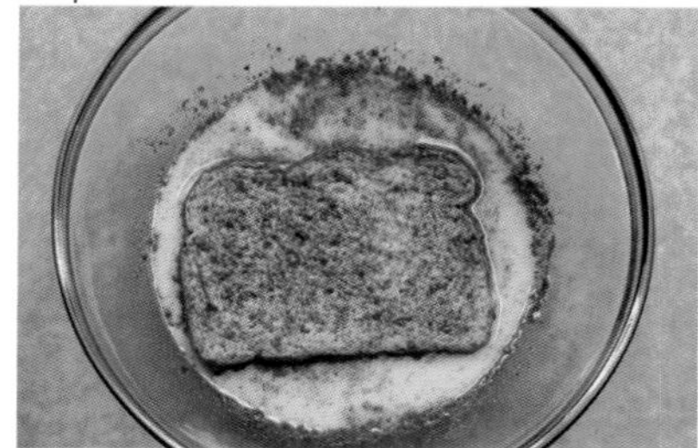

Step 3

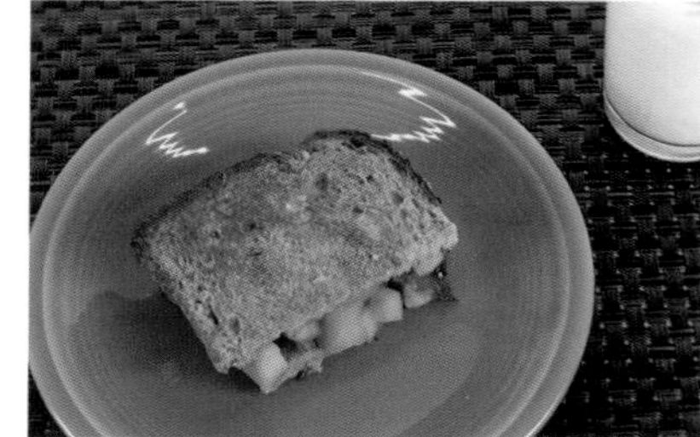

Creditable breakfast

Strawberry or Banana-Stuffed French Toast

Prep time - 15 minutes
Cook time - 25 minutes
Total time - 40 minutes

Bake in oven

Yield -
3 French toast sandwiches

Ingredients

2 tablespoons butter
2 tablespoons brown sugar
3 cups fresh or frozen strawberries or 3 cups bananas, sliced —if strawberries are frozen, thawed and drained
2 eggs
½ cup milk
½ teaspoon vanilla extract
½ teaspoon ground cinnamon
6 slices whole grain bread

Directions

1. Preheat oven to 375 degrees. Line baking sheet with parchment paper or foil, or coat with cooking spray.
2. In a mixing bowl, combine brown sugar with the strawberries or bananas; set aside.
3. Whisk eggs, milk, vanilla and cinnamon in a wide, shallow bowl until well combined.
4. Dip bread in egg mixture, moistening both sides.
5. Lay 3 slices of the dipped bread on baking sheet, leaving a small space between slices. Top each with one-third of the strawberries or bananas, followed by a slice of dipped bread.
6. Bake until golden brown, 25-30 minutes. Rotate pan about halfway through baking. French toast is done when a toothpick inserted into the center comes out clean.

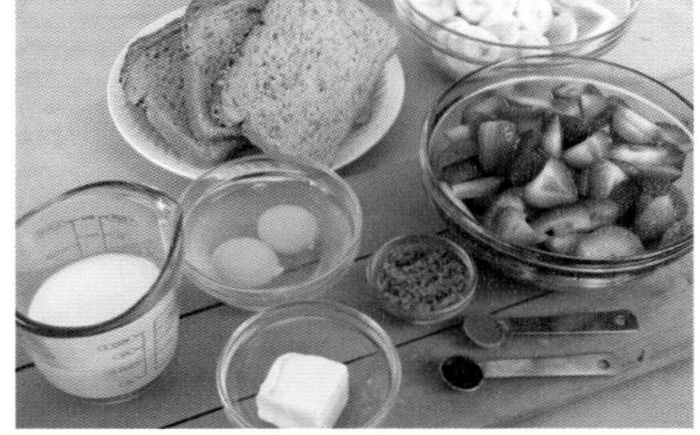
Ingredients

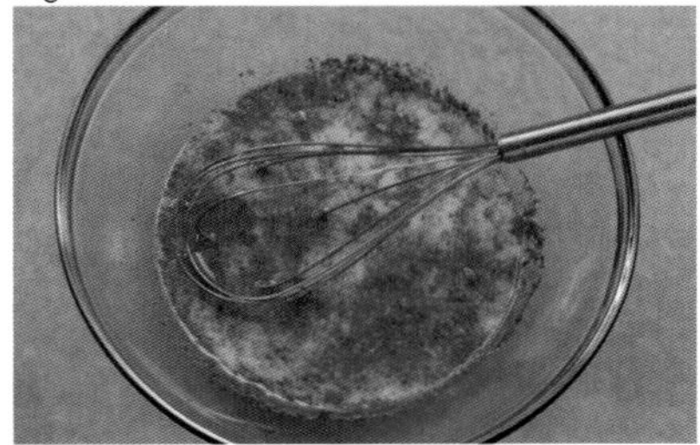
Step 2

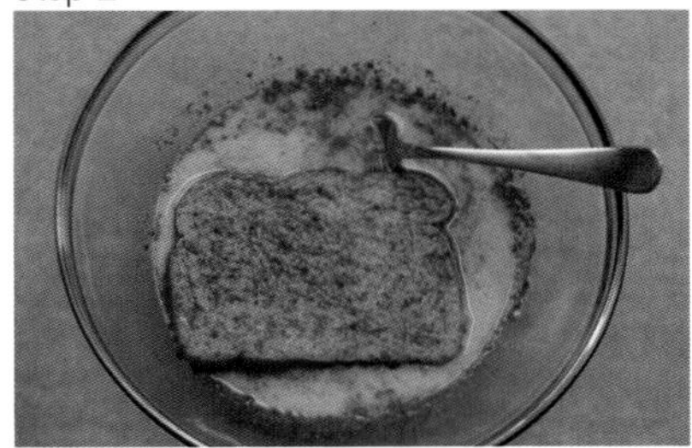
Step 4

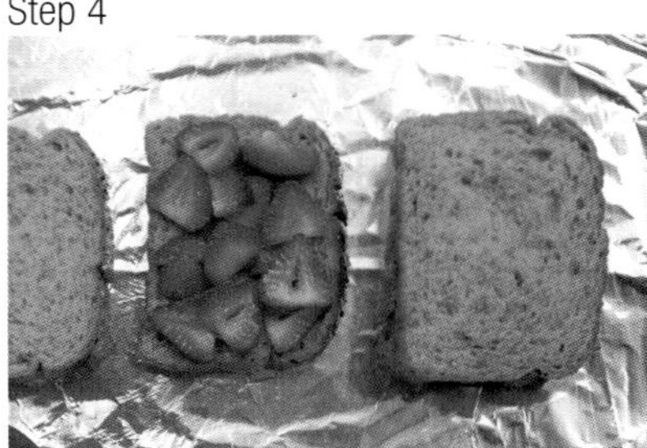
Step 5

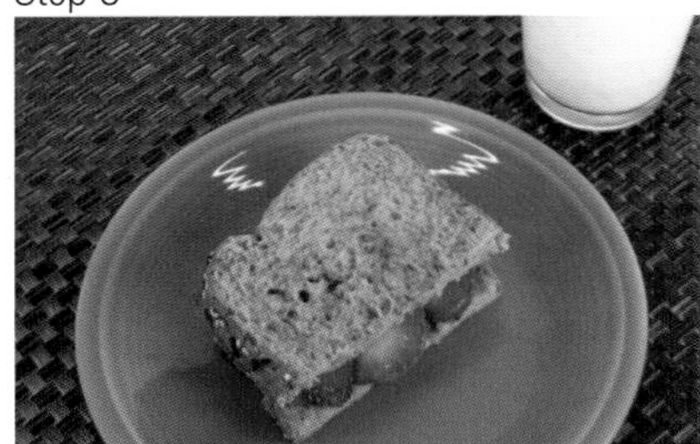
Creditable breakfast

Strawberry or Banana-Stuffed French Toast
provides G/B and FR at breakfast

	Toddler	Pre-School	School Age
Stuffed French Toast	1/2 sandwich	1/2 sandwich	1 sandwich
Milk	1/2 cup	3/4 cup	1 cup

Granola Master Recipe

Prep time - 10 minutes
Cook time - 30 minutes
Total time - 40 minutes

Bake in oven

Yield - 1 cup

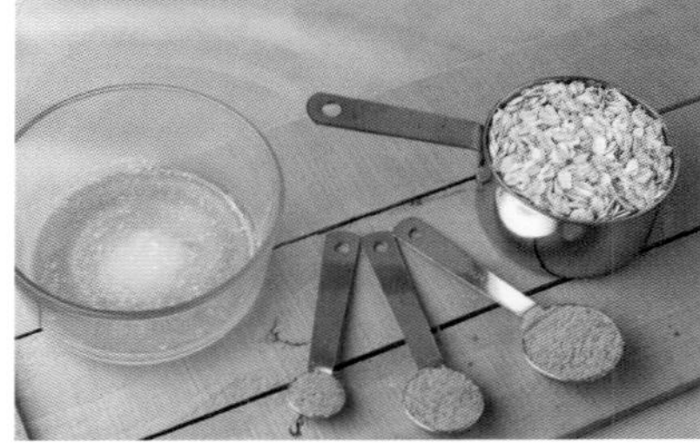
Ingredients

Ingredients

1 cup rolled oats

1½ tablespoons melted butter

1½ tablespoons brown sugar

Directions

1. Preheat oven to 350 degrees. Line a baking sheet with parchment paper or foil.
2. In a small bowl, combine the melted butter and brown sugar.
3. Put oats in a medium bowl. Pour the butter/sugar mixture over the oats and mix well.
4. Spread the granola in a single layer on baking sheet.
5. Bake for 30 minutes, stirring halfway through baking. Remove from oven and cool.

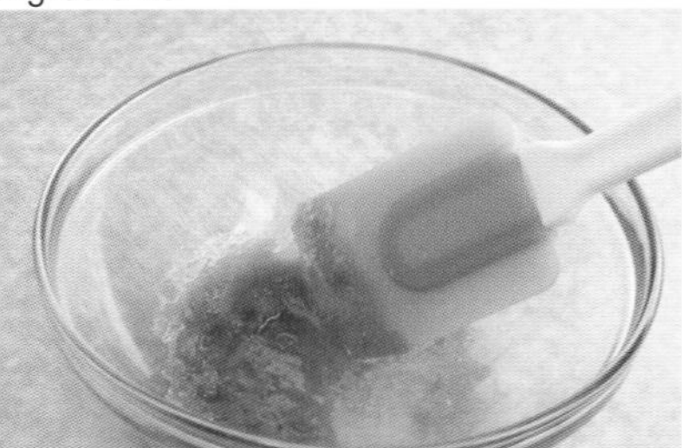
Step 2

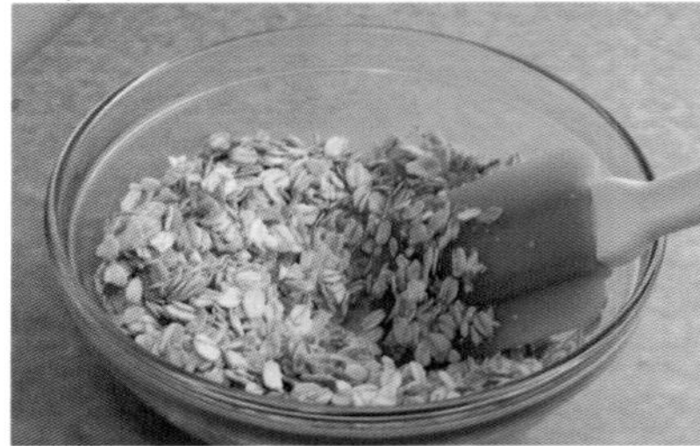
Step 3

Variations
Cinnamon Granola
Good Morning Granola
Ginger Granola
Golden Granola Bars

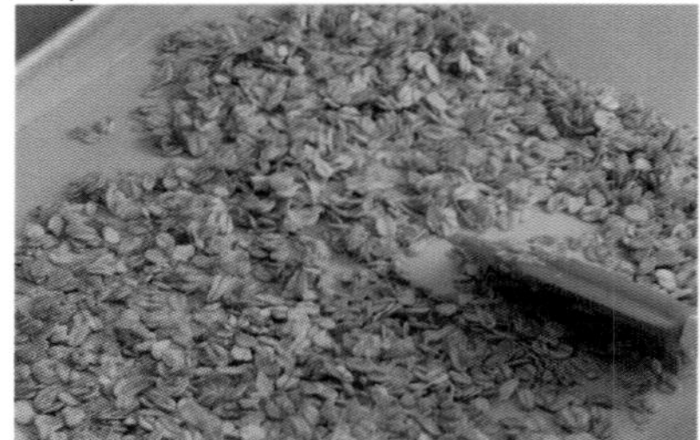
Step 4

Granola provides G/B at breakfast or snack			
	Toddler	Pre-School	School Age
Granola	1/2 oz. or 1/8 cup	1/2 oz. or 1/8 cup	1 oz. or 1/4 cup
Fruit	1/4 cup	1/2 cup	1/2 cup
Milk	1/2 cup	3/4 cup	1 cup

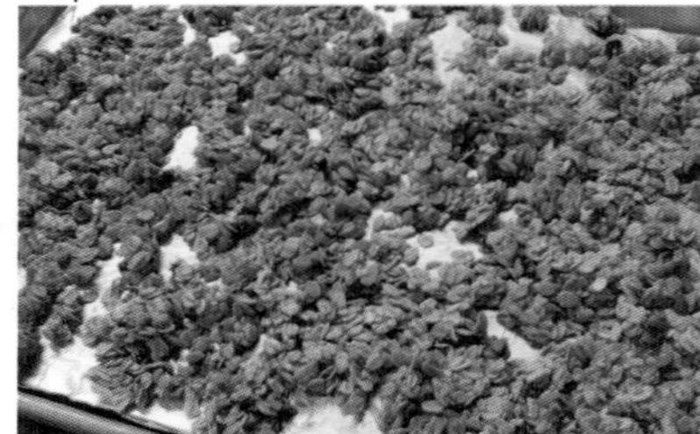
Step 5

Variations

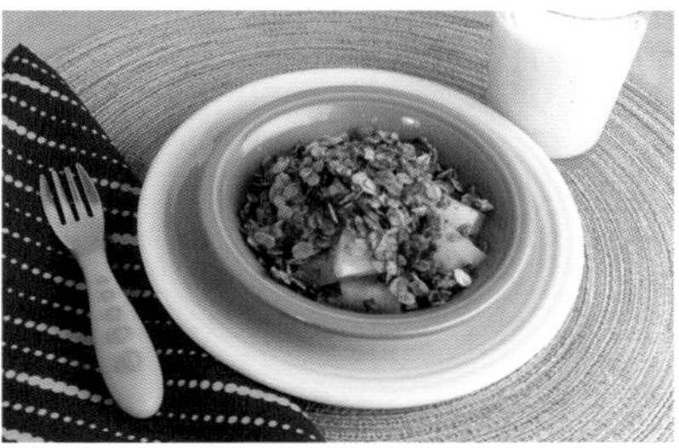
Cinnamon Granola

Cinnamon Granola

Add to the Master Recipe ingredients:
1½ teaspoons ground cinnamon

Follow Master Recipe directions, plus:
In Step 3, add the cinnamon to the butter and brown sugar.

For a creditable breakfast, serve with pineapple and milk.

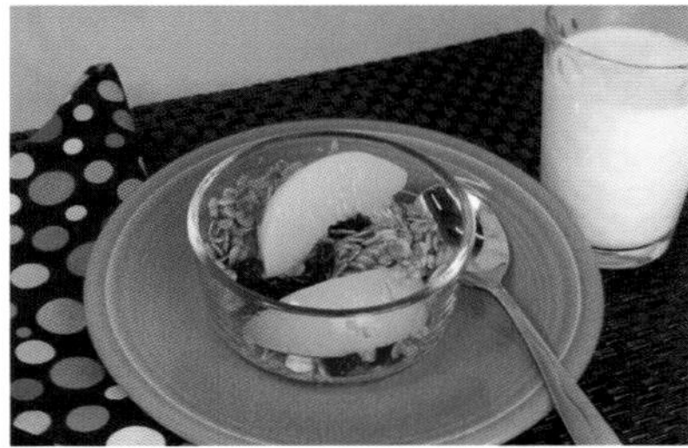
Good Morning Granola

Good Morning Granola

Add to the Master Recipe ingredients:
¼ cup raisins

Follow Master Recipe directions, plus add Step 6:
6. After baking, stir in the raisins.

For a creditable breakfast, serve with peaches and milk.

Granola Variations
provide G/B at breakfast or snack

	Toddler	Pre-School	School Age
Granola	1/2 oz. or 1/8 cup	1/2 oz. or 1/8 cup	1 oz. or 1/4 cup
Fruit	1/4 cup	1/2 cup	1/2 cup
Milk	1/2 cup	3/4 cup	1 cup

Tip *- The longer granola bakes, the crunchier it gets.*

Ginger Granola

Prep time - 10 minutes
Cook time - 30 minutes
Total time - 40 minutes

Bake in oven

Yield - 1¼ cups

Ingredients

1 cup rolled oats
¼ cup walnuts, chopped
¼ teaspoon ground ginger
¼ teaspoon ground cinnamon
2 tablespoons brown sugar
2 tablespoons melted butter
⅛ teaspoon salt

Directions

1. Preheat oven to 350 degrees. Line a baking sheet with parchment paper or foil.
2. In a medium bowl, thoroughly combine all the ingredients.
3. Spread the granola in a single layer on baking sheet.
4. Bake for 30 minutes, stirring halfway through baking. Remove from oven and cool.

Ginger Granola provides G/B at breakfast or snack			
	Toddler	Pre-School	School Age
Granola	1/2 oz. or 1/8 cup	1/2 oz. or 1/8 cup	1 oz. or 1/4 cup
Apples	1/4 cup	1/2 cup	1/2 cup
Milk	1/2 cup	3/4 cup	1 cup

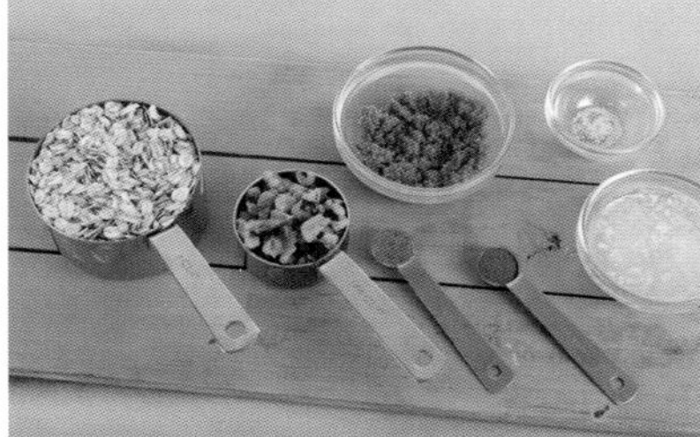

Ingredients

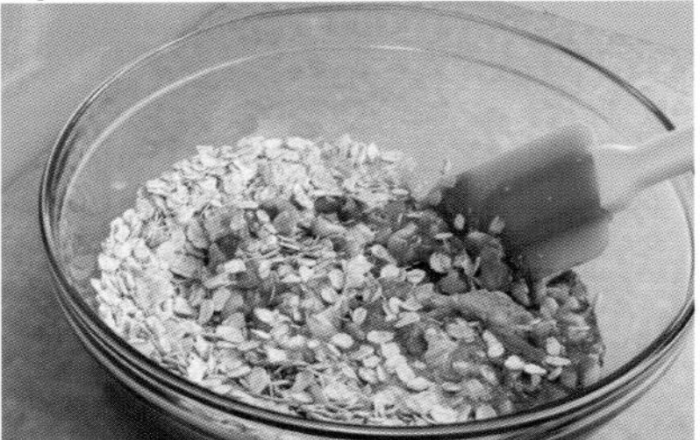

Step 2

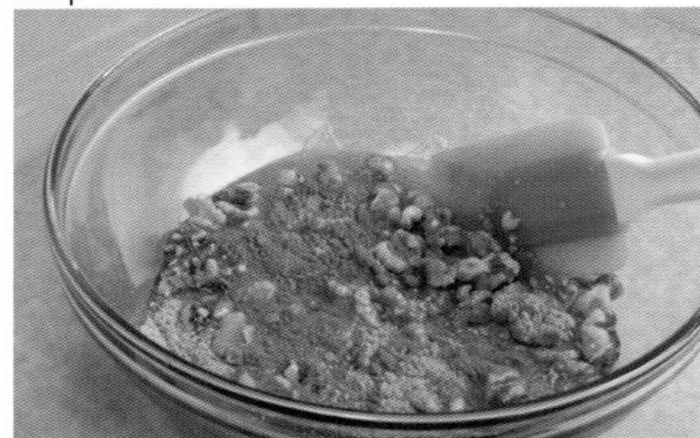

Step 2

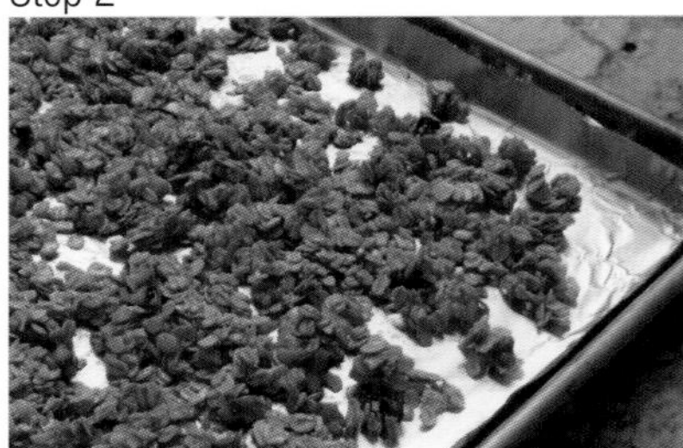

Step 3

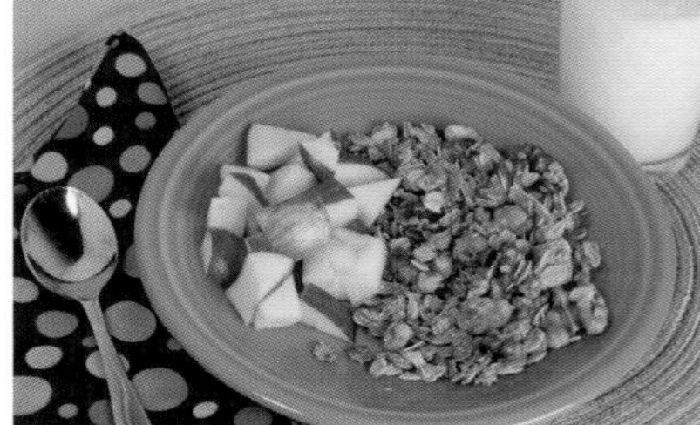

Creditable breakfast

Golden Granola Bars

Prep time - 15 minutes
Cook time - 20 minutes
Total time - 35 minutes

Bake in oven

Yield - 16 bars

Ingredients

¾ cup butter, softened
½ cup brown sugar, packed
2 teaspoons vanilla extract
1 egg
2 teaspoons ground cinnamon
4 cups quick-cooking oats
1 teaspoon baking powder

Directions

1. Preheat oven to 375 degrees. Line a 9x13-inch baking pan with foil or parchment paper.
2. In a medium bowl, cream the butter, sugar, vanilla and egg until fluffy.
3. In a separate bowl, combine the cinnamon, oats and baking powder. Add to the butter mixture and combine thoroughly.
4. Press mixture evenly into the lined baking pan.
5. Bake until lightly browned, about 20-25 minutes. Rotate pan about halfway through baking time.
6. Remove from oven and flatten bars again, using the bottom of a measuring cup or similar tool.
7. Cut into 16 pieces while hot, but let cool before removing from baking dish.

Golden Granola Bars provide G/B at breakfast			
	Toddler	Pre-School	School Age
Granola Bar	1/2 bar	1/2 bar	1 bar
Oranges	1/4 cup	1/2 cup	1/2 cup
Milk	1/2 cup	3/4 cup	1 cup

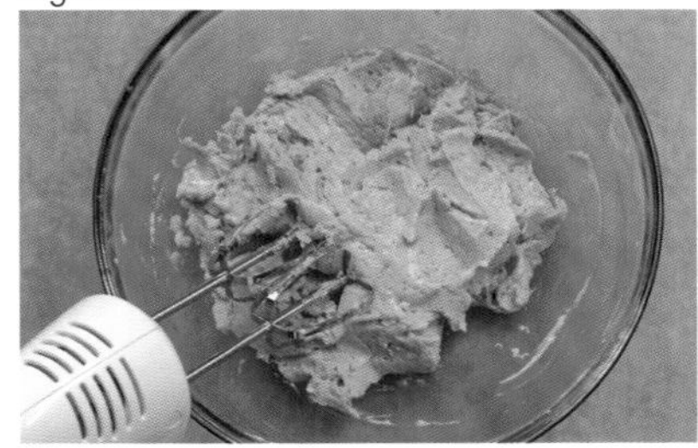

Ingredients

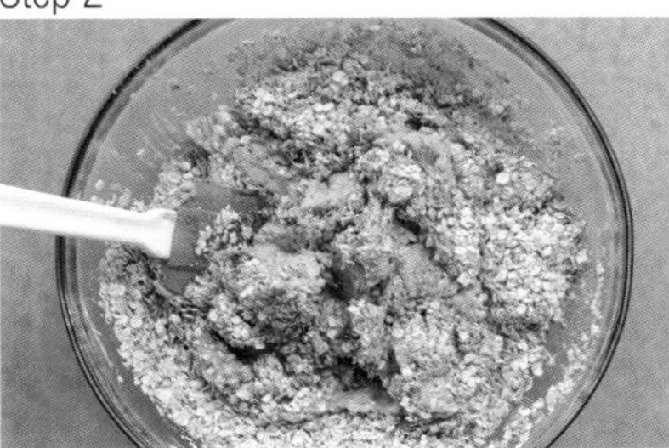

Step 2

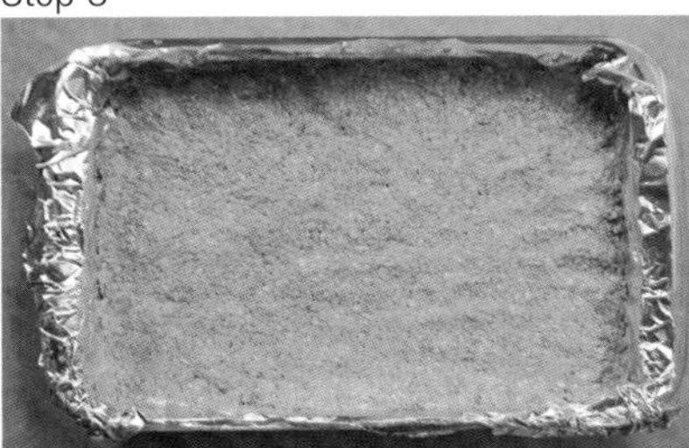

Step 3

Step 4

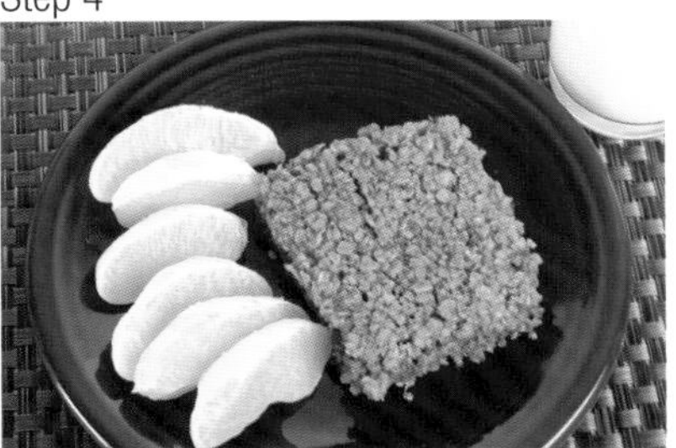

Creditable breakfast

Muffin Master Recipe

Prep time - 15 minutes
Cook time - 20 minutes
Total time - 35 minutes

Bake in oven

Yield -12 muffins

Ingredients

2 cups whole wheat flour
1 tablespoon baking powder
½ teaspoon salt
¼ cup sugar
1 egg
1 cup milk
¼ cup vegetable oil

Directions

1. Preheat oven to 375 degrees. Grease muffin pans or use paper liners.
2. In a bowl, mix the flour, baking powder, salt and sugar.
3. In another bowl, whisk together the egg, milk and oil.
4. Add the egg mixture to the flour mixture, stirring until flour is just moistened. Batter should be lumpy.
5. Spoon batter into the muffin cups, filling each two-thirds full. Bake for 20 to 25 minutes, until muffins spring back when lightly pressed.

Variations
Apple Muffins
Banana-Chocolate Chip Muffins
Cinnamon Muffins
Gingerbread Muffins
Jam Muffins
Peachy Keen Muffins
Pumpkin Muffins
Strawberry Muffins

Muffins provide G/B at breakfast			
	Toddler	Pre-School	School Age
Muffins	1/2 oz. or 1/2 muffin	1/2 oz. or 1/2 muffin	1 oz. or 1 muffin
Fruit	1/4 cup	1/2 cup	1/2 cup
Milk	1/2 cup	3/4 cup	1 cup

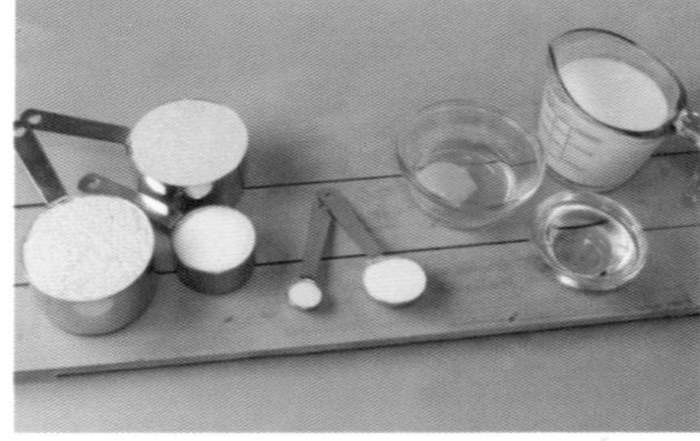
Ingredients

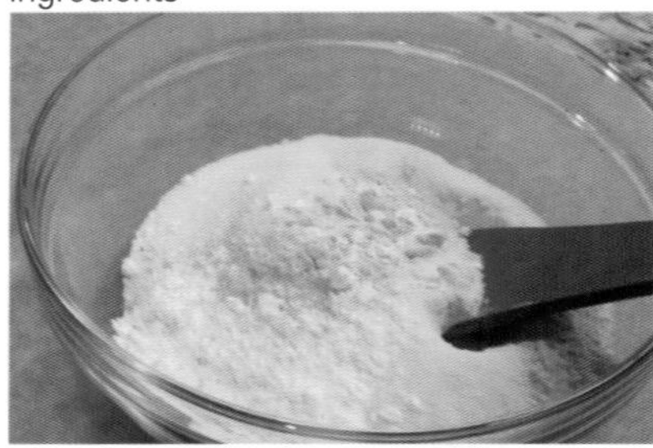
Step 2

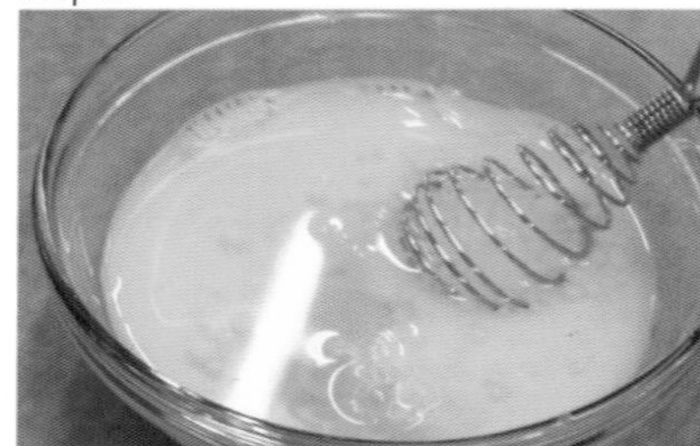
Step 3

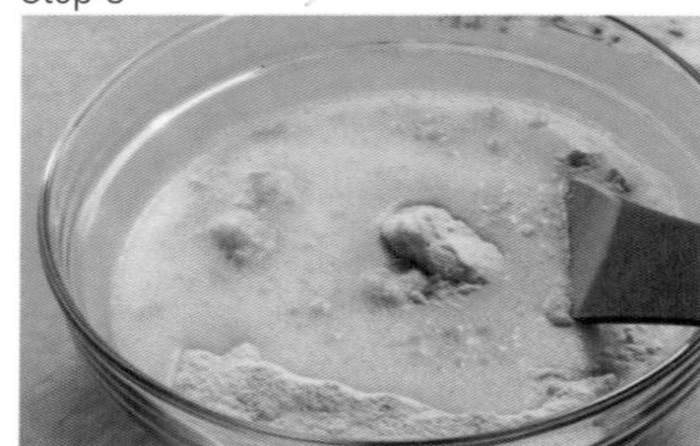
Step 4

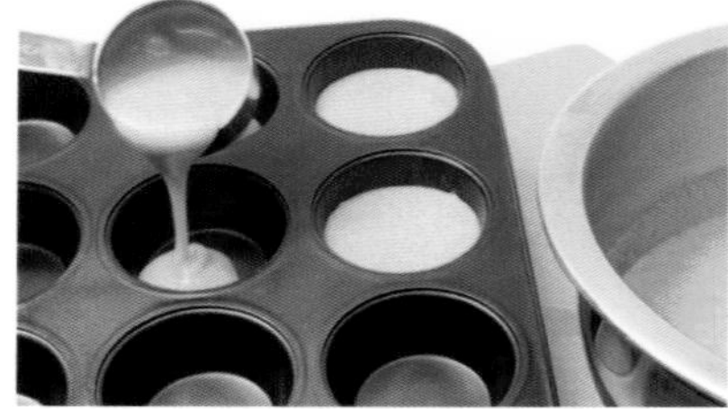
Step 5

Variations

Apple Muffins

Add to the Master Recipe ingredients:
1½ cups apples, finely chopped

Follow Master Recipe directions, plus:
In Step 3, whisk eggs, then stir in chopped apples.

For a creditable breakfast, serve with peaches and milk.

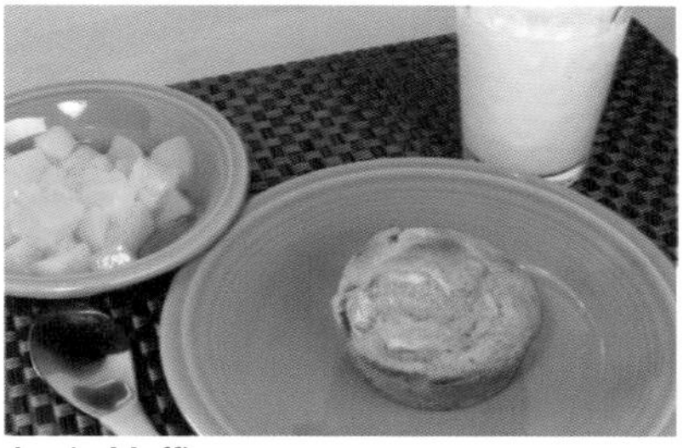
Apple Muffins

Banana-Chocolate Chip Muffins

Add to the Master Recipe ingredients:
1½ cups bananas, mashed
¼ cup mini chocolate chips

Follow Master Recipe directions, plus:
In Step 3, whisk eggs, then stir in bananas and chocolate chips.

For a creditable breakfast, serve with bananas and milk.

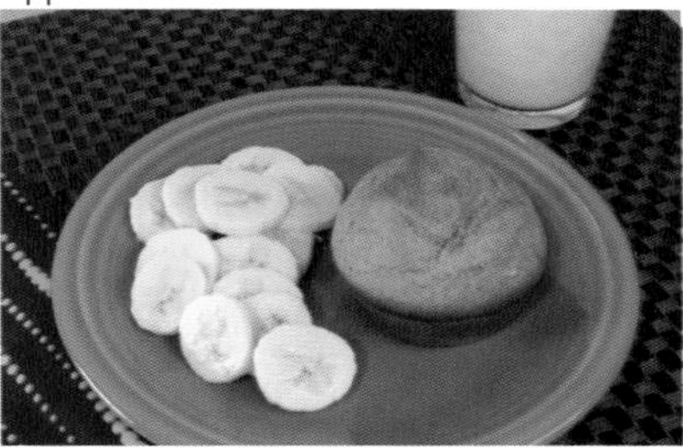
Banana Chocolate Chip Muffins

Cinnamon Muffins

Add to the Master Recipe ingredients:
1 teaspoon ground cinnamon

Follow Master Recipe directions, plus:
In Step 2, add cinnamon to dry ingredients.

For a creditable breakfast, serve with applesauce and milk.

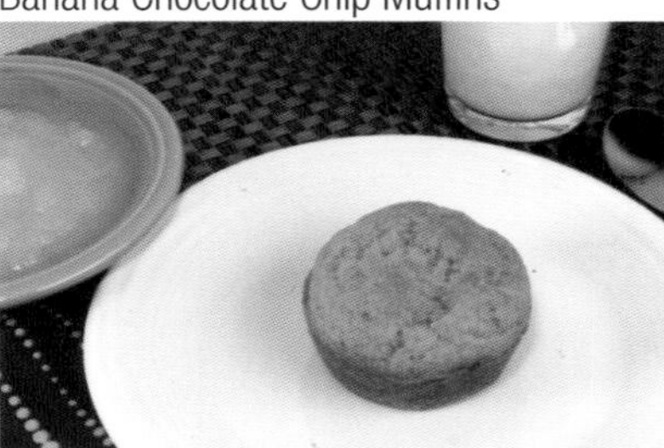
Cinnamon Muffins

Gingerbread Muffins

Add to the Master Recipe ingredients:
½ teapoon ground cinnamon
½ teaspoon ground ginger
2 teaspoons molasses
½ teaspoon vanilla extract

Follow Master Recipe directions, plus:
In Step 2, add cinnamon and ginger to the flour mixture.
In Step 3, whisk molasses and vanilla with the egg.

For a creditable breakfast, serve with applesauce and milk.

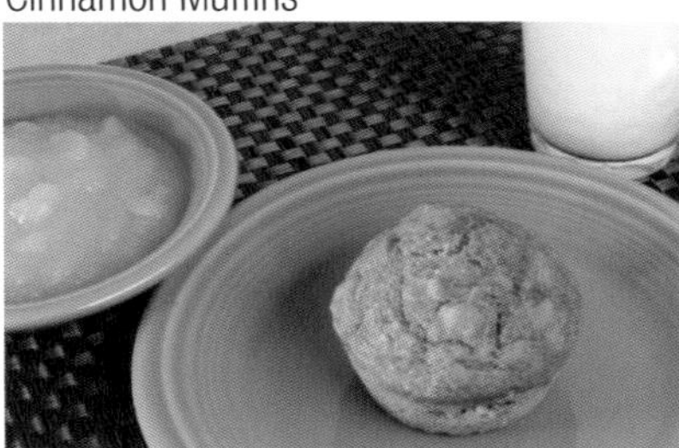
Gingerbread Muffins

Variations

Jam Muffins

Add to the Master Recipe ingredients:
½ cup jelly or jam, any flavor

Follow Master Recipe directions, plus:
In Step 3, add jam and whisk with the egg and milk.

For a creditable breakfast, serve with melon and milk.

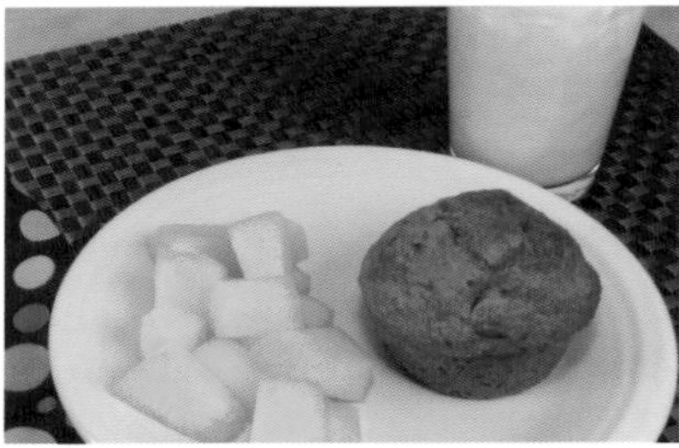
Jam Muffins

Peachy Keen Muffins

Add to the Master Recipe ingredients:
1½ cups peaches, finely chopped

Follow Master Recipe directions, plus:
In Step 3, whisk the egg and milk, then stir in peaches.

For a creditable breakfast, serve with pears and milk.

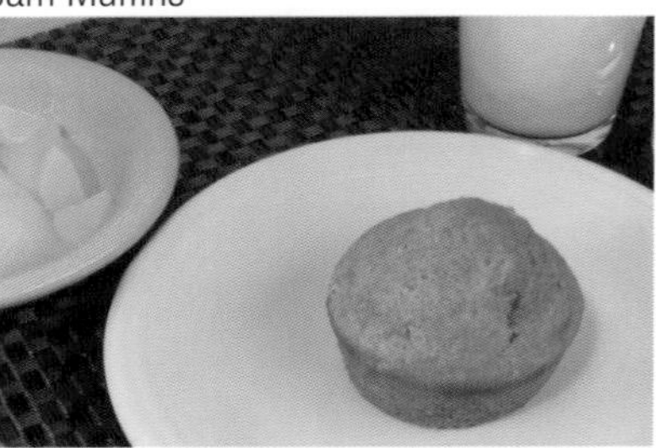
Peachy Keen Muffins

Pumpkin Muffins

Add to the Master Recipe ingredients:
½ teaspoon ground allspice
½ teaspoon ground cinnamon
½ cup canned pumpkin

Follow Master Recipe directions, plus:
In Step 2, add allspice and cinnamon to the flour mixture.
In Step 3, whisk the egg and milk, then stir in pumpkin.

For a creditable breakfast, serve with applesauce and milk.

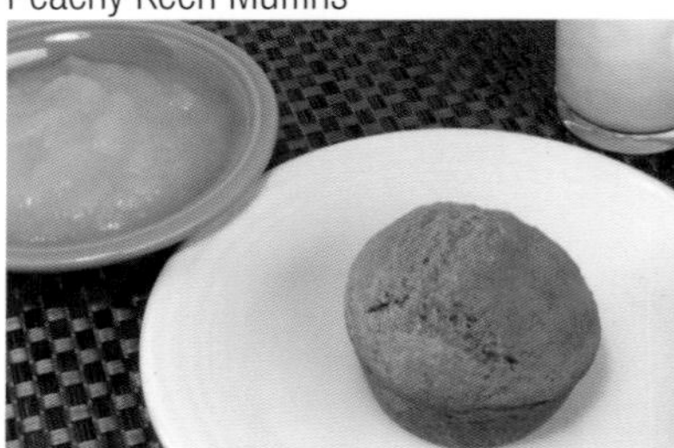
Pumpkin Muffins

Strawberry Muffins

Add to the Master Recipe ingredients:
½ cup strawberries, finely chopped

Follow Master Recipe directions, plus:
In Step 3, whisk the egg and milk, then stir in strawberries.

For a creditable breakfast, serve with strawberries and milk.

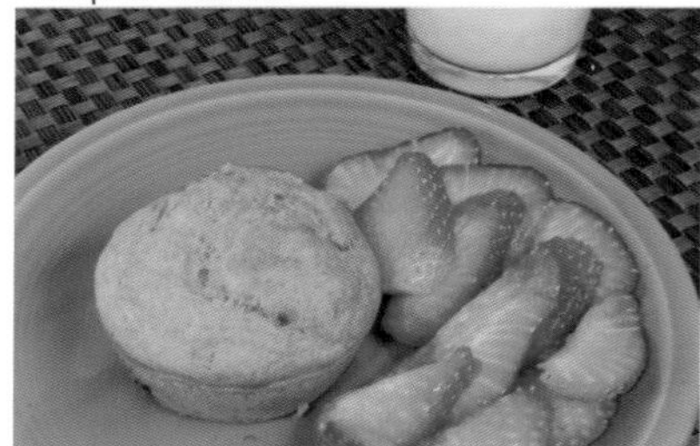
Strawberry Muffins

Oatmeal Master Recipe

Prep time - 15 minutes
Cook time - 10 minutes
Total time - 25 minutes

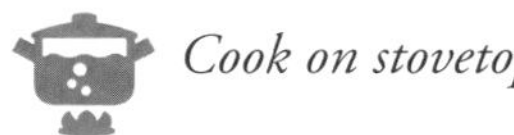

Cook on stovetop

Yield - 2 cups

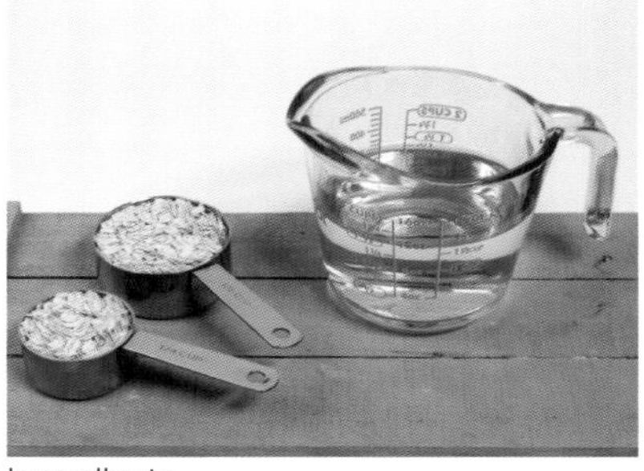

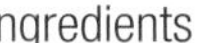

Ingredients

Ingredients

1½ cups water

1 cup rolled oats

Directions

1. In a medium saucepan, bring water to a boil.
2. Stir in oats.
3. Reduce heat and simmer, uncovered, for 10 minutes, stirring occasionally.
4. Remove pan from the heat. If desired, cover and let stand for 2 minutes before serving.
5. If adding fruit, after oatmeal is cooked, remove from heat and stir in fruit. Let sit for 2 minutes before serving to heat the fruit through.

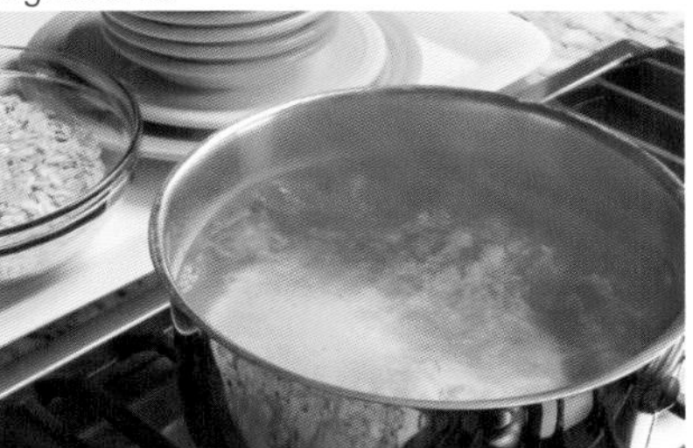

Step 1

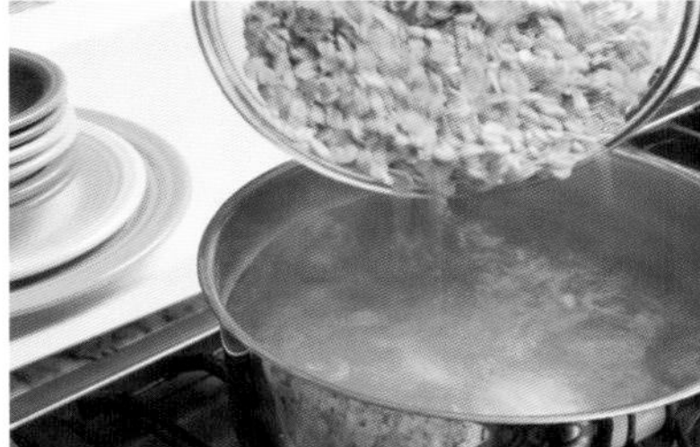

Step 2

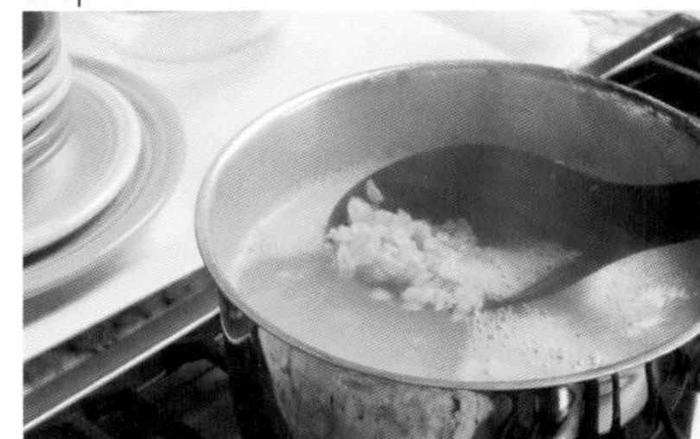

Step 3

Variations

Apple-Cinnamon Oatmeal
Banana Oatmeal
Peach Oatmeal
Sweet Strawberry Oatmeal

Tips: For creamier oatmeal, heat the water and oats together. For added nutrition, substitute milk for the water.

Oatmeal provides G/B at breakfast			
	Toddler	Pre-School	School Age
Oatmeal	1/4 cup	1/4 cup	1/2 cup
Fruit	1/4 cup	1/2 cup	1/2 cup
Milk	1/2 cup	3/4 cup	1 cup

Variations

Directions for all variations:

Follow Master Recipe directions, plus:

When oatmeal is cooked, remove from heat and stir in fruit and cinnamon. Allow to sit for 2 minutes before serving to heat the fruit through.

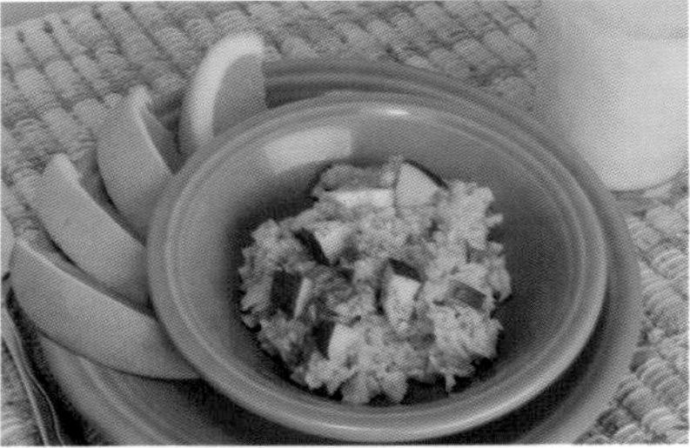
Apple-Cinnamon Oatmeal

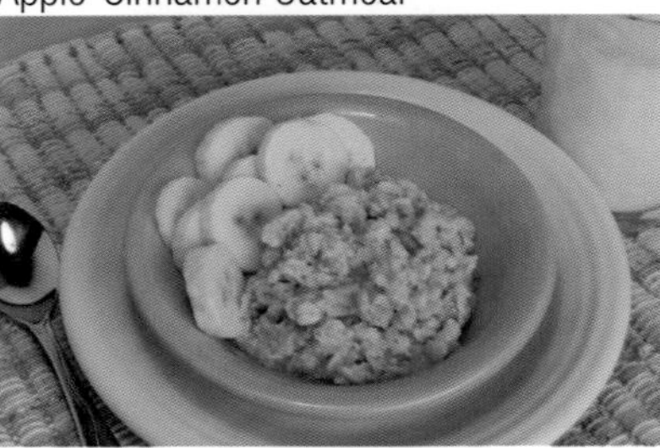
Banana Oatmeal

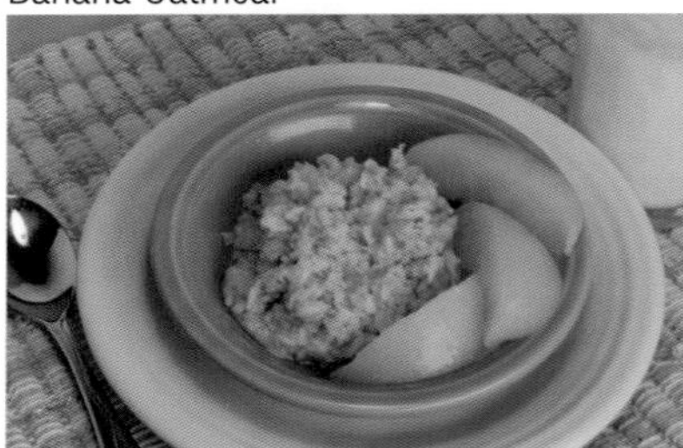
Peach Oatmeal

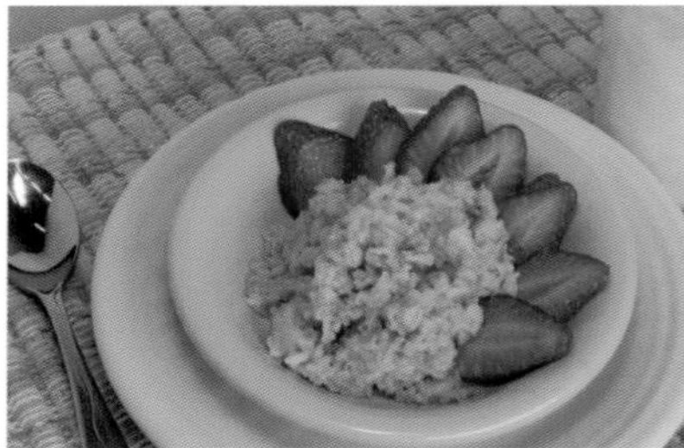
Sweet Strawberry Oatmeal

Apple-Cinnamon Oatmeal

Add to the Master Recipe ingredients:
3 cups apples, chopped small
1 teaspoon ground cinnamon

For a creditable breakfast, serve with oranges and milk.

Banana Oatmeal

Add to the Master Recipe ingredients:
3 cups bananas, sliced
1 teaspoon ground cinnamon

For a creditable breakfast, serve with milk.

Peach Oatmeal

Add to the Master Recipe ingredients:
3 cups peaches, drained and sliced
1 teaspoon ground cinnamon

For a creditable breakfast, serve with milk.

Sweet Strawberry Oatmeal

Add to the Master Recipe ingredients:
3 cups strawberries, sliced
1 teaspoon ground cinnamon

For a creditable breakfast, serve with milk.

Oatmeal Variations provide G/B at breakfast			
	Toddler	Pre-School	School Age
Oatmeal	1/4 cup	1/4 cup	1/2 cup
Fruit	1/4 cup	1/2 cup	1/2 cup
Milk	1/2 cup	3/4 cup	1 cup

Pancake Master Recipe

Prep time - 10 minutes
Cook time - 5 minutes
Total time - 15 minutes

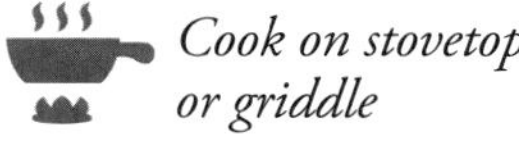

Cook on stovetop or griddle

Yield - 6 pancakes

Ingredients

¾ cup whole wheat flour
1 teaspoon baking powder
⅛ teaspoon salt
1 egg
¾ cup milk
Butter for pan, optional

Directions

1. In a bowl, mix together dry ingredients.
2. In separate bowl, whisk egg and milk until just mixed. Pour egg mixture into dry ingredients, stirring gently. Batter will be thick.
3. Heat a large skillet over medium heat or set griddle to medium. Add butter, as needed.
4. Pour ¼ cup batter per pancake into pan/griddle. Cook until bubbles form on top, about 2-3 minutes.
5. Carefully flip pancakes and cook until browned on the second side, 2-3 more minutes.
6. If making multiple batches of pancakes, hold the cooked pancakes in a warm oven until all are cooked.

Variations

Banana Pancakes
Just Peachy Pancakes
Pumpkin Pancakes
Silver Dollar Griddlecakes

Pancakes provide G/B at breakfast			
	Toddler	Pre-School	School Age
Pancakes	1/2 oz. or 1/2 pancake	1/2 oz. or 1/2 pancake	1 oz. or 1 pancake
Fruit	1/4 cup	1/2 cup	1/2 cup
Milk	1/2 cup	3/4 cup	1 cup

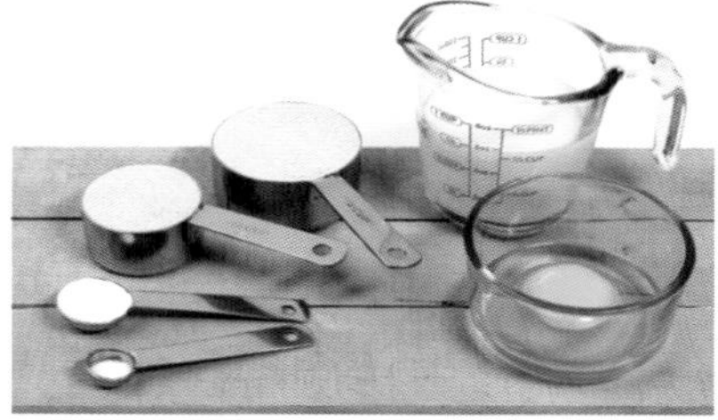

Ingredients

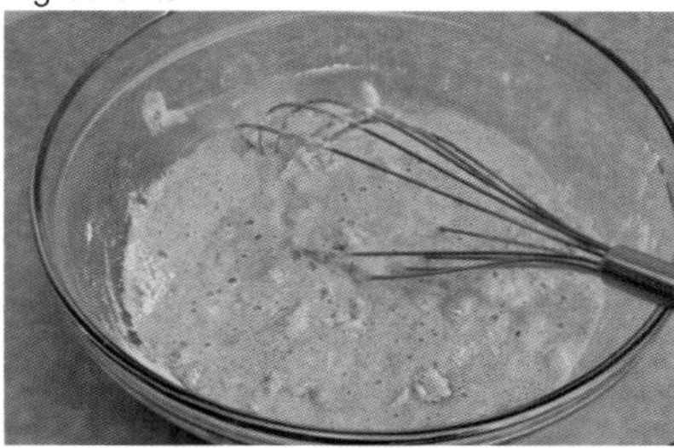

Step 2

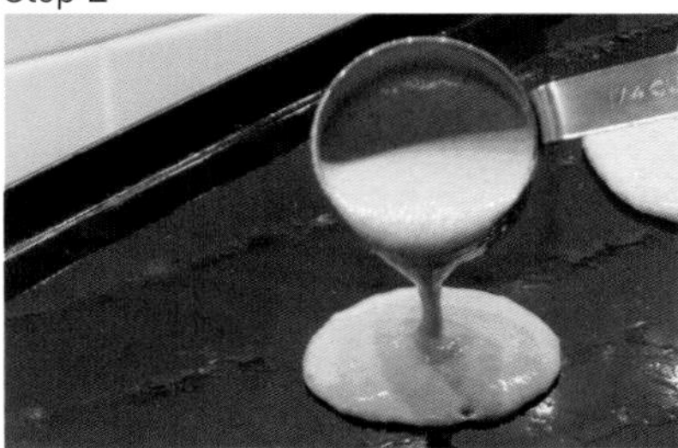

Step 4

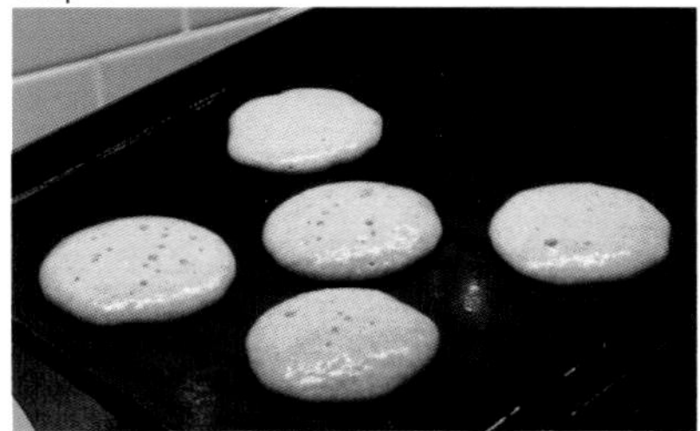

Step 4

Variations

Banana Pancakes

Add to the Master Recipe ingredients:

1 cup sliced bananas

Follow Master Recipe directions and substitute Step 4 below:

Cook for 30 seconds and then gently press two slices of banana on top of each cooking pancake. Continue cooking until bubbles form on top, about 2-3 minutes.

For a creditable breakfast, serve with bananas and milk.

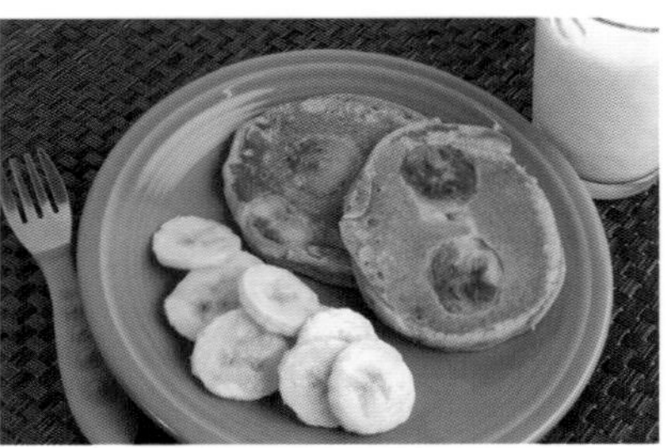

Banana Pancakes

Just Peachy Pancakes

Add to the Master Recipe ingredients:

2 cups peaches, finely chopped

¼ teaspoon ground cinnamon

Follow Master Recipe directions, plus:

Combine peaches with cinnamon. To serve, spoon ⅓ cup peaches over each pancake.

For a creditable breakfast, serve with peaches and milk.

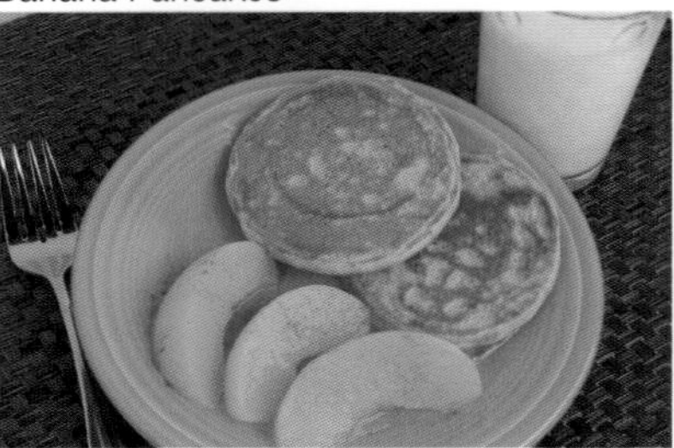

Just Peachy Pancakes

Pumpkin Pancakes

Add to the Master Recipe ingredients:

½ teaspoon allspice

½ teaspoon ground cinnamon

½ cup canned pumpkin

Follow Master Recipe directions, plus:

1. Mix allspice and cinnamon with the dry ingredients.
2. Whisk egg and milk, then stir in pumpkin.

For a creditable breakfast, serve with cinnamon apple chunks and milk.

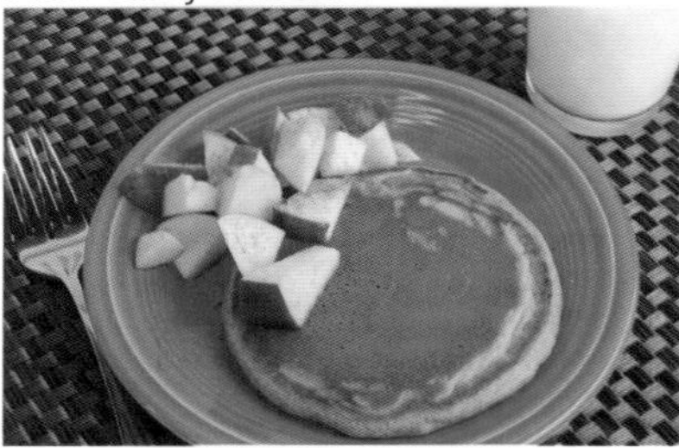

Pumpkin Pancakes

Silver Dollar Griddlecakes

Use Master Recipe ingredients

Follow Master Recipe directions, but in Step 3:

Use 2 tablespoons batter for each Silver Dollar pancake.

For a creditable breakfast, serve with grapes and milk.

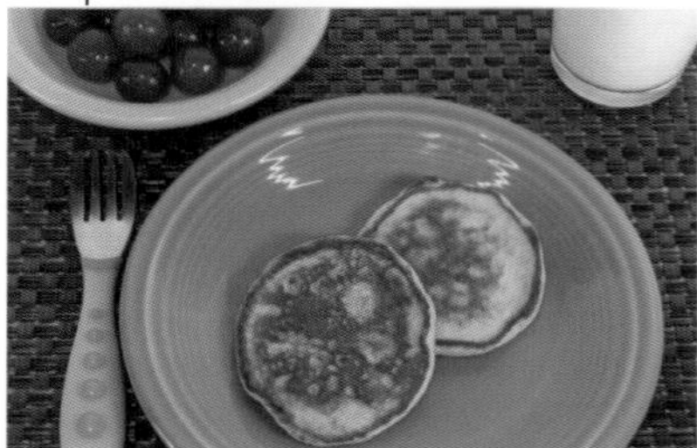

Silver Dollar Griddlecakes

***Tip** - Make pancakes ahead of time. Cool completely, then wrap in plastic and freeze for up to 6 months. To reheat, microwave on high for 1-2 minutes or wrap in foil and heat in 350 degree oven until warmed through.*

Carrot Cake Baked Oatmeal

Prep time - 20 minutes
Cook time - 30 minutes
Total time - 50 minutes

Bake in oven

Yield - 24 squares

Ingredients

2¼ cups rolled oats
½ cup raisins
1½ teaspoons pumpkin pie spice
1 teaspoon baking powder
¼ teaspoon salt
2½ cups milk
3 tablespoons brown sugar
2 tablespoons melted butter
2½ cups carrots, shredded

Directions

1. Preheat oven to 375 degrees. Grease an 8x11-inch oven-proof casserole dish or coat with cooking spray.
2. In a large bowl, stir together the rolled oats, raisins, pumpkin pie spice, baking powder and salt.
3. In a separate bowl, whisk together the milk, brown sugar and melted butter. Stir in the shredded carrots.
4. Add the wet ingredients to the dry ingredients and stir until combined. Pour mixture into casserole dish and smooth the top surface.
5. Bake, uncovered, until lightly golden along the edge, about 30-35 minutes.
6. Remove from heat and set aside to cool. The oatmeal will firm up as it cools. Cut into 24 squares.

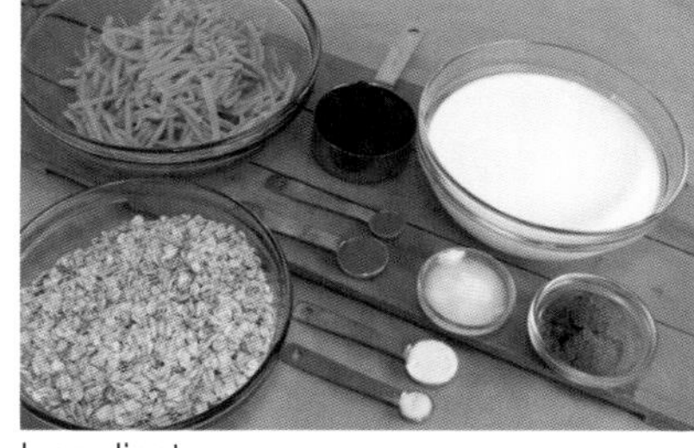

Ingredients

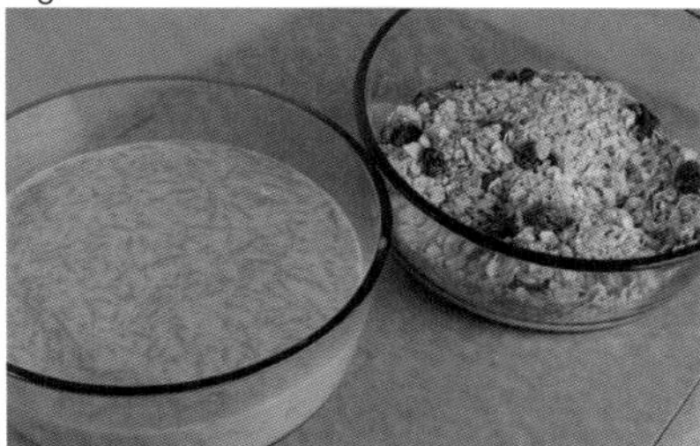

Step 2

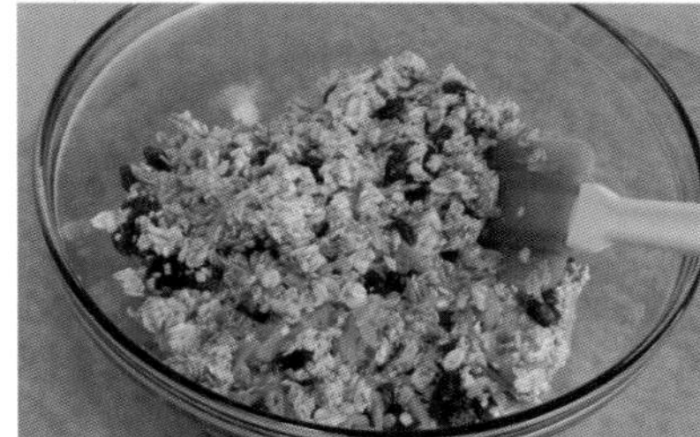

Step 4

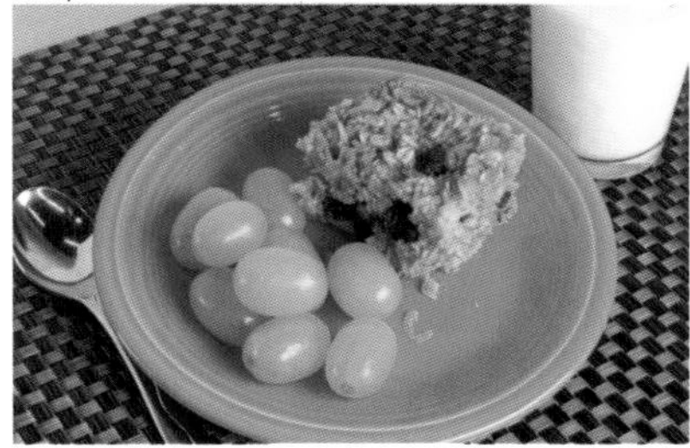

Creditable breakfast

Carrot Cake Baked Oatmeal provides G/B at breakfast			
	Toddler	Pre-School	School Age
Baked Oatmeal	1 square	1 square	2 squares
Grapes	1/4 cup	1/2 cup	1/2 cup
Milk	1/2 cup	3/4 cup	1 cup

Cinnamon Pita Chips & Fruit Salsa

Prep time - 20 minutes
Cook time - 5 minutes
Total time - 25 minutes

Bake in oven

Yield - 18 pita chips

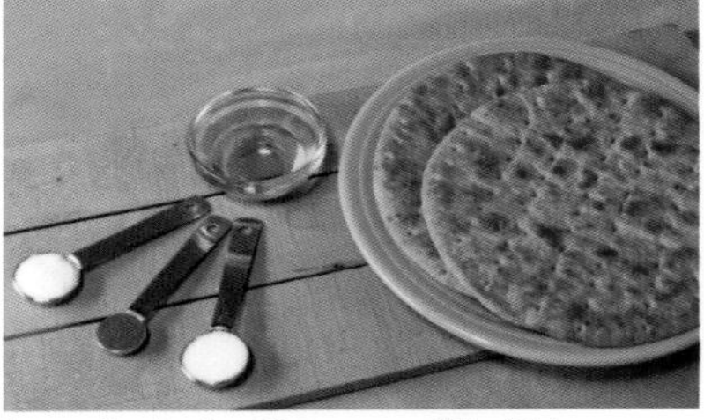

Ingredients for Cinnamon Pita Chips

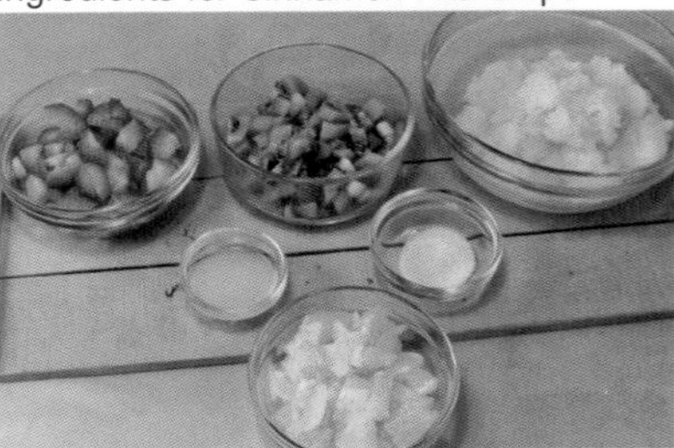

Ingredients for Fruit Salsa

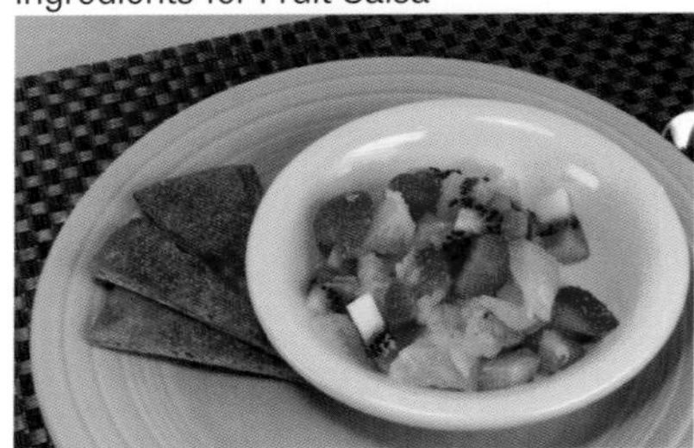

Creditable breakfast

Ingredients

3 whole wheat pita rounds, at least 1½ ounces each
1 tablespoon vegetable oil
1 tablespoon sugar
¾ teaspoon ground cinnamon

Directions

1. Preheat oven to 400 degrees. Line a baking sheet with foil or parchment paper.
2. Brush one side of each pita with oil.
3. In a small bowl, combine sugar and cinnamon; sprinkle evenly on the oiled side of each pita round.
4. Cut each pita into 6 triangles and place on baking sheet, cinnamon side up. Bake until triangles are crispy, 5-8 minutes.
5. Serve with Fruit Salsa.

Fruit Salsa

Yield - 4 cups

Ingredients

1 cup fresh strawberries, finely chopped
1 cup fresh navel oranges, peeled and finely chopped
3 medium kiwi fruit, peeled and finely chopped
1 cup unsweetened crushed pineapple, drained
1 tablespoon lemon juice
1½ teaspoons sugar

Directions

1. In a small bowl, combine all ingredients.
2. Cover and refrigerate until serving time.

Cinnamon Pita Chips & Fruit Salsa provides G/B and FR at breakfast			
	Toddler	Pre-School	School Age
Pita Chips	1/2 oz. or 2 chips	1/2 oz. or 2 chips	1 oz. or 4 chips
Fruit Salsa	1/4 cup	1/2 cup	1/2 cup
Milk	1/2 cup	3/4 cup	1 cup

Cinnamon Swirl Bread

Prep time - 20 minutes
Cook time - 35 minutes
Total time - 55 minutes

Bake in oven

Yield - 1 loaf

Ingredients for Streusel

¼ cup sugar
2 teaspoons ground cinnamon

Ingredients for Bread

2 cups whole wheat flour
4 teaspoons baking powder
½ teaspoon salt
⅔ cup sugar
2 eggs
1 cup milk
¼ cup vegetable oil

Directions

1. Preheat oven to 350 degrees. Grease a 9x5-inch loaf pan.
2. In a small bowl, mix together the streusel ingredients.
3. In a large bowl, combine flour, baking powder, salt and ⅔ cup sugar. In a small bowl, whisk together the egg, milk and oil.
4. Add the wet ingredients to the dry ingredients and stir just until moistened.
5. Pour half of the batter into the pan and sprinkle it with half of the streusel. Repeat with the remaining batter and streusel. Draw a knife through batter to marble.
6. Bake until golden brown and firm and a toothpick inserted in the center comes out clean, about 35-40 minutes.
7. Cool in pan for 10 minutes before removing loaf. Place on a wire rack to cool completely. Cut into 16 slices.

Cinnamon Swirl Bread
provides G/B at breakfast

	Toddler	Pre-School	School Age
Cinnamon Bread	1/2 oz. or 1/2 slice	1/2 oz. or 1/2 slice	1 oz. or 1 slice
Cinn. Applesauce	1/4 cup	1/2 cup	1/2 cup
Milk	1/2 cup	3/4 cup	1 cup

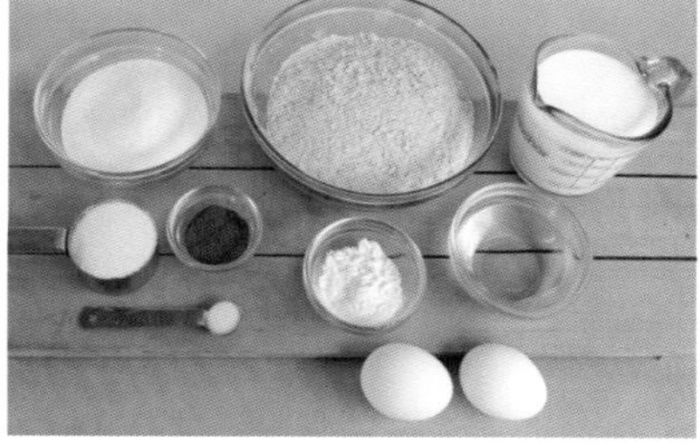

Ingredients

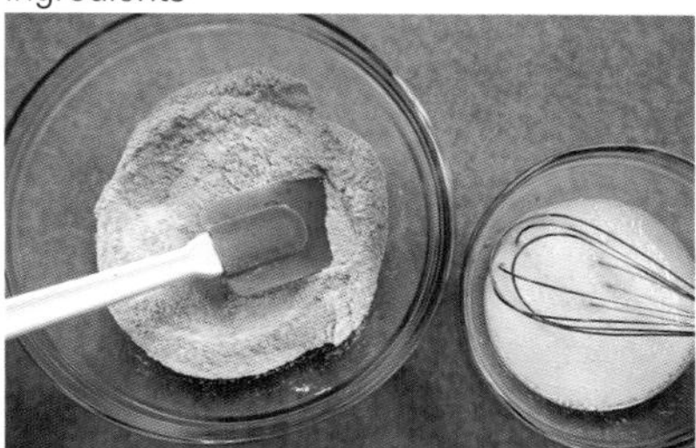

Step 3

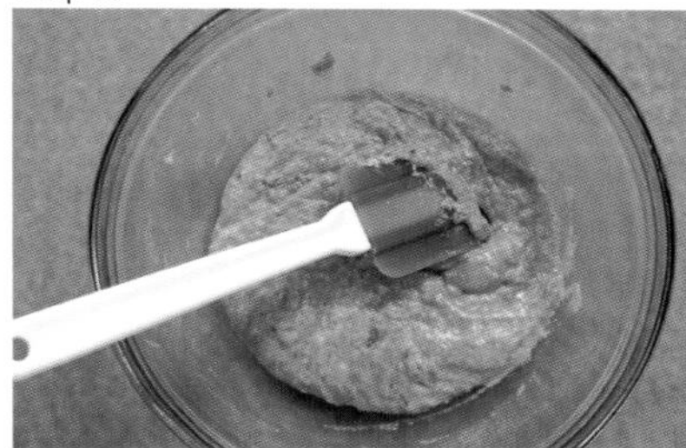

Step 4

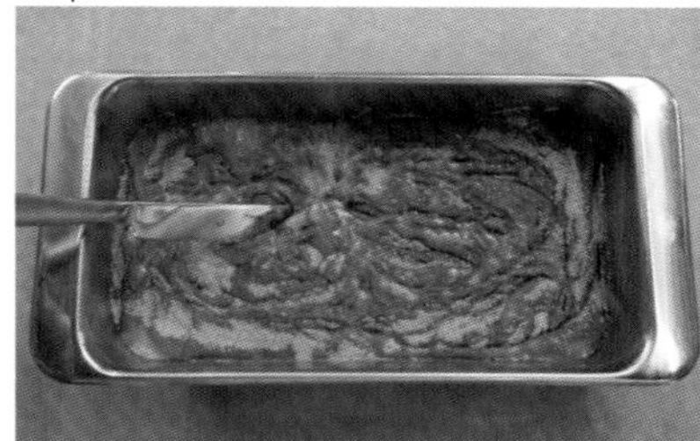

Step 5

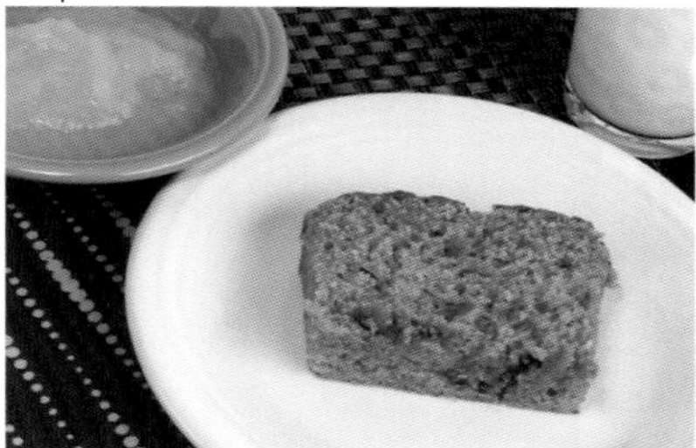

Creditable breakfast

Cinnamon Tortilla Chips

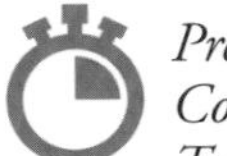

Prep time - 10 minutes
Cook time - 5 minutes
Total time - 15 minutes

Bake in oven

Yield - 18 chips

Ingredients

3 6-inch whole wheat tortillas
1 tablespoon vegetable oil
2 teaspoons sugar
½ teaspoon ground cinnamon

Directions

1. Preheat oven to 400 degrees. Line a baking sheet with foil or parchment paper.
2. Place tortillas on work surface and brush one side of each with oil.
3. In a small bowl, combine sugar and cinnamon; sprinkle evenly on the oiled side of the tortillas.
4. Cut each tortilla into 6 triangles.
5. Place triangles on baking sheet, cinnamon side up.
6. Bake until triangles are crispy, about 5-8 minutes.

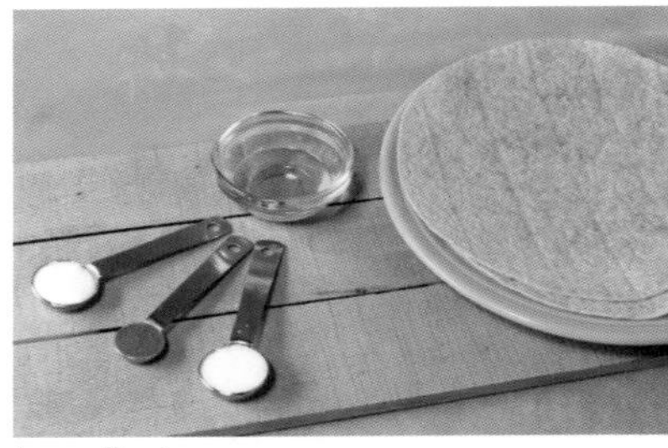

Ingredients

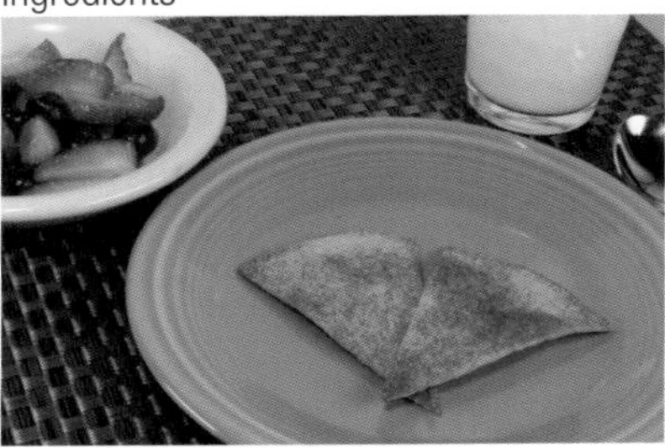

Creditable breakfast

Cinnamon Tortilla Chips provide G/B at breakfast			
	Toddler	Pre-School	School Age
Tortilla Chips	1/2 oz. or 2 chips	1/2 oz. or 2 chips	1 oz. or 4 chips
Diced Berries	1/4 cup	1/2 cup	1/2 cup
Milk	1/2 cup	3/4 cup	1 cup

Oatmeal-Chocolate Chip Breakfast Treats

Prep time - 15 minutes
Cook time - 15 minutes
Total time - 30 minutes

Bake in oven

Yield - 18 treats

Ingredients

2 medium ripe bananas
1¼ cups quick-cooking oats
¼ cup mini chocolate chips

Directions

1. Preheat oven to 375 degrees. Grease a baking sheet or coat with cooking spray.
2. In a bowl, mash the bananas.
3. Add the oats and chocolate chips and combine well.
4. Drop one heaping tablespoon of batter on the baking sheet for each treat.
5. Bake for 15 minutes.

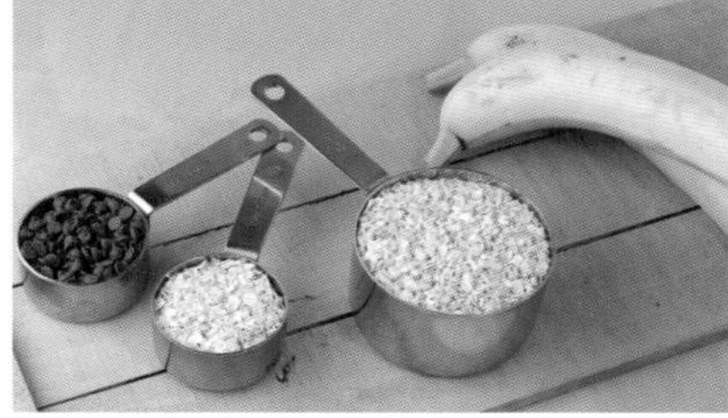

Ingredients

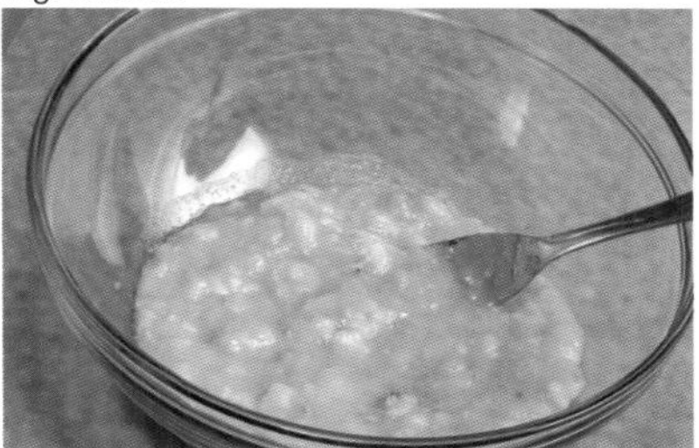

Step 2

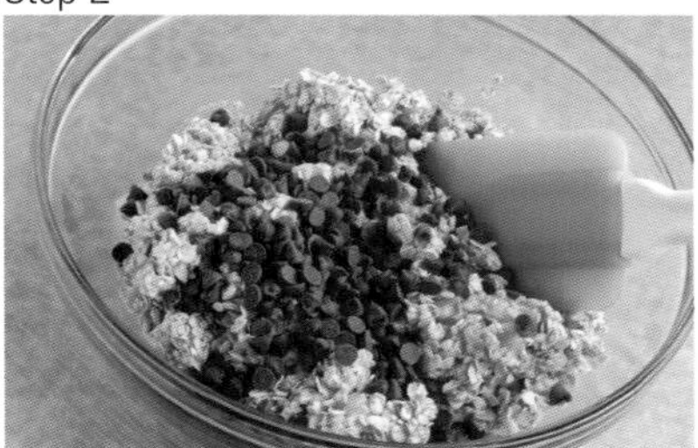

Step 3

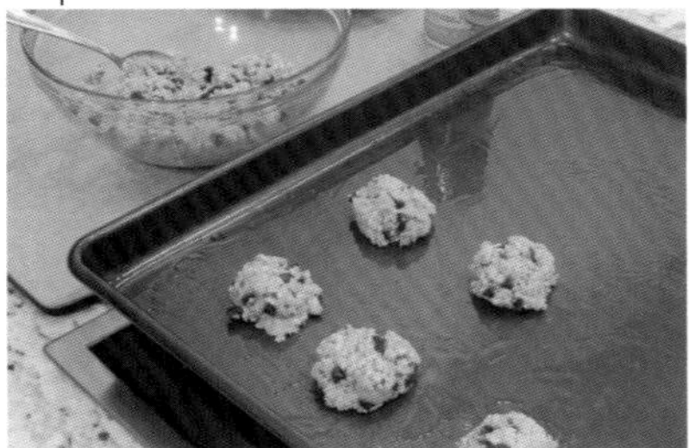

Step 4

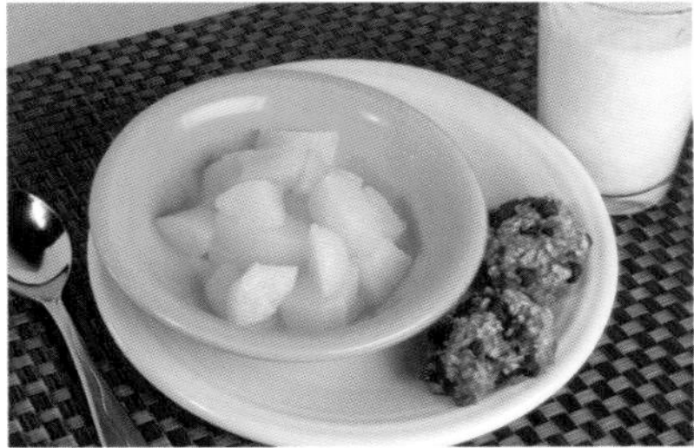

Creditable breakfast

Oatmeal-Chocolate Chip Breakfast Treats
provide G/B at breakfast

	Toddler	Pre-School	School Age
Breakfast Treats	3 treats	3 treats	6 treats
Pears	1/4 cup	1/2 cup	1/2 cup
Milk	1/2 cup	3/4 cup	1 cup

Pumpkin Bread

Prep time - 20 minutes
Cook time - 35 minutes
Total time - 55 minutes

Bake in oven

Yield - 1 loaf

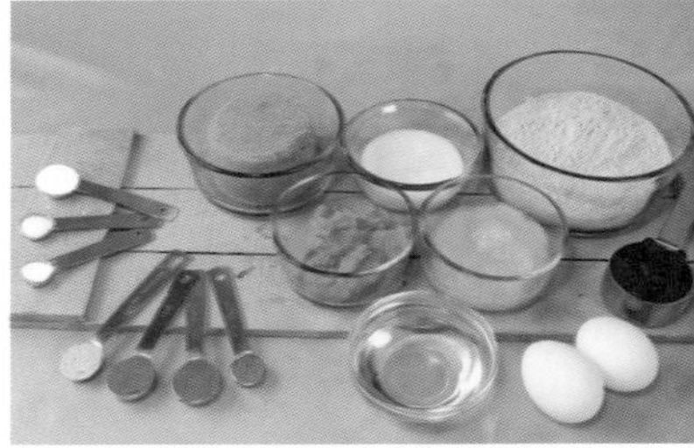
Ingredients

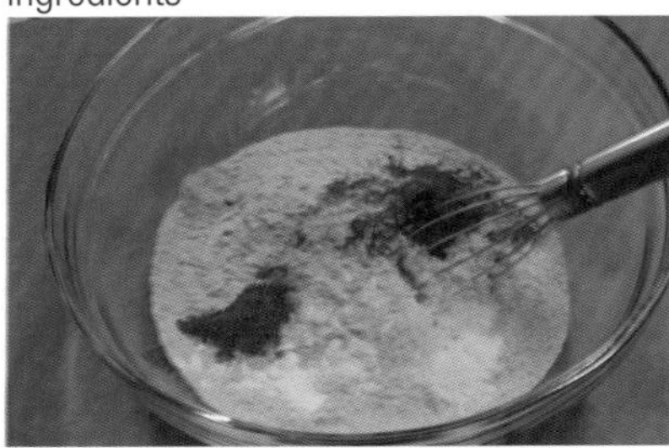
Step 2

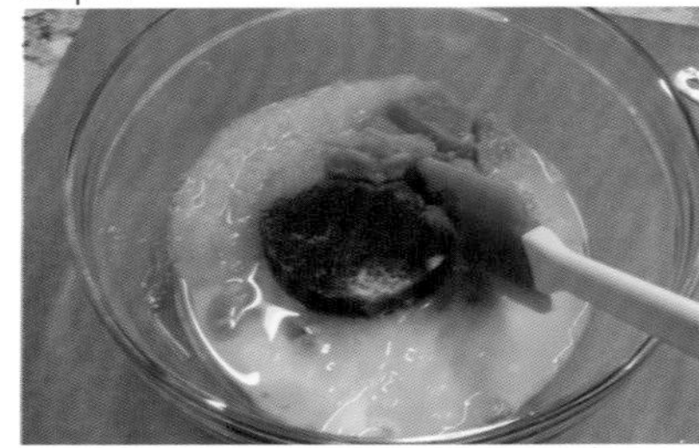
Step 3

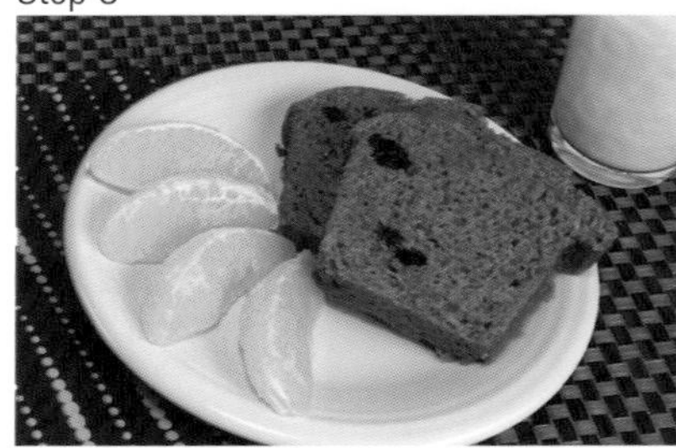
Creditable breakfast

Ingredients

2 cups whole wheat flour
1 teaspoon baking powder
¼ teaspoon baking soda
½ teaspoon salt
2 teaspoons ground cinnamon
½ teaspoon ground nutmeg
½ teaspoon ground ginger
½ cup brown sugar
¼ cup vegetable oil
½ cup unsweetened applesauce
¾ cup canned pumpkin
⅓ cup buttermilk
2 eggs, slightly beaten
½ cup raisins

Directions

1. Preheat oven to 350 degrees. Grease a 9x5-inch loaf pan.
2. Whisk together flour, baking powder, baking soda, salt and spices.
3. Combine brown sugar, oil, applesauce, pumpkin, buttermilk and eggs; mix until well blended.
4. Pour the pumpkin mixture into the dry ingredients and stir until combined. Fold in the raisins.
5. Pour batter into loaf pan and bake 35-40 minutes, until toothpick inserted in the center comes out clean.
6. Cool in pan for 15 minutes. Remove loaf and place on a wire rack to cool completely. Cut into 16 slices.

Pumpkin Bread provides G/B at breakfast			
	Toddler	Pre-School	School Age
Pumpkin Bread	1/2 oz. or 1/2 slice	1/2 oz. or 1/2 slice	1 oz. or 1 slice
Oranges	1/4 cup	1/2 cup	1/2 cup
Milk	1/2 cup	3/4 cup	1 cup

Strawberry Sunshine Bread

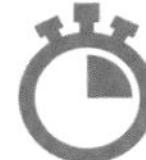

Prep time - 20 minutes
Cook time - 50 minutes
Total time - 70 minutes

Bake in oven

Yield - 1 loaf

Ingredients

2½ cups whole wheat flour
2 teaspoons baking powder
½ teaspoon salt
½ cup butter, softened
½ cup sugar
2 eggs
1 teaspoon vanilla
4 teaspoons orange zest
1 cup milk
½ cup orange juice, freshly squeezed
2 cups strawberries, finely chopped

Directions

1. Preheat oven to 350 degrees. Grease a 9x5-inch loaf pan.
2. In mixing bowl, combine flour, baking powder and salt.
3. In a separate bowl, beat butter and sugar vigorously by hand, about 1 minute. Add eggs one at a time, beating thoroughly each time. Then beat in the vanilla and orange zest.
4. In a small bowl, combine the milk and orange juice. Pour half into the creamed butter, beating until well mixed.
5. Next, stir into the creamed butter half of the dry ingredients followed by the remaining milk mixture and dry ingredients. Combine well after each addition. Fold strawberries into batter.
6. Pour batter into loaf pan. Bake until top is golden brown and a toothpick inserted in center of loaf comes out clean, about 50-55 minutes.
7. Cool in pan for 15 minutes. Remove loaf and place on a wire rack to cool completely. Cut into 16 slices.

Strawberry Sunshine Bread provides G/B at breakfast			
	Toddler	Pre-School	School Age
Strawberry Bread	1/2 oz. or 1/2 slice	1/2 oz. or 1/2 slice	1 oz. or 1 slice
Oranges	1/4 cup	1/2 cup	1/2 cup
Milk	1/2 cup	3/4 cup	1 cup

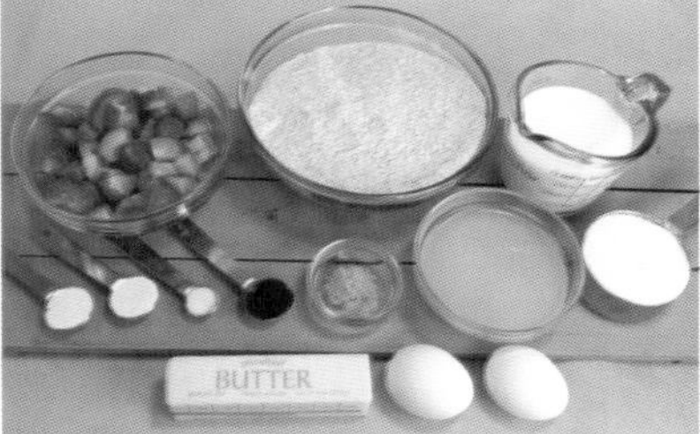

Ingredients

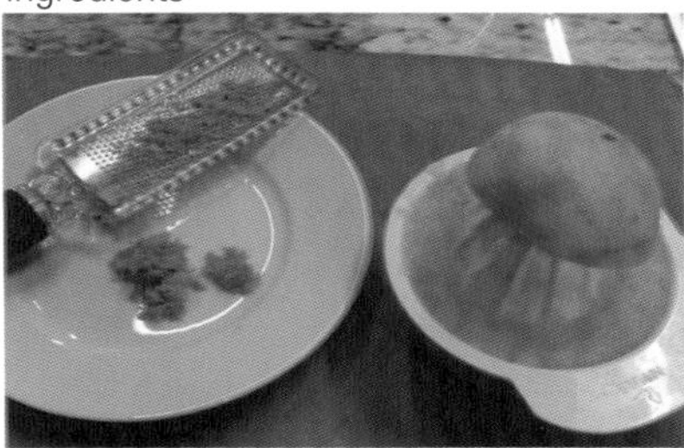
Zest and juice from the oranges

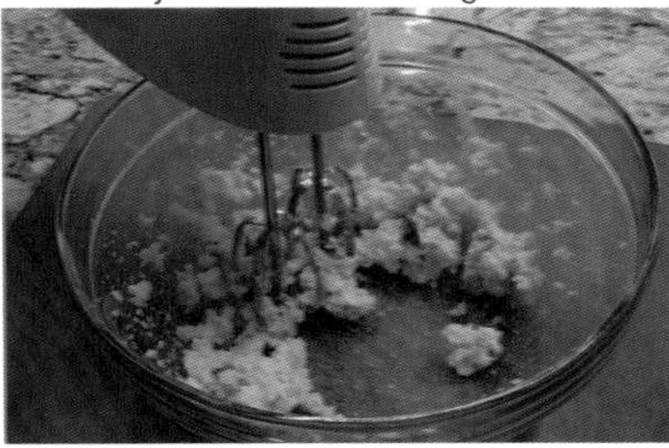
Step 2

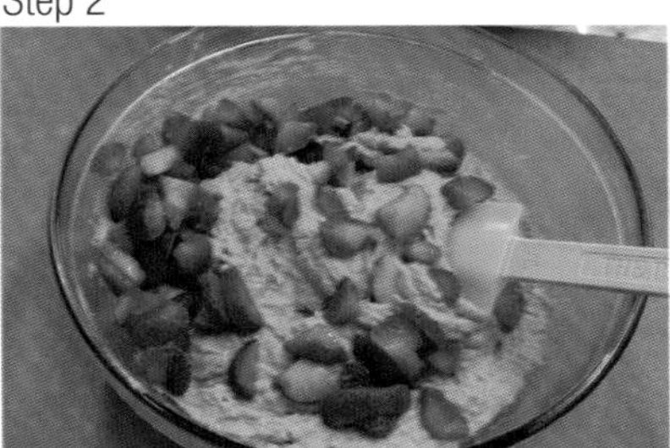
Step 4

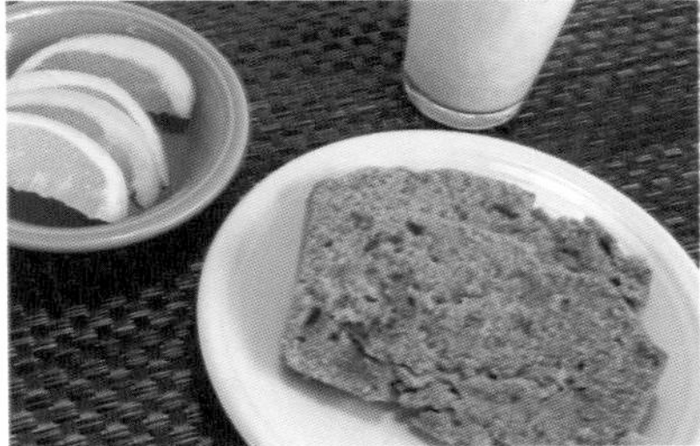
Creditable breakfast

English Muffin Breakfast Pizza

Prep time - 15 minutes
Cook time - 5 minutes
Total time - 15 minutes

Toast in toaster or in oven

Yield - 6 rounds

Ingredients

3 whole wheat English muffins, at least 1½ ounces each —split into 6 rounds
2 cups strawberries, sliced
1 cup bananas, sliced
1½ cups cottage cheese

Directions

1. Toast split English muffins. If using toasting in oven, preheat oven to 350 degrees. Toast muffins on a baking sheet until golden, about 5 minutes.
2. Lay toasted muffins in a row on the work surface.
3. Mix together the banana and strawberry slices.
4. Spread ¼ cup cottage cheese and ¼ cup fruit on each muffin. Serve remaining fruit on side.

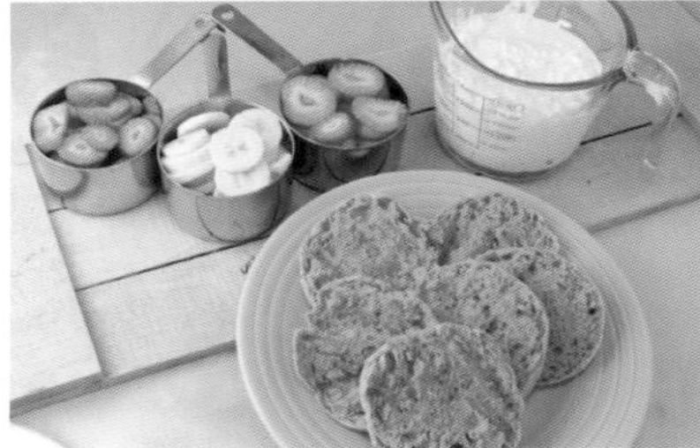

Ingredients

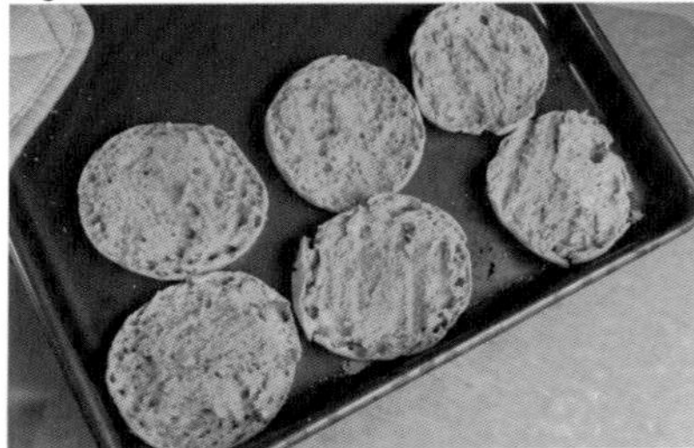

Step 1

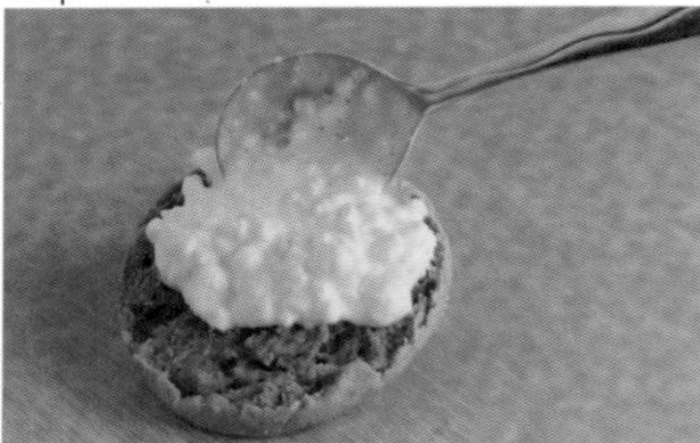

Step 3

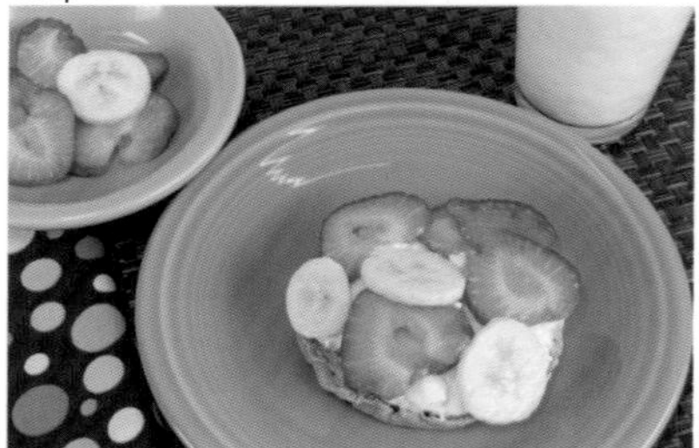

Creditable breakfast

English Muffin Breakfast Pizza
provides G/B and FR at breakfast

	Toddler	Pre-School	School Age
Breakfast Pizza	1 round	1 round	2 rounds
Extra Fruit	-	1/4 cup	1/4 cup
Milk	1/2 cup	3/4 cup	1 cup

English Muffin Egg Sandwich

Prep time - 15 minutes
Cook time - 10 minutes
Total time - 25 minutes

Bake in oven

Yield - 6 open-faced sandwiches

Ingredients

6 eggs
⅛ teaspoon salt
⅛ teaspoon black pepper
3 whole wheat English muffins, at least 1½ ounces each —split into 6 rounds
6 ounces turkey ham, thinly sliced
⅜ cup (1½ ounces) shredded cheddar cheese

Directions

1. Preheat oven to 350 degrees. Grease a 6-cup muffin pan or 6 ramekins and place on a baking sheet.
2. Crack one egg into each cup or ramekin. Pierce egg yolk with a fork and beat very slightly. Season with salt and pepper.
3. Bake eggs until set, about 10-15 minutes.
4. While the eggs are baking, toast the English muffins in the oven for 3-5 minutes.
5. Remove eggs from oven and allow to cool slightly. To remove egg, run a knife around the edge.
6. To assemble, top each English muffin with 1 ounce turkey ham, 1 egg and 1 tablespoon cheese.

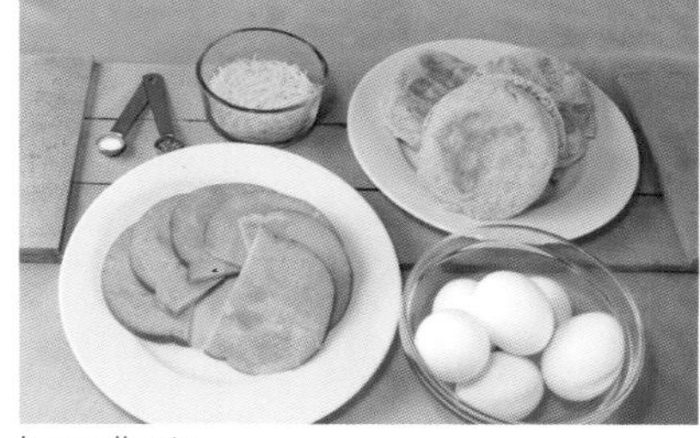

Ingredients

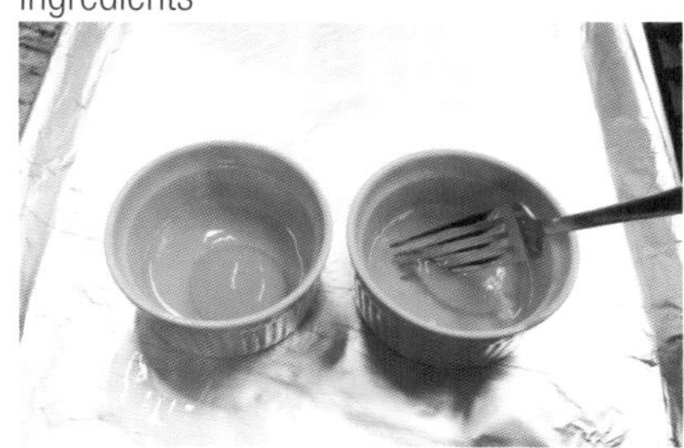

Step 2

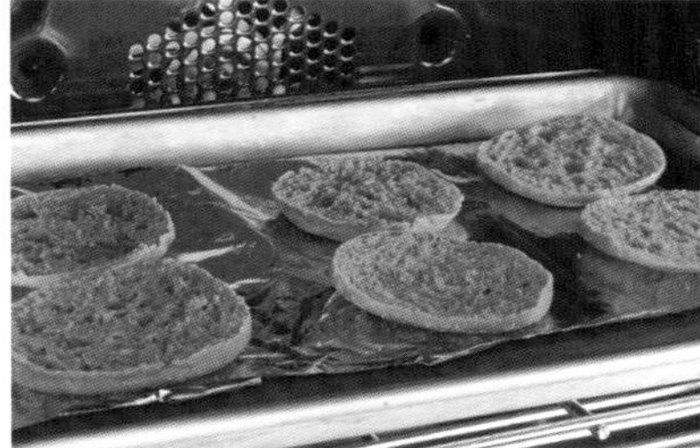

Step 4

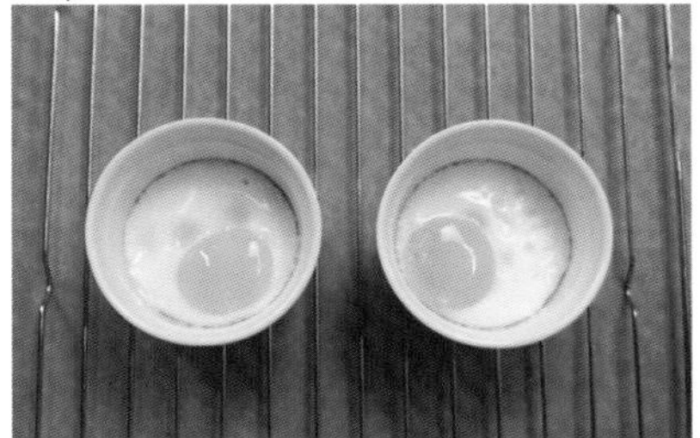

Step 5

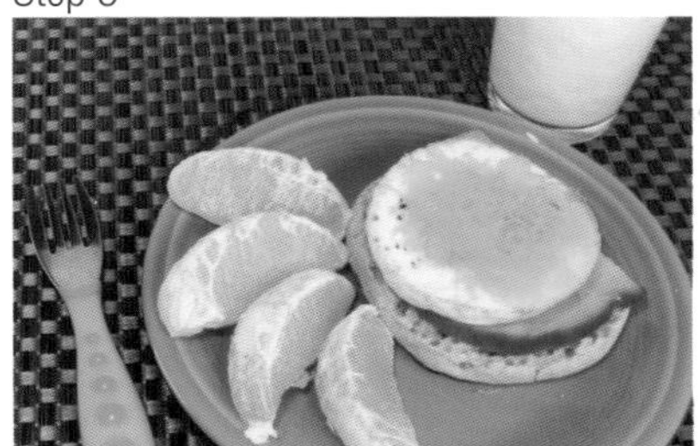

Creditable breakfast

English Muffin Egg Sandwich
provides G/B at breakfast

	Toddler	Pre-School	School Age
Egg Sandwich	1 sandwich	1 sandwich	2 sandwiches
Oranges	1/4 cup	1/2 cup	1/2 cup
Milk	1/2 cup	3/4 cup	1 cup

Ham & Veggie Omelet

Prep time - 15 minutes
Cook time - 10 minutes
Total time - 25 minutes

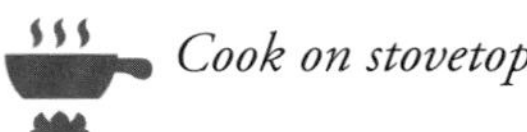

Cook on stovetop

Yield - 6 omelet slices

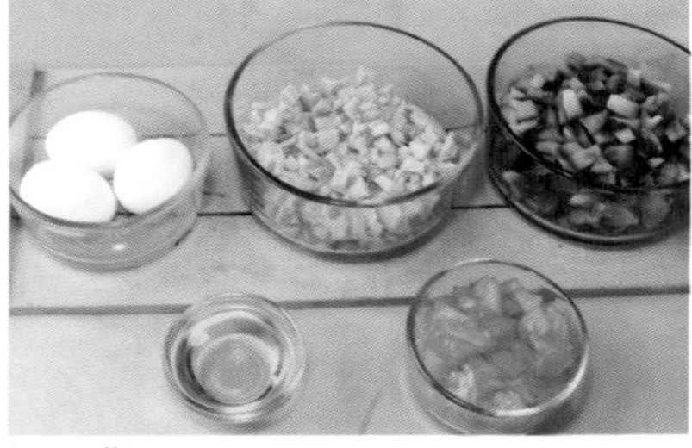

Ingredients

Ingredients

2 tablespoons vegetable oil, divided
6 ounces turkey ham, diced
3 cups green peppers, diced
1½ cups tomatoes, diced
3 eggs

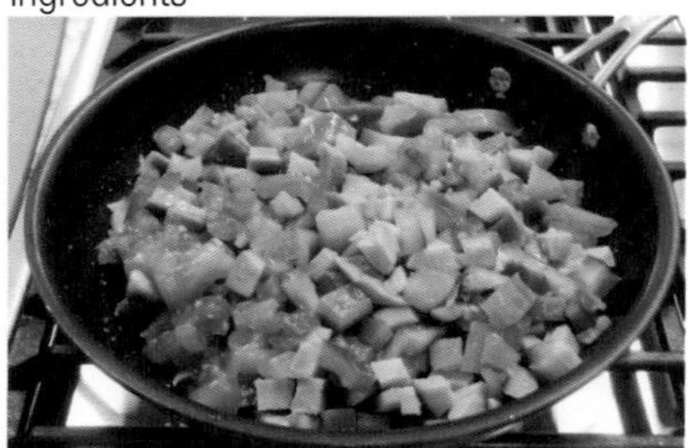

Step 2

Directions

1. Heat oil in a large skillet over medium heat.
2. Add ham, green peppers and tomatoes; sauté until green peppers are tender, about 5 minutes. Remove from heat and place in a bowl.
3. In another bowl, whisk eggs.
4. Starting with a clean skillet, heat remaining oil over medium heat, tilting pan to coat evenly. Once oil is hot, add the eggs. As eggs cook, use a spatula to lift the edges of the eggs, allowing the uncooked egg to flow underneath and cook. Repeat as needed.
5. When eggs are set, about 5 minutes, spoon the sautéed vegetables onto one side of the eggs.
6. Remove from heat; fold the eggs over the filling and slide omelet onto a plate. Cut into 6 portions.

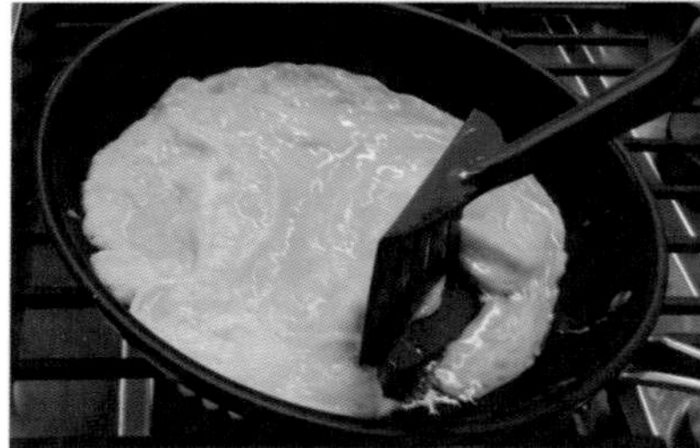

Step 5

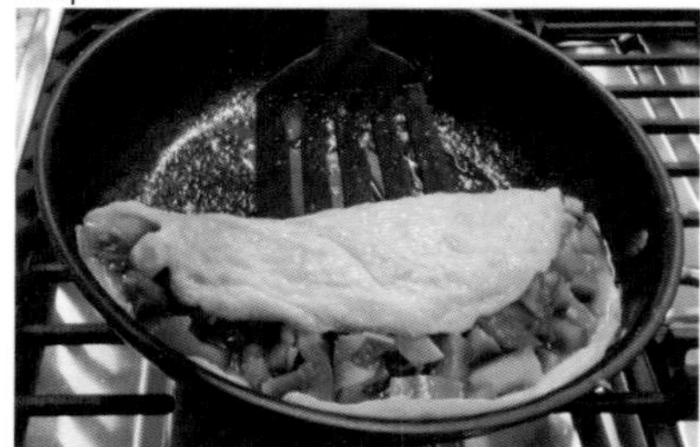

Step 6

Ham & Veggie Omelet provides M/MA and VEG at breakfast			
	Toddler	Pre-School	School Age
Omelet	1/2 slice	1 slice	1 slice
Toast	1/2 oz. or 1/2 slice	1/2 oz. or 1/2 slice	1 oz. or 1 slice
Milk	1/2 cup	3/4 cup	1 cup

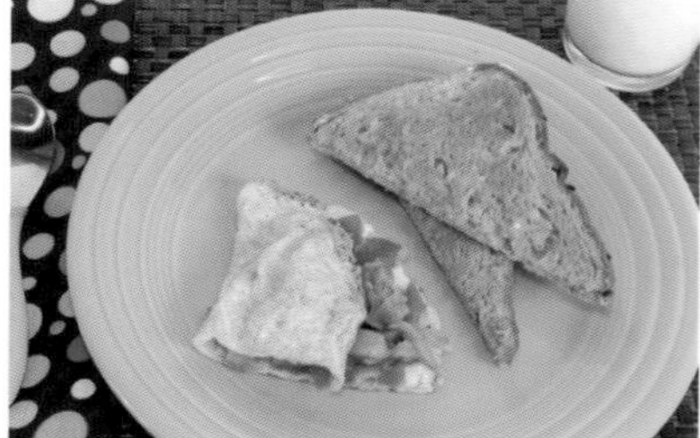

Creditable breakfast

Ham & Veggie Frittata

Prep time - 15 minutes
Cook time - 15 minutes
Total time - 30 minutes

Cook on stovetop and bake in oven

Yield - 6 wedges

Ingredients

3 eggs
2 tablespoons vegetable oil
6 ounces turkey ham, diced
½ cup onions, diced
½ cup green peppers, diced

Directions

1. Position rack at top of oven and preheat to 450 degrees.
2. Whisk eggs and set aside.
3. Heat oil in a large, ovenproof skillet over medium heat. Sauté turkey ham, onions and peppers until peppers are tender, about 5 minutes.
4. Pour egg mixture over the sautéed vegetables and place pan in oven.
5. Bake until lightly browned and firm to the touch, about 10-15 minutes. Cut into 6 wedges.

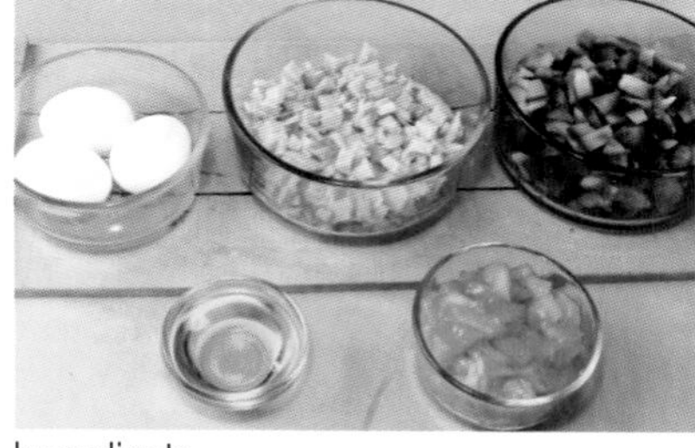

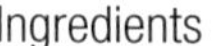
Ingredients

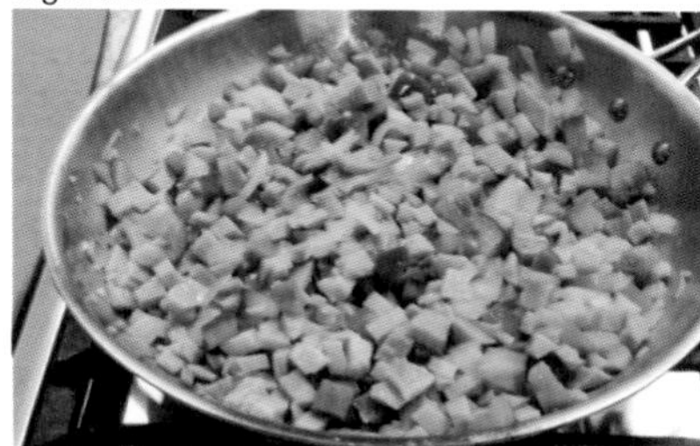
Step 3

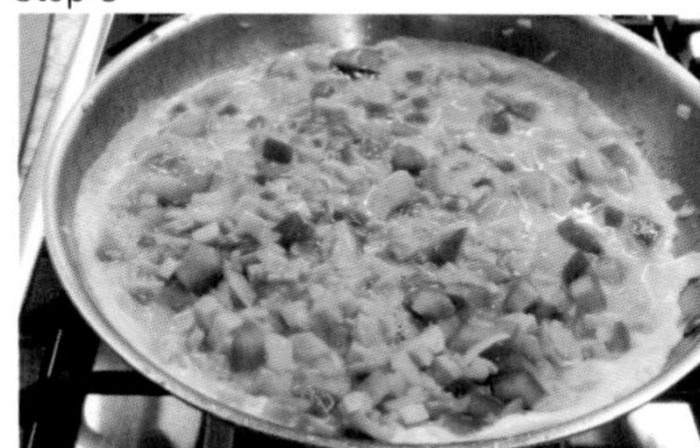
Step 4

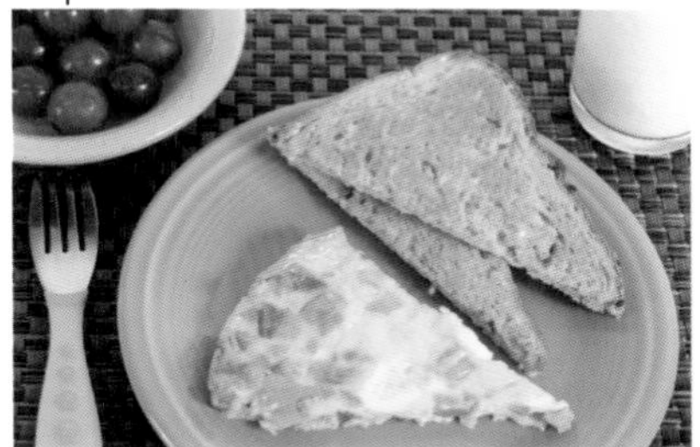
Creditable breakfast

Ham & Veggie Frittata provides M/MA at breakfast			
	Toddler	Pre-School	School Age
Frittata	1/2 wedge	1 wedge	1 wedge
Toast	1/2 oz. or 1/2 slice	1/2 oz. or 1/2 slice	1 oz. or 1 slice
Grapes	1/4 cup	1/2 cup	1/2 cup
Milk	1/2 cup	3/4 cup	1 cup

Veggie Omelet

Prep time - 15 minutes
Cook time - 10 minutes
Total time - 25 minutes

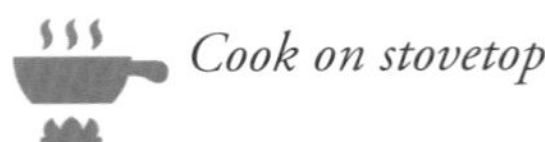

Cook on stovetop

Yield - 6 omelet slices

Ingredients

2 tablespoons vegetable oil, divided
½ cup onions, diced
3 cups green peppers, diced
1½ cups tomatoes, diced
3 eggs
⅛ teaspoon salt
⅛ teaspoon pepper
1½ cups (6 ounces) shredded sharp cheddar cheese

Directions

1. Heat 1 tablespoon of the oil in a large skillet over medium heat.
2. Add green peppers and onions and cook 2 minutes. Add the tomatoes and sauté until peppers are tender, about 3 minutes. Remove from heat and place in a bowl.
3. In another bowl, whisk eggs with the salt and pepper.
4. Starting with a clean skillet, heat remaining oil over medium heat, tilting pan to coat evenly. Once oil is hot, add eggs. As eggs cook, use a spatula to lift the edges of the eggs, allowing the uncooked egg to flow underneath and cook. Repeat as needed.
5. When eggs are set, about 5 minutes, spoon the sautéed vegetables and cheese onto one side of the eggs.
6. Remove from heat; fold eggs over the vegetables and slide omelet onto a plate. Cut into 6 portions.

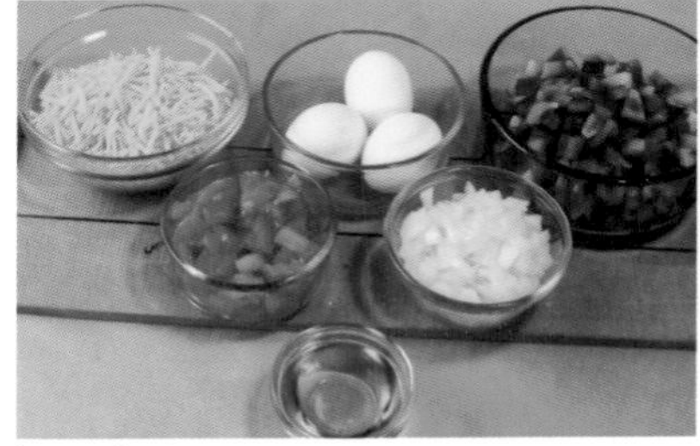

Ingredients

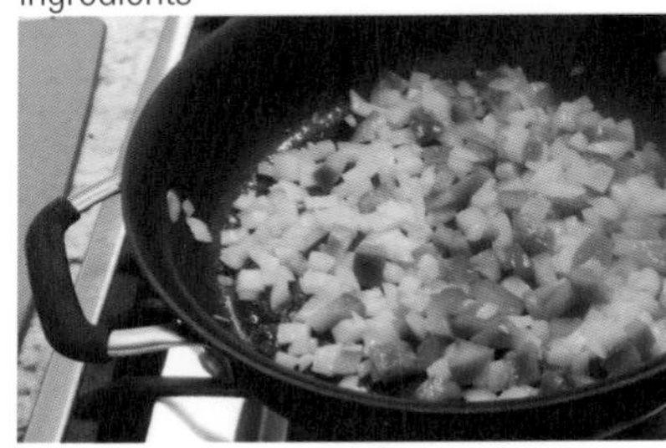

Step 2

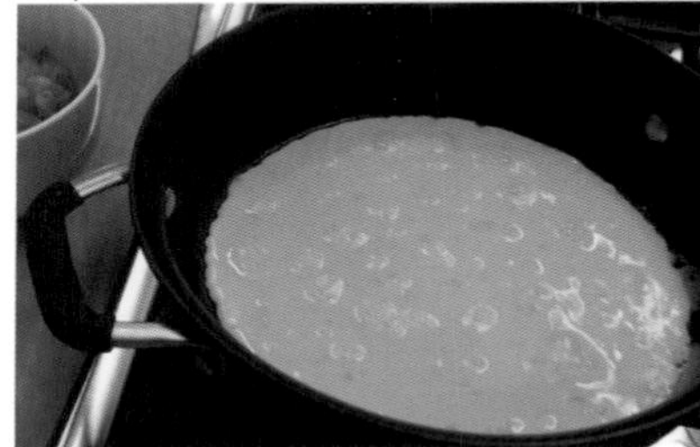

Step 5

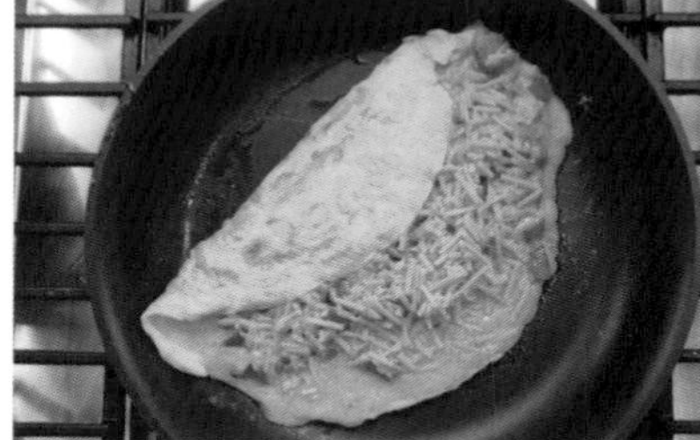

Step 7

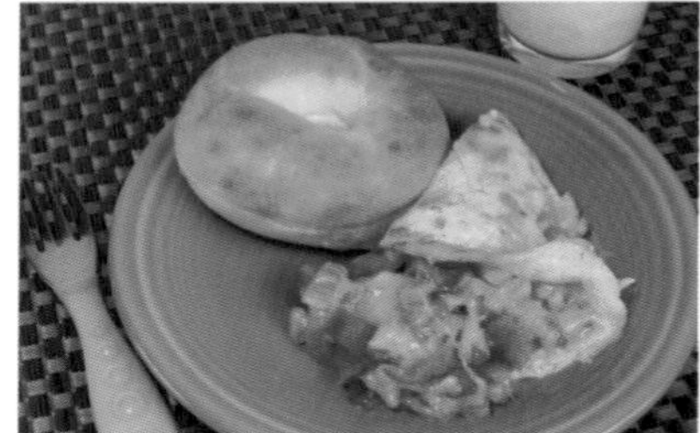

Creditable breakfast

Veggie Omelet provides VEG at breakfast			
	Toddler	Pre-School	School Age
Veggie Omelet	1/2 slice	1 slice	1 slice
Mini-Bagel	1/2 oz. or 1/2 bagel	1/2 oz. or 1/2 bagel	1 oz. or 1 bagel
Milk	1/2 cup	3/4 cup	1 cup

Breakfast Burritos

Prep time - 15 minutes
Cook time - 10 minutes
Total time - 25 minutes

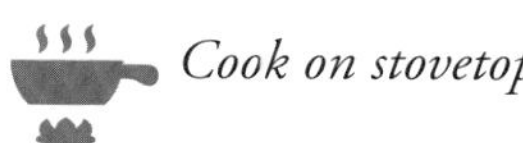

Cook on stovetop

Yield - 3 burritos

Ingredients

6 eggs
1 tablespoon butter
2 cups black beans, rinsed and drained
3 8-inch whole wheat tortillas
⅜ cup (1½ ounces) shredded mozzarella cheese
1 cup salsa

Directions

1. In a bowl, whisk eggs.
2. Heat butter in a large skillet over medium heat. When butter foams, add eggs and cook until firm to the touch, about 5 minutes.
3. When eggs are done, turn heat to low and stir in the black beans. Heat through, stirring occasionally, about 5 minutes.
4. Lay tortillas on work surface. Sprinkle each with 2 tablespoons of cheese. Then place ⅔ cup of the eggs and ⅓ cup salsa down the middle of each tortilla.
5. Roll tortillas over the filling.
6. To serve, cut each burrito in half.

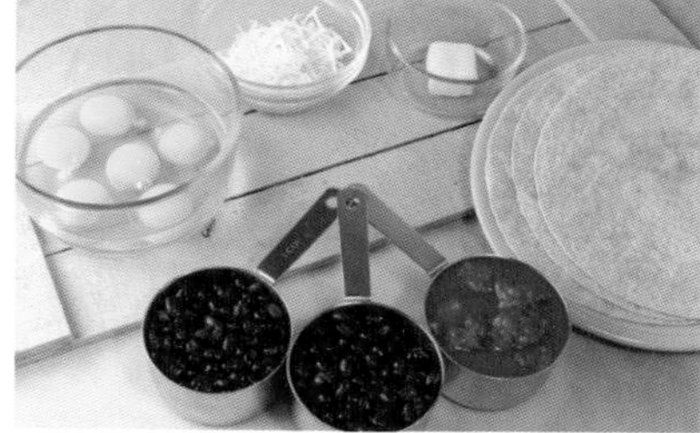

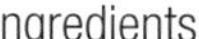

Ingredients

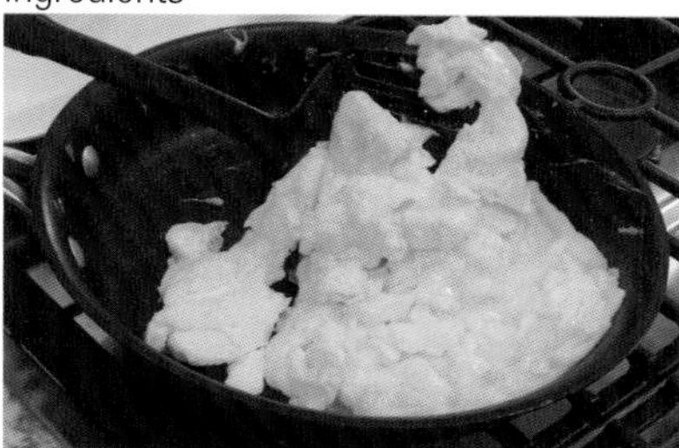

Step 2

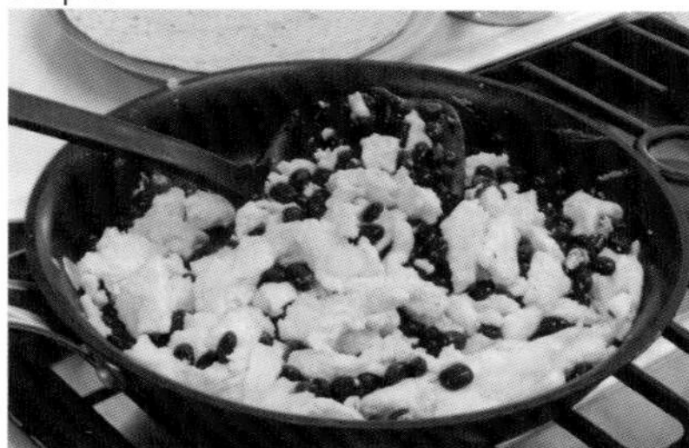

Step 3

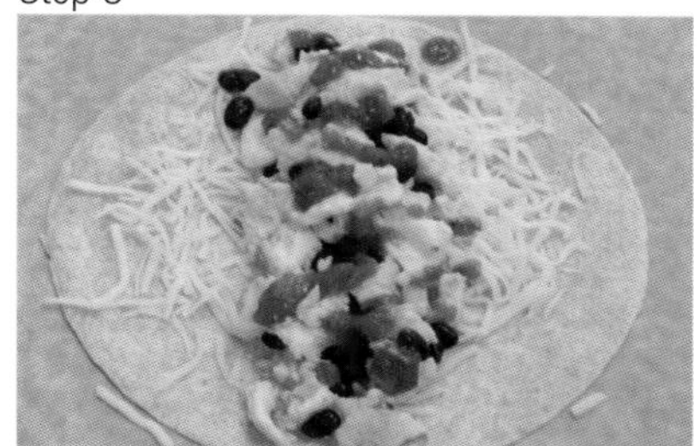

Step 4

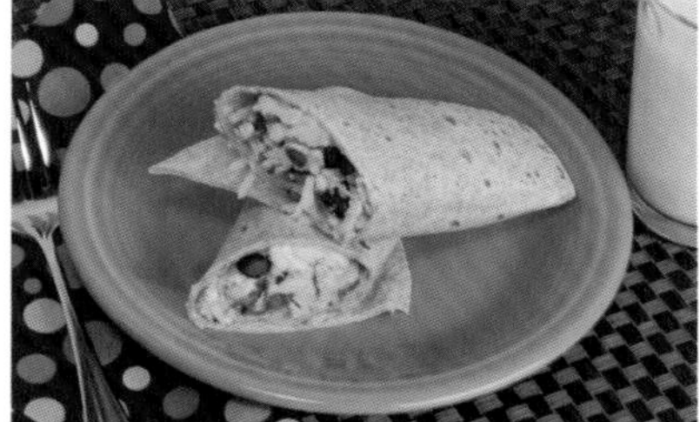

Creditable breakfast

Breakfast Burritos provide G/B and VEG at breakfast			
	Toddler	Pre-School	School Age
Burritos	1/2 burrito	1/2 burrito	1 burrito
Milk	1/2 cup	3/4 cup	1 cup

Breakfast Quesadillas

Prep time - 15 minutes
Cook time - 10 minutes
Total time - 25 minutes

Cook on stovetop and bake in oven

Yield - 3 quesadillas

Ingredients

2 tablespoons vegetable oil, divided
3 eggs
2¼ cups salsa, divided
3 tablespoons (¾ ounce) shredded cheddar cheese
¾ cup black beans, rinsed and drained
3 6-inch whole grain tortillas

Directions

1. Preheat oven to 400 degrees. Line a baking sheet with foil or parchment paper.
2. In a bowl, whisk eggs.
3. Heat 1 tablespoon of oil in a large skillet over medium heat. Once hot, add eggs and cook until firm to the touch, about 5 minutes; remove from heat.
4. Brush one side of each tortilla with the remaining oil and place on baking sheet, oiled side down.
5. Top one half of each tortilla with ¼ cup black beans, ¼ cup egg, 1 tablespoon cheese and ¼ cup salsa. Reserve remaining salsa. Fold tortilla in half.
6. Bake quesadillas until cheese is melted and tortillas become lightly crisp, about 5-8 minutes.
7. Cut each quesadilla in half. Serve with ¼ cup of salsa.

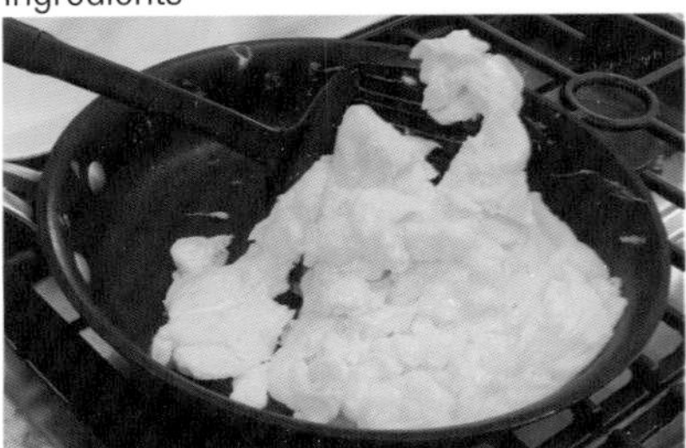

Ingredients

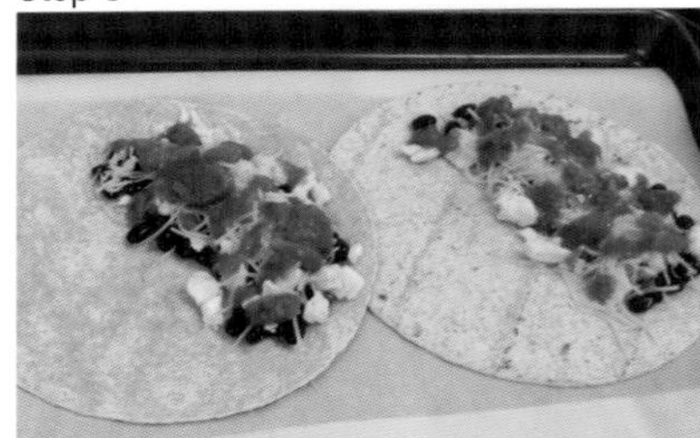

Step 3

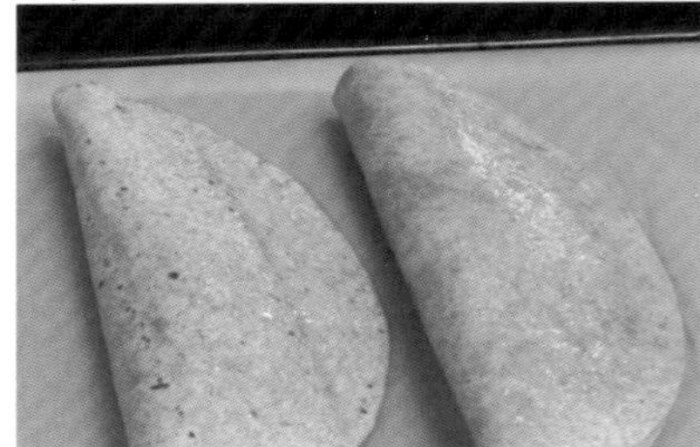

Step 5

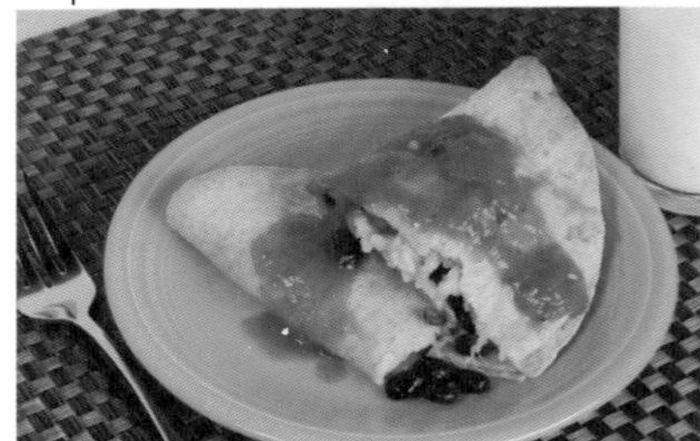

Step 6

Creditable breakfast

Breakfast Quesadillas provide G/B and VEG at breakfast			
	Toddler	Pre-School	School Age
Quesadillas	1/2 quesadilla	1/2 quesadilla	1 quesadilla
Milk	1/2 cup	3/4 cup	1 cup

Breakfast Tostadas

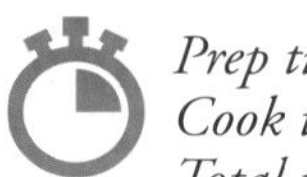

Prep time - 15 minutes
Cook time - 10 minutes
Total time - 25 minutes

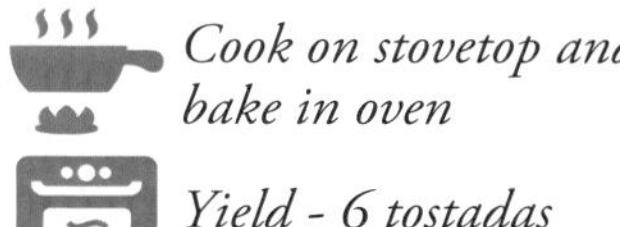

Cook on stovetop and bake in oven

Yield - 6 tostadas

Ingredients

6 eggs
⅛ teaspoon salt
⅛ teaspoon black pepper
2 tablespoons vegetable oil
6 6-inch whole grain corn tortillas
1 cup refried beans
½ cup (2 ounces) shredded sharp cheddar cheese
¼ cup green onions, chopped (optional)
½ cup salsa
¼ cup sour cream

Directions

1. Position rack at top of oven and preheat to 400 degrees. Line a baking sheet with parchment paper or foil.
2. In a bowl, whisk eggs, salt and pepper.
3. Heat large skillet over medium heat. Add the oil and tilt pan to coat evenly. Add eggs and cook, stirring frequently, until eggs are cooked and firm to the touch, about 5 minutes.
4. Arrange tortillas on baking sheet. Spread 2 tablespoons refried beans on each tortilla, all the way to the edges. Top with the eggs, 2 tablespoons cheese and a sprinkling of green onions.
5. Bake tostadas until cheese melts, about 5 minutes.
6. Remove from oven and top each tostada with 1 tablespoon salsa and ½ tablespoon sour cream.

Breakfast Tostadas
provide G/B at breakfast

	Toddler	Pre-School	School Age
Tostadas	1 tostada	1 tostada	2 tostadas
Oranges	1/4 cup	1/2 cup	1/2 cup
Milk	1/2 cup	3/4 cup	1 cup

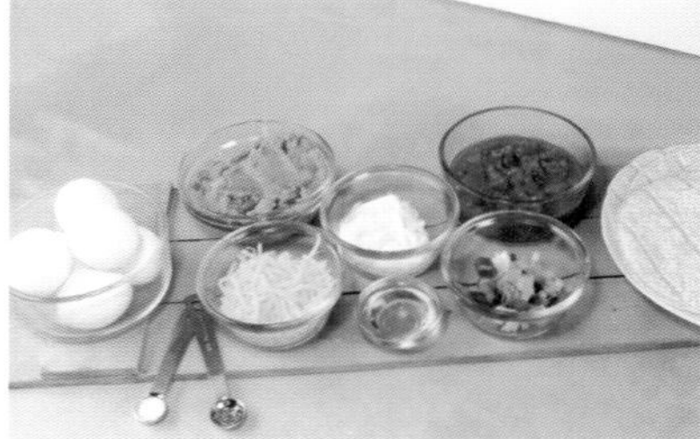

Ingredients

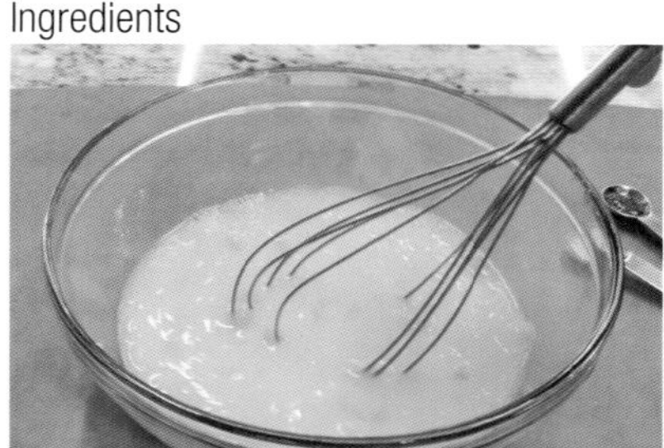

Step 2

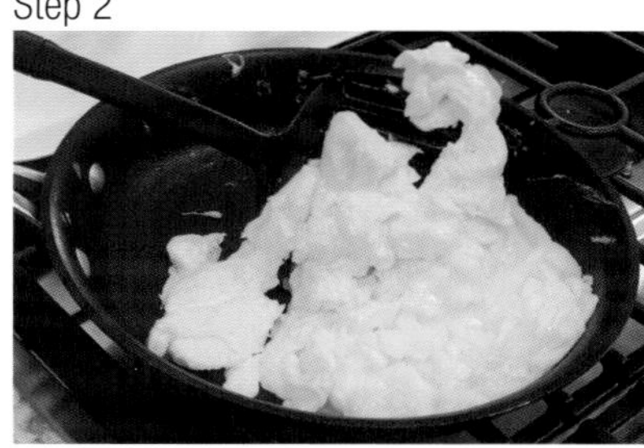

Step 3

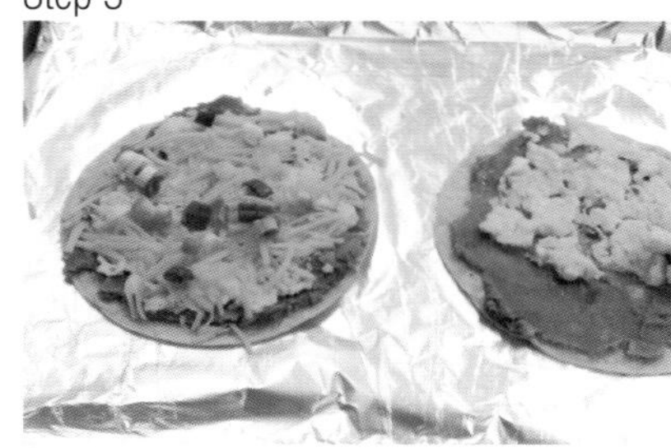

Step 4

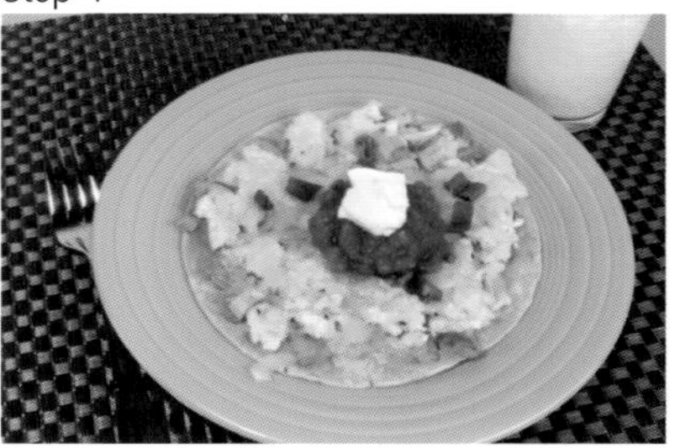

Creditable breakfast

Lunch

Apple, Cheddar & Ham Salad

Prep time - 15 minutes
Cook time - 0 minutes
Total time - 15 minutes

No cook, no bake

Yield - 5 cups

Ingredients

½ cup plain yogurt
1 teaspoon sugar
1½ cups red apples, cored and diced
1 cup (4 ounces) shredded cheddar cheese
5 ounces turkey ham, finely diced
1½ cups lettuce, chopped

Directions

1. Make dressing by combining the yogurt and sugar.
2. In a bowl, combine apples, cheese, turkey ham and lettuce.
3. Pour yogurt dressing over salad and toss to coat evenly.

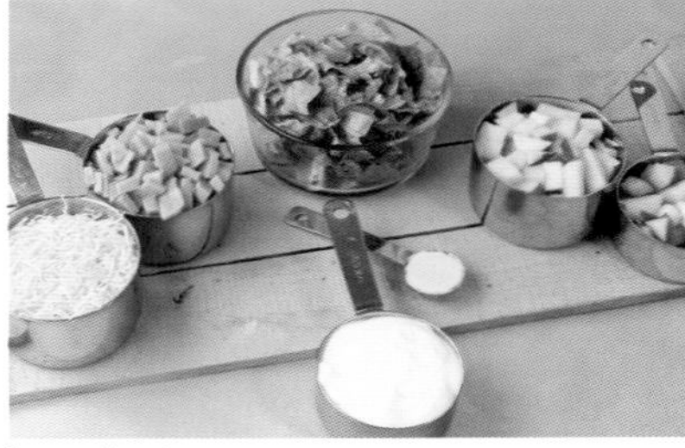

Ingredients

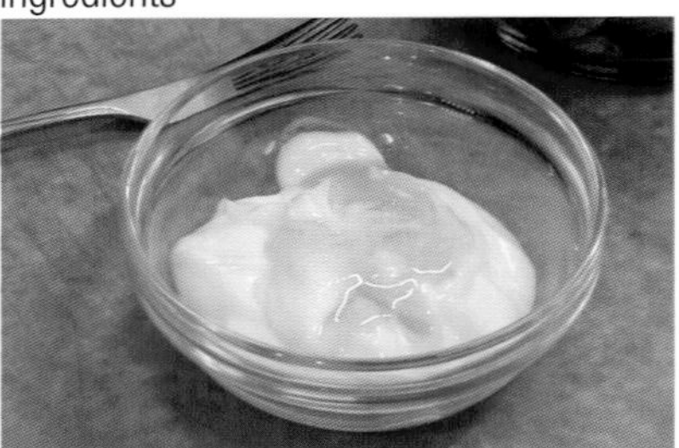

Step 1

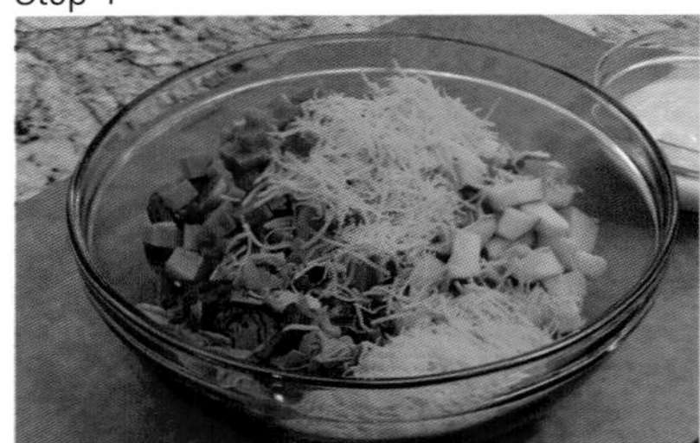

Step 2

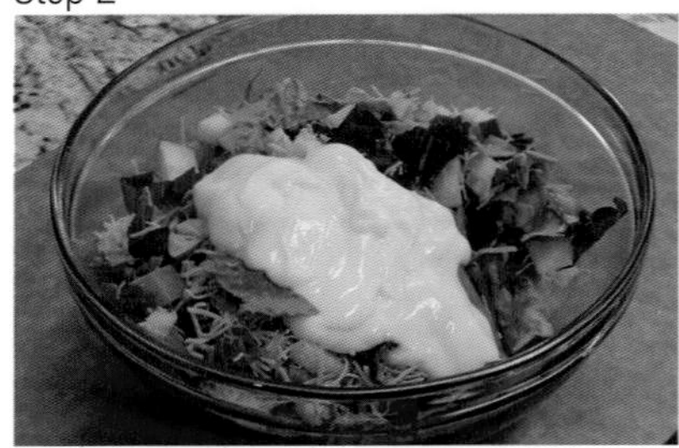

Step 3

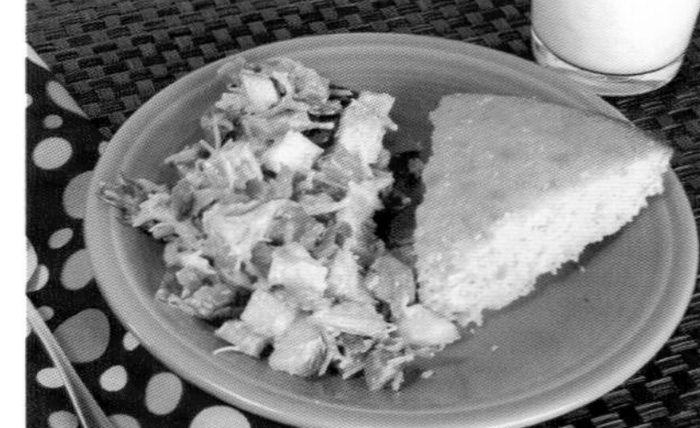

Creditable lunch/supper

Apple Cheddar Ham Salad provides M/MA, VEG and FR at lunch/supper			
	Toddler	Pre-School	School Age
Apple Ham Salad	1/2 cup	3/4 cup	1 cup
Cornbread	3/4 ounce	3/4 ounce	1-1/4 ounces
Milk	1/2 cup	3/4 cup	1 cup

Honey Mustard Chicken Salad

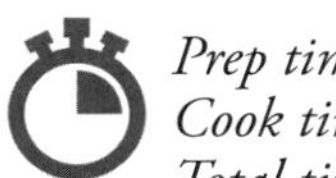

Prep time - 15 minutes
Cook time - 0 minutes
Total time - 15 minutes

No cook, no bake

Yield - 4 cups

Ingredients

3 tablespoons honey mustard
3 tablespoons mayonnaise
¼ cup plain yogurt, optional
9 ounces cooked chicken, diced or shredded
1½ cups celery, finely diced
1½ cups apples, finely diced

Directions

1. Make dressing by combining the honey mustard, mayonnaise and yogurt.
2. In a large bowl, toss the chicken, celery and apples.
3. Pour dressing over salad and toss.

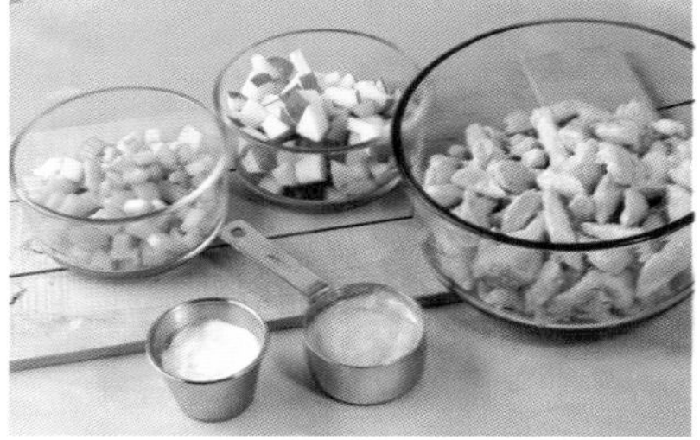

Ingredients

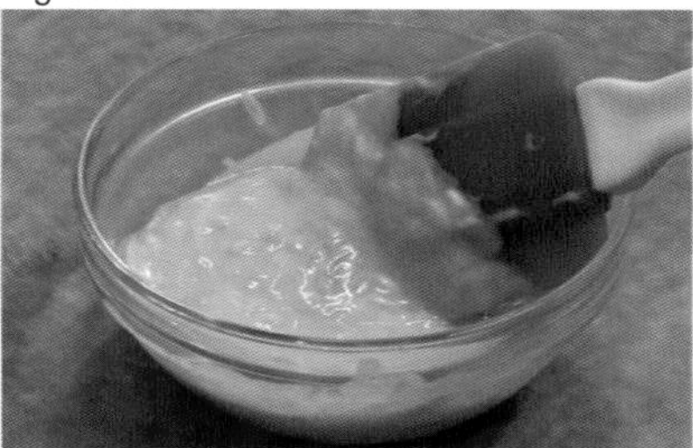

Step 1

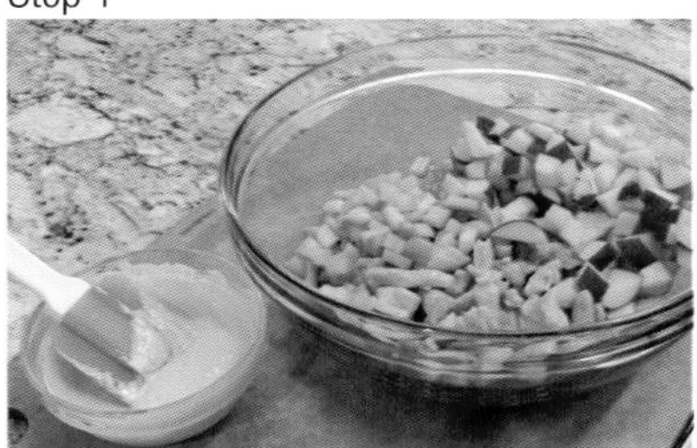

Step 2

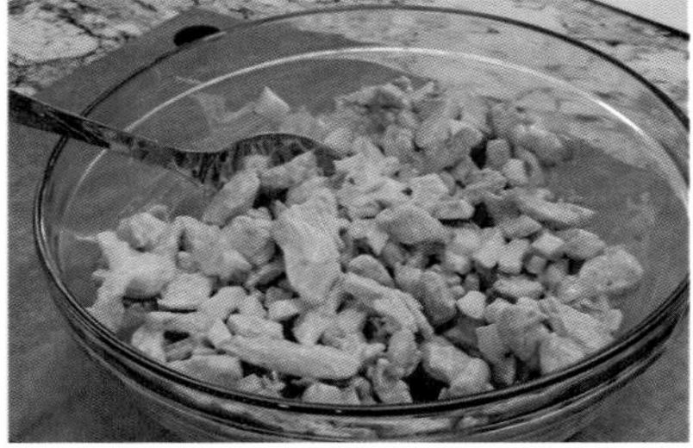

Step 3

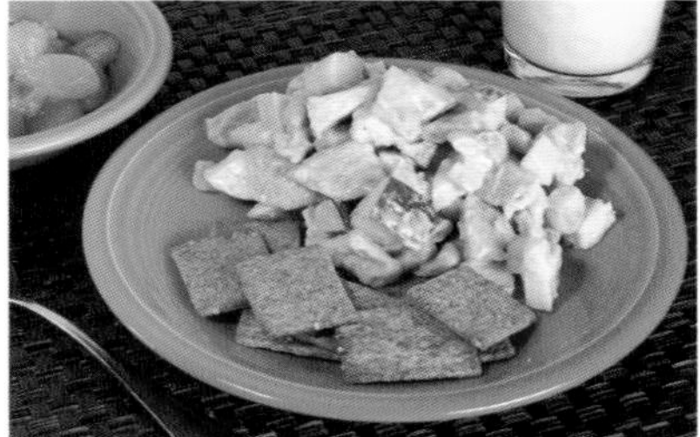

Creditable lunch/supper

Honey Mustard Chicken Salad provides M/MA and 1/2 serving of VEG and FR at lunch/supper			
	Toddler	Pre-School	School Age
Chicken Salad	2/3 cup	2/3 cup	1-1/3 cups
Crackers	1/2 ounce	1/2 ounce	3/4 ounce
Mandarin Oranges	1/8 cup	1/4 cup	1/4 cup
Milk	1/2 cup	3/4 cup	1 cup

Pizza Soup

Prep time - 15 minutes
Cook time - 30 minutes
Total time - 45 minutes

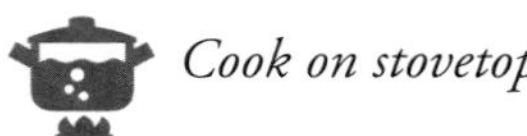

Cook on stovetop

Yield - 5 cups

Ingredients

2 tablespoons vegetable oil
½ cup fresh mushrooms, sliced
½ cup onions, chopped
1 cup red or green bell peppers, chopped
1 14½-ounce can diced tomatoes, with juice
1 pound ground beef, at least 80% lean or chopped roast beef
1 cup beef stock
½ teaspoon dried oregano
1 cup (4 ounces) shredded mozzarella cheese

Directions

1. Heat oil in a large saucepan over medium heat. Add onions, mushrooms and peppers and cook until softened, but not browned, about 5 minutes.
2. Add the ground beef and oregano and cook until beef is almost cooked through, about 5 minutes.
3. Add the tomatoes and stock. Heat to a simmer and cook for 20 minutes until beef reaches temperature of 160 degrees.
4. To serve, pour soup into bowls and sprinkle each with 2 tablespoons of cheese.

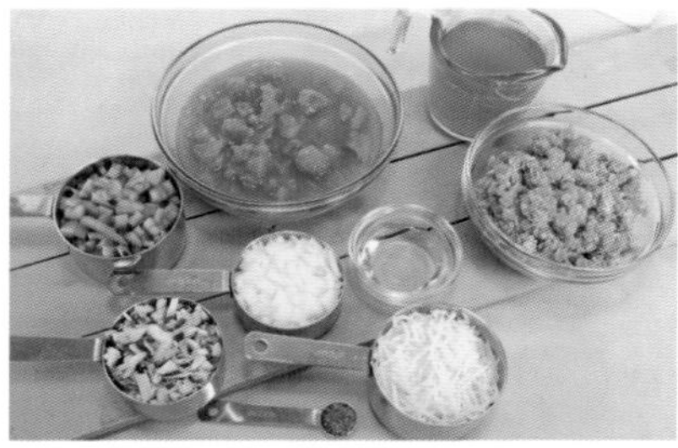

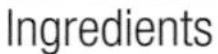

Ingredients

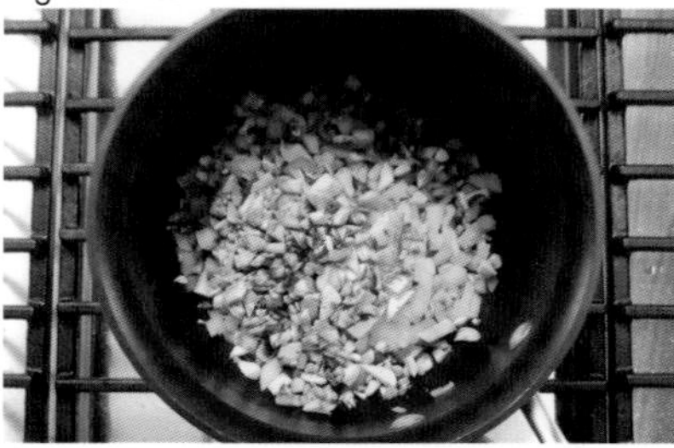

Step 1

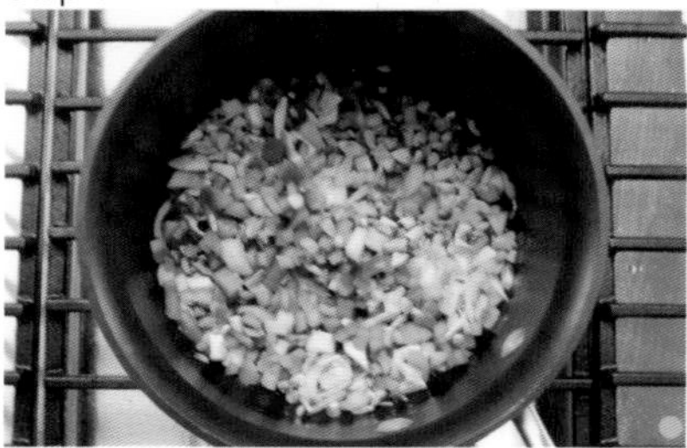

Step 2

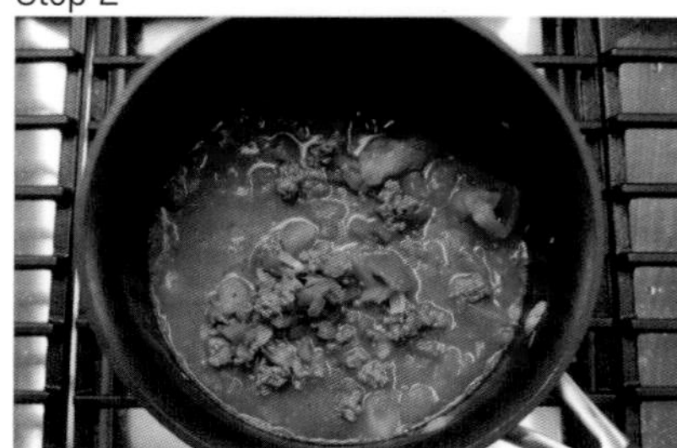

Step 3

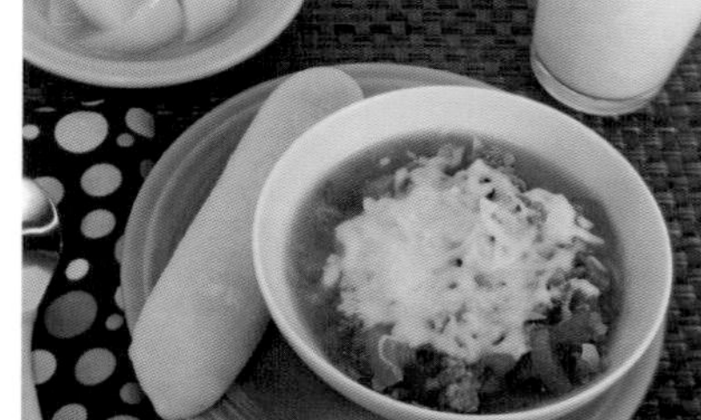

Creditable lunch/supper

Pizza Soup provides M/MA and VEG at lunch/supper			
	Toddler	Pre-School	School Age
Pizza Soup	1/2 cup	3/4 cup	1 cup
Breadsticks	1/2 ounce	1/2 ounce	1 ounce
Peaches	1/8 cup	1/4 cup	1/4 cup
Milk	1/2 cup	3/4 cup	1 cup

Potato & Corn Chowder

Prep time - 15 minutes
Cook time - 25 minutes
Total time - 40 minutes

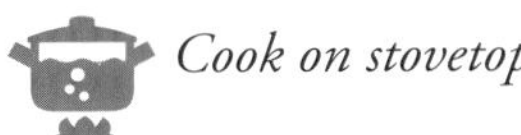

Cook on stovetop

Yield - 6 cups

Ingredients

1 tablespoon vegetable oil
½ cup onions, chopped
3 cups chicken broth
2 cups potatoes, finely diced
1 cup frozen whole kernel corn
¾ cup milk, divided
½ teaspoon salt
¼ teaspoon pepper
2 tablespoons cornstarch

Directions

1. Heat oil in large saucepan over medium heat. Add onions and cook until tender, about 5 minutes.
2. Add broth and potatoes and bring to a boil. Reduce heat, cover and simmer until potatoes are cooked through, about 15 minutes.
3. Stir in the corn, ¼ cup of the milk, salt and pepper.
4. In a small bowl, whisk cornstarch and the remaining ½ cup milk until smooth.
5. Stir cornstarch mixture into soup and return to a boil. Reduce heat and simmer, stirring frequently, until thickened, about 5 minutes.

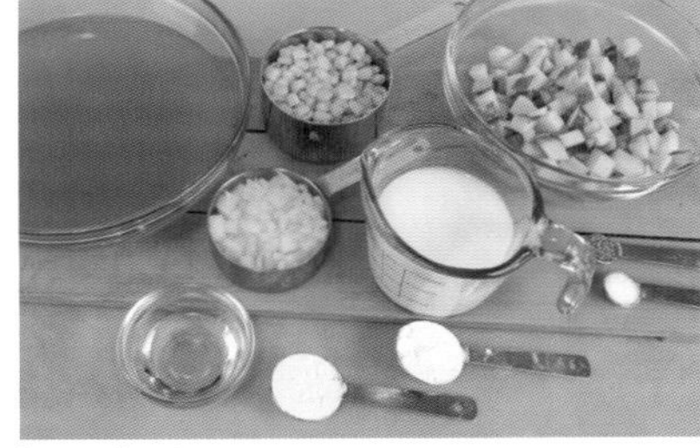

Ingredients

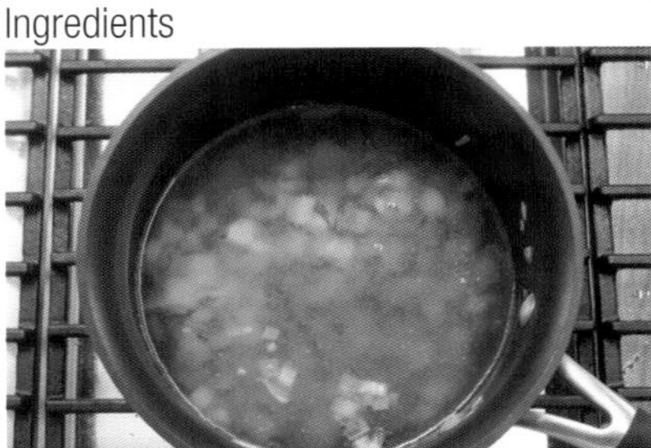

Step 2

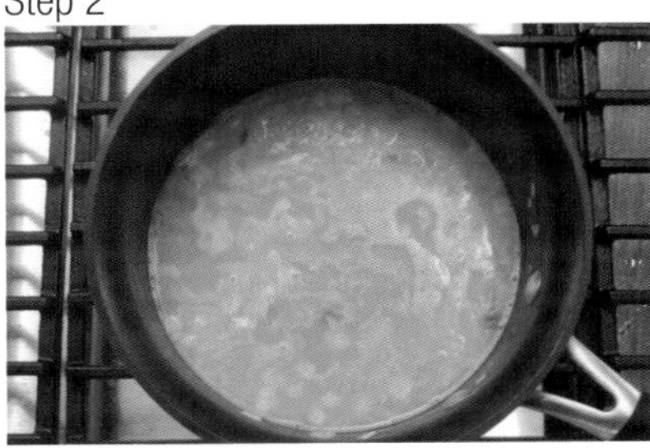

Step 3

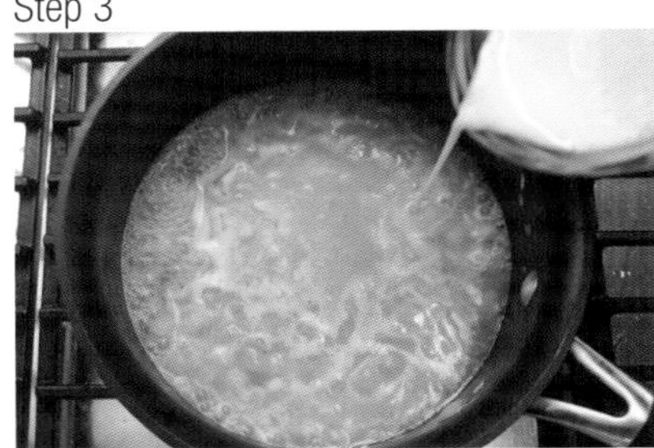

Step 5

Potato & Corn Chowder provides VEG at lunch/supper			
	Toddler	Pre-School	School Age
Chowder	2/3 cup	1 cup	1-1/3 cups
Roast Beef Sandwich	1/2 sandwich	1/2 sandwich	1 sandwich
Tropical Fruit	1/8 cup	1/4 cup	1/4 cup
Milk	1/2 cup	3/4 cup	1 cup

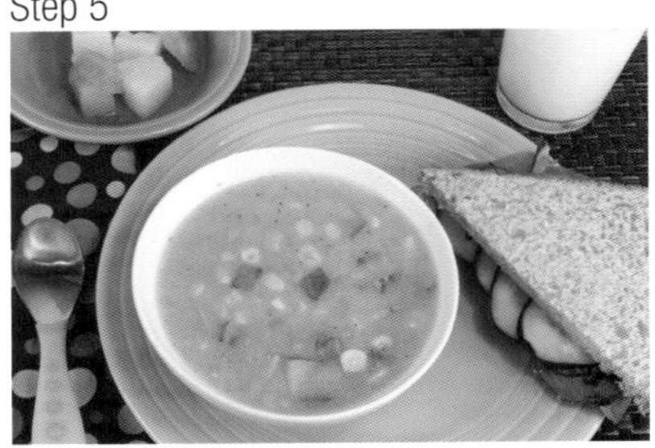

Creditable lunch/supper

Primo Pasta Salad

Prep time - 20 minutes
Cook time - 10 minutes
Total time - 30 minutes

Cook on stovetop

Yield - 6 cups

Ingredients

3 ounces (1¼ cups) whole grain rotini (spiral) pasta
Water for boiling pasta
12 ounces cooked chicken, diced
1½ cups fresh tomatoes, diced
1½ cups carrots, finely shredded
3 tablespoons vegetable oil
¼ cup grated Parmesan cheese

Directions

1. Cook pasta according to package directions, around 10 minutes. Drain and cool.
2. In a large bowl, mix together the chicken and vegetables.
3. When the pasta is cooled, add it to the chicken and vegetables.
4. Drizzle oil and sprinkle Parmesan cheese over all. Toss well to coat.

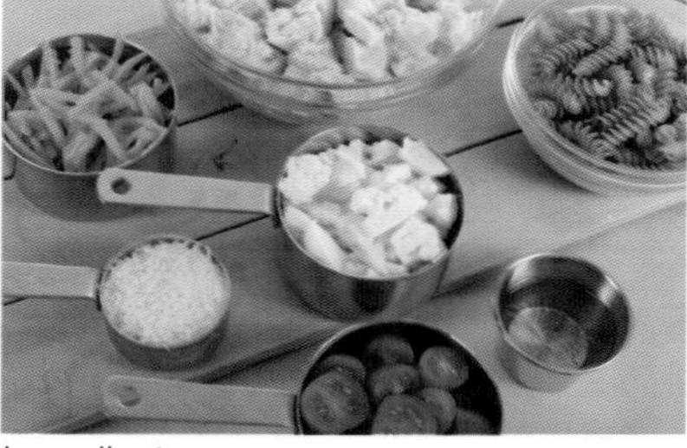

Ingredients

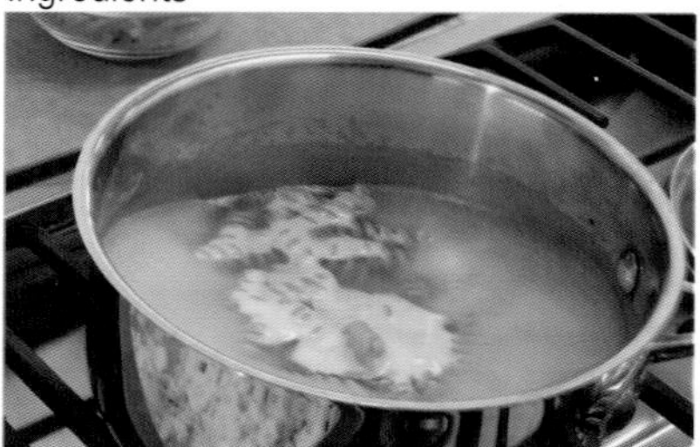

Step 1

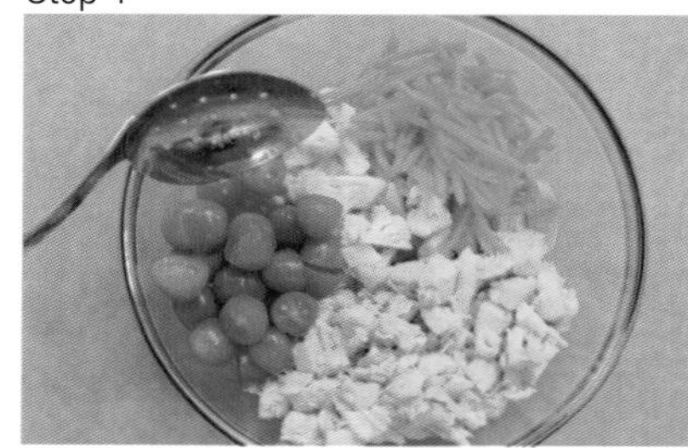

Step 2

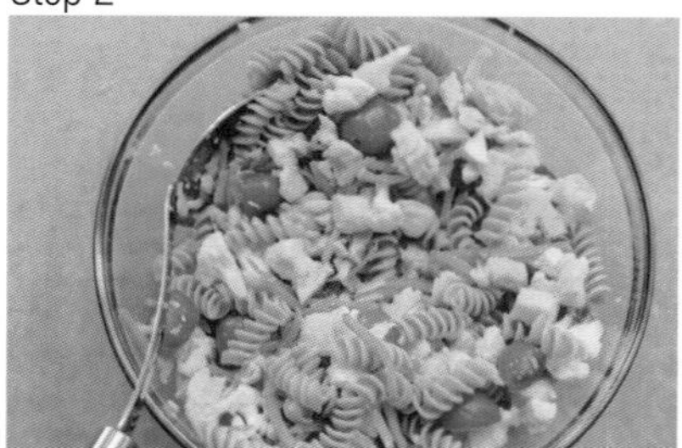

Step 4

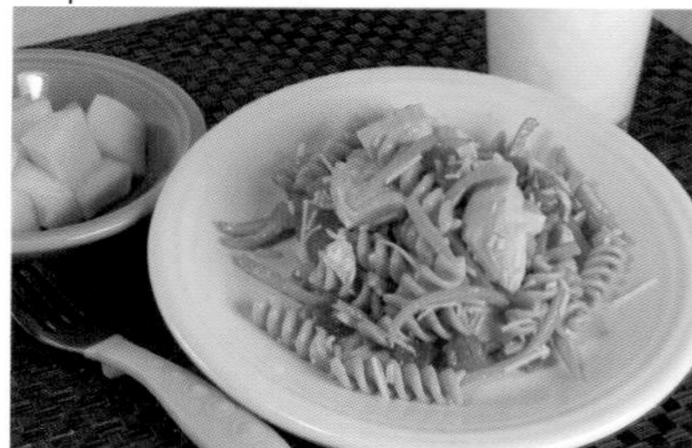

Creditable lunch/supper

Primo Pasta Salad provides G/B, M/MA and VEG at lunch/supper			
	Toddler	Pre-School	School Age
Pasta Salad	1 cup	1 cup	1-1/2 cups
Melon	1/8 cup	1/4 cup	1/4 cup
Milk	1/2 cup	3/4 cup	1 cup

Southwest Chicken Salad

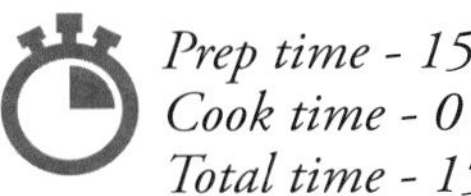

Prep time - 15 minutes
Cook time - 0 minutes
Total time - 15 minutes

No cook, no bake

Yield - 3 cups

Ingredients

½ cup sour cream
6 tablespoons lemon juice
½ teaspoon chili powder
¼ teaspoon salt, or to taste
6 ounces cooked chicken, diced
1 cup black beans, rinsed and drained
1½ cups romaine lettuce, shredded
¾ cup (3 ounces) shredded cheddar cheese

Directions

1. In a small bowl, make the dressing by whisking together the sour cream, lemon juice, chili powder and salt.
2. In another bowl, combine the chicken and black beans. Pour dressing over the chicken and toss to coat.
3. To serve, place lettuce on each plate. Top with the chicken salad and sprinkle with 2 tablespoons cheese.

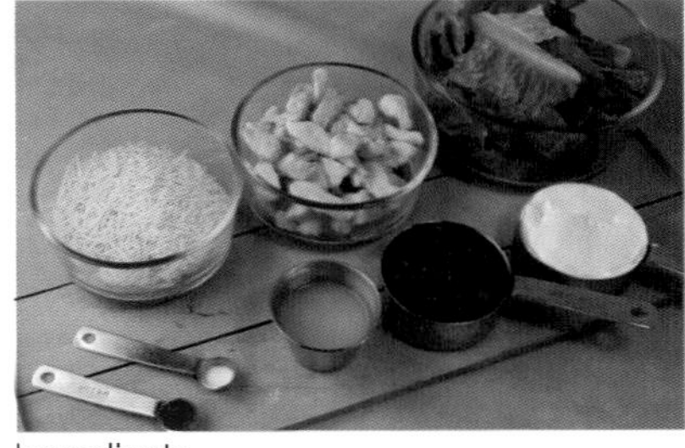

Ingredients

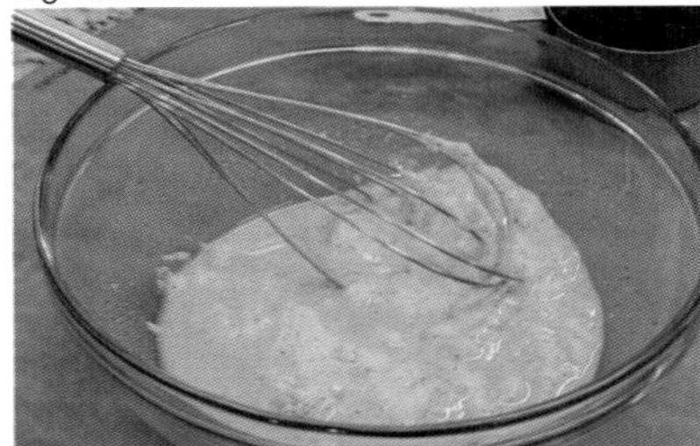

Step 1

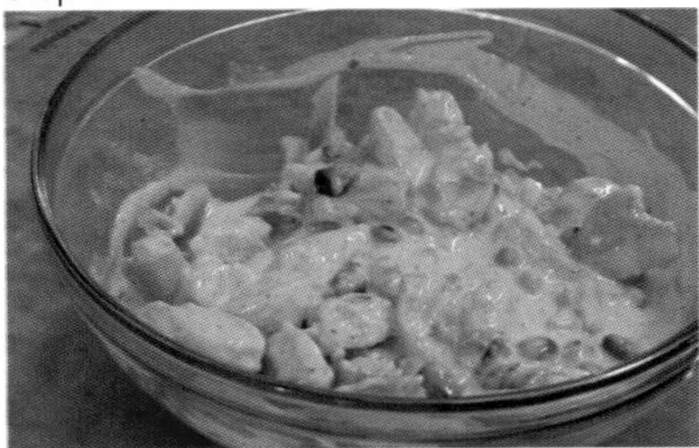

Step 2

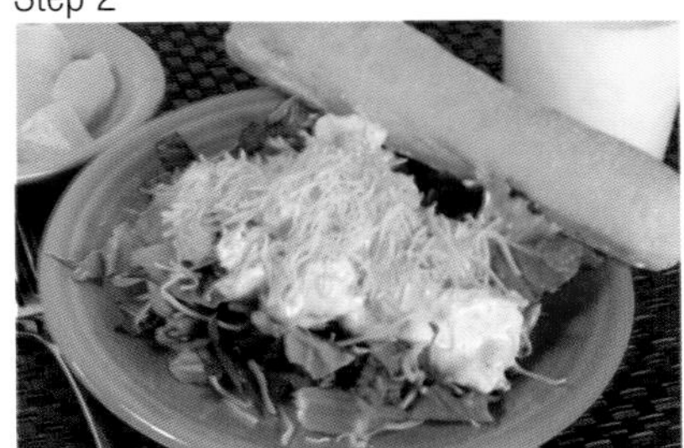

Creditable lunch/supper

Southwest Chicken Salad
provides M/MA and VEG at lunch/supper

	Toddler	Pre-School	School Age
Chicken Salad	1/3 cup	1/2 cup	2/3 cup
Lettuce	1/8 cup	1/4 cup	1/2 cup
Breadsticks	1/2 ounce	1/2 ounce	1 ounce
Tropical Fruit	1/8 cup	1/4 cup	1/4 cup
Milk	1/2 cup	3/4 cup	1 cup

Squash Soup

Prep time - 20 minutes
Cook time - 50 minutes
Total time - 70 minutes

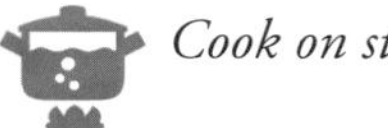

Cook on stovetop

Yield - 9 cups

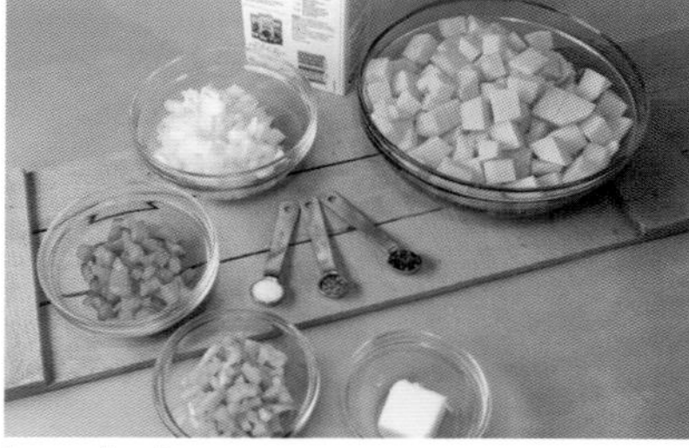
Ingredients

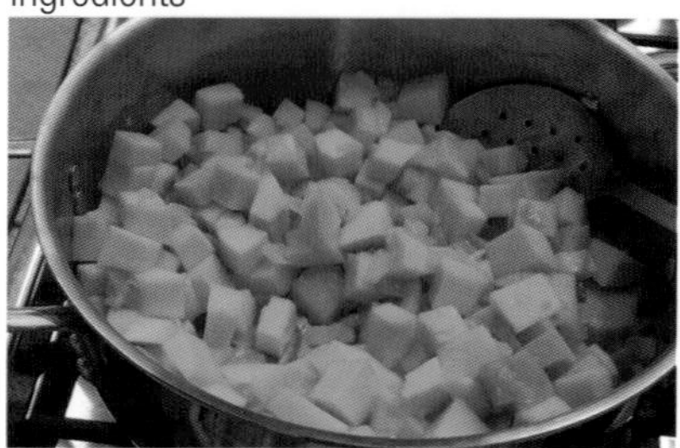
Step 2

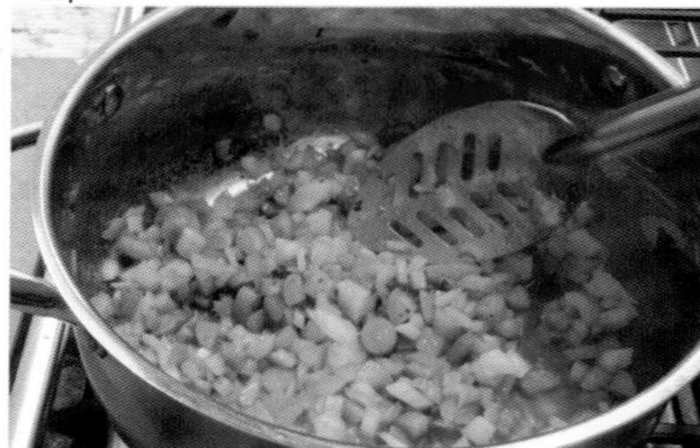
Step 2

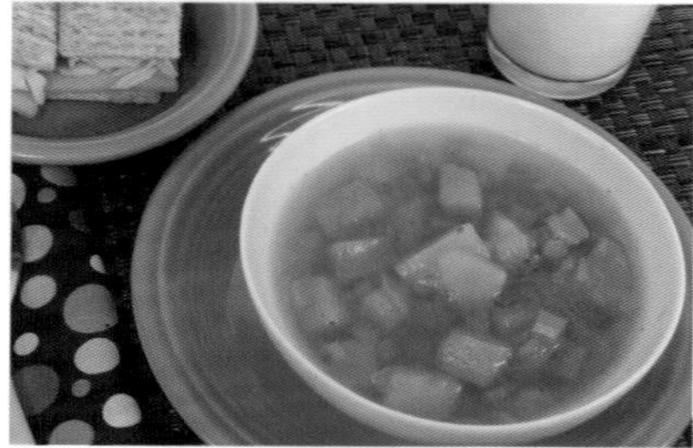
Creditable lunch/supper

Ingredients

2 tablespoons butter
1 cup onions, chopped
½ cup celery, chopped
½ cup carrots, peeled and chopped
4 cups butternut squash, (about 1 medium)
—peeled, seeded and cubed
4 cups vegetable broth
½ teaspoon dried parsley
½ teaspoon salt
¼ teaspoon black pepper

Directions

1. Melt the butter in a large soup pot over medium heat.
2. Add the squash, onions, celery, carrots, parsley, salt and pepper. Cook, stirring occasionally, until lightly browned, about 10 minutes.
3. Add the broth and bring to a boil. Reduce heat, cover and simmer until all vegetables are tender, about 40 minutes.

Batch Cooking Recipe *- Make ahead, freeze and reheat.*
This recipe provides 20 ¼-cup servings of VEG.

Squash Soup provides VEG at lunch/supper			
	Toddler	Pre-School	School Age
Squash Soup	3/4 cup	3/4 cup	1-1/4 cups
Crackerwiches	2	2	3
Pears	1/8 cup	1/4 cup	1/4 cup
Milk	1/2 cup	3/4 cup	1 cup

Recipe for Crackerwiches is on page 170.

Three-Bean Turkey Chili

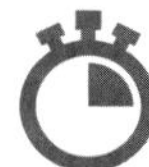

Prep time - 20 minutes
Cook time - 3 hours, 10 min.
Total time - 3½ hours

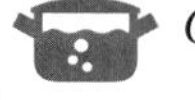

Cook in slow cooker

Yield - 12 cups

Ingredients

1 pound ground turkey
3 cups diced tomatoes, with juice
2 cups chunky salsa
1¾ cups black beans, rinsed and drained
1¾ cups kidney beans, rinsed and drained
1¾ cups great northern beans, rinsed and drained
1 teaspoon chili powder
1 teaspoon ground cumin
¾ cup (3 ounces) shredded cheddar cheese

Directions

1. Cook ground turkey in a skillet over medium-high heat, stirring occasionally, until no longer pink, about 10 minutes.
2. Add turkey to slow cooker with all remaining ingredients except the cheese.
3. Stir well and cover. Cook on high for 3 to 4 hours or on low for 5 to 6 hours, stirring occasionally
4. To serve, top each bowl of soup with 2 tablespoons cheese.

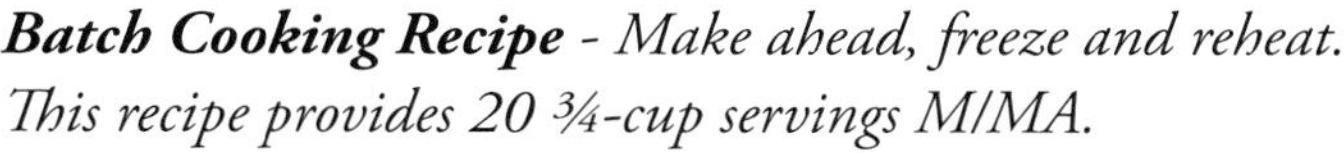

***Batch Cooking Recipe** - Make ahead, freeze and reheat.*
This recipe provides 20 ¾-cup servings M/MA.

Three-Bean Turkey Chili provides M/MA and VEG at lunch/supper			
	Toddler	Pre-School	School Age
Turkey Chili	1/2 cup	3/4 cup	1 cup
Breadsticks	1/2 ounce	1/2 ounce	1 ounce
Pears	1/8 cup	1/4 cup	1/4 cup
Milk	1/2 cup	3/4 cup	1 cup

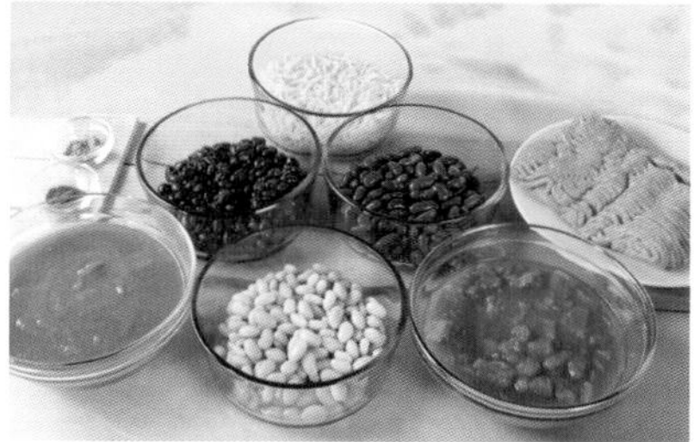

Ingredients

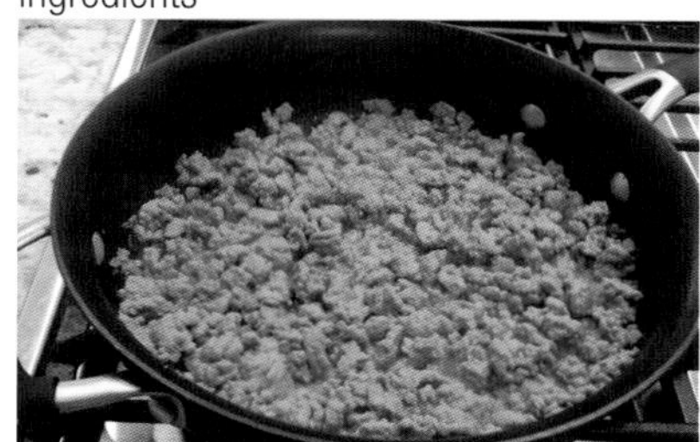

Step 1

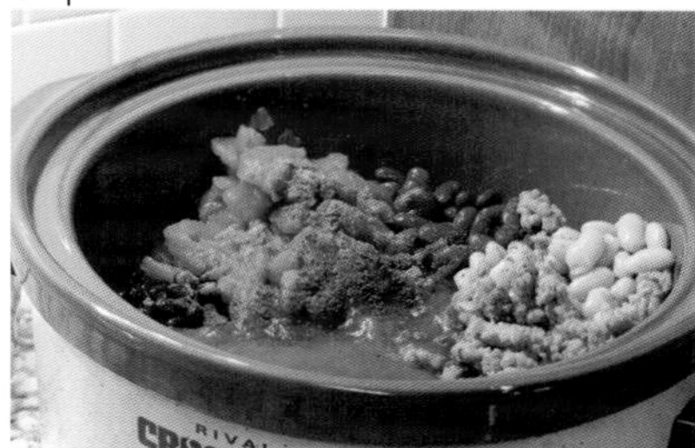

Step 2

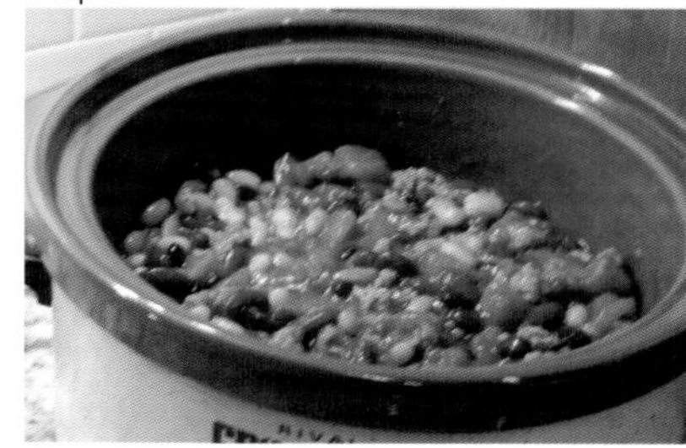

Step 3

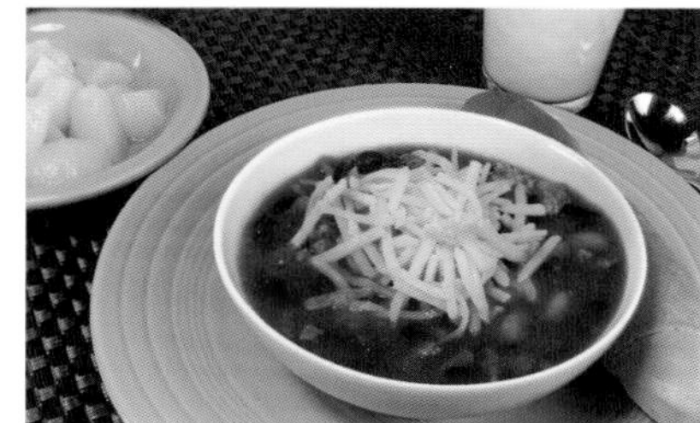

Creditable lunch/supper

Two-Bean Veggie Chili

Prep time - 15 minutes
Cook time - 15 minutes
Total time - 30 minutes

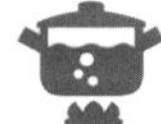

Cook on stovetop

Yield - 8 cups

Ingredients

1¾ cups beans in chili sauce
1¾ cups cannellini beans, rinsed and drained
1½ cups diced tomatoes, with juice
1½ cups tomato-vegetable juice
1½ cups frozen whole kernel corn
1 cup green peppers, cut into 1-inch long strips
2 teaspoons chili powder

Directions

1. In a large soup pot over medium heat, stir together all the beans and vegetables.
2. Add chili powder and bring to a boil.
3. Reduce heat to medium-low, cover and simmer 15 minutes, stirring occasionally.

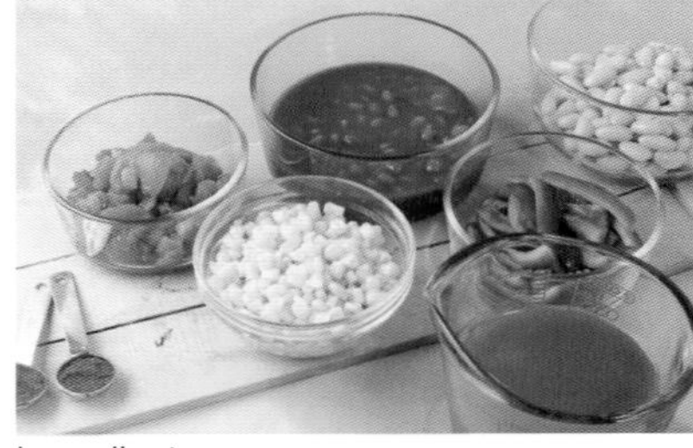

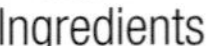

Ingredients

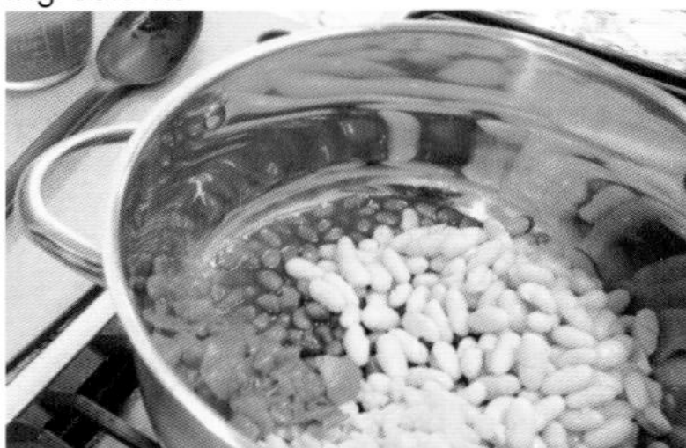

Step 1

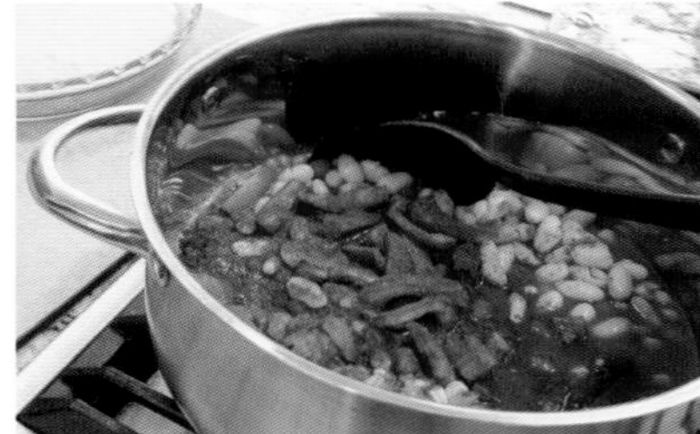

Step 2

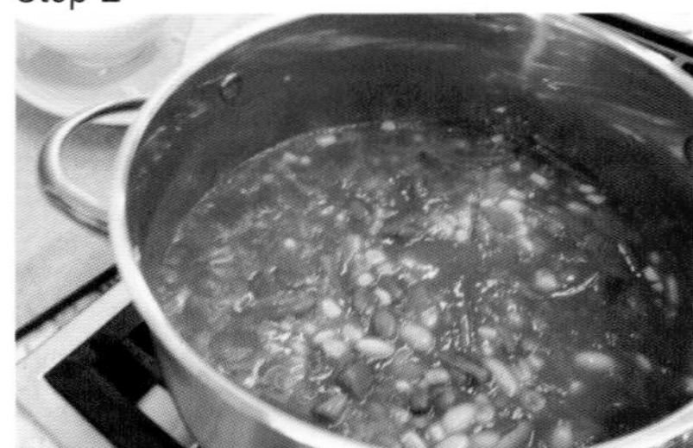

Step 3

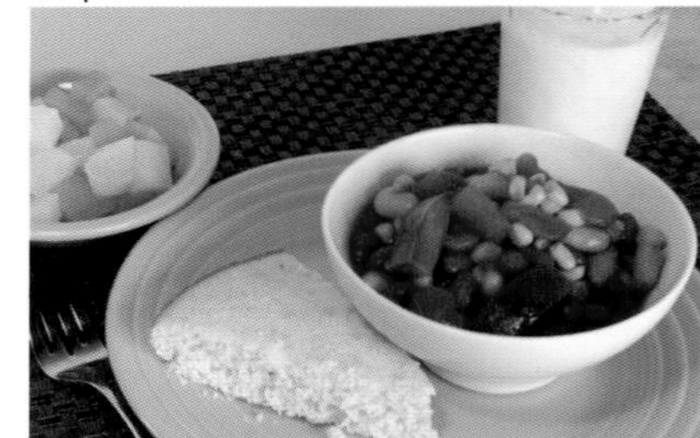

Creditable lunch/supper

Two-Bean Veggie Chili provides M/MA and VEG at lunch/supper			
	Toddler	Pre-School	School Age
Veggie Chili	2/3 cup	1 cup	1-1/3 cups
Cornbread	3/4 ounce	3/4 ounce	1-1/4 ounces
Tropical Fruit	1/8 cup	1/4 cup	1/4 cup
Milk	1/2 cup	3/4 cup	1 cup

Vegetable Beef Soup

Prep time - 15 minutes
Cook time - 45 minutes
Total time - 60 minutes

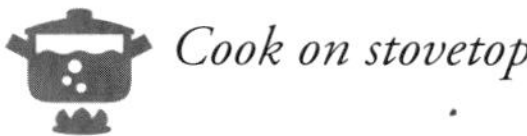

Cook on stovetop

Yield - 6 cups

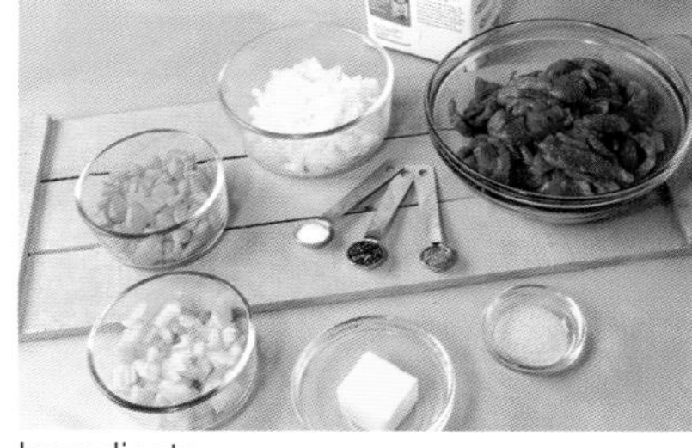

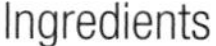

Ingredients

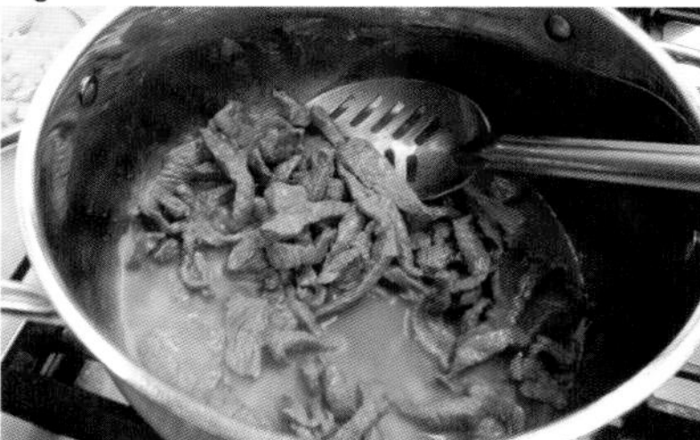

Step 1

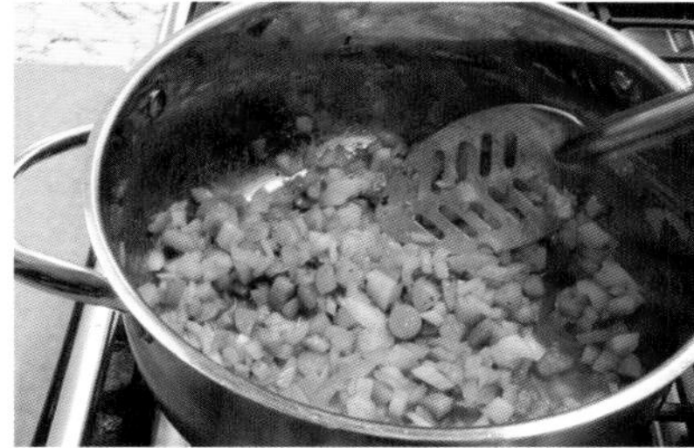

Step 2

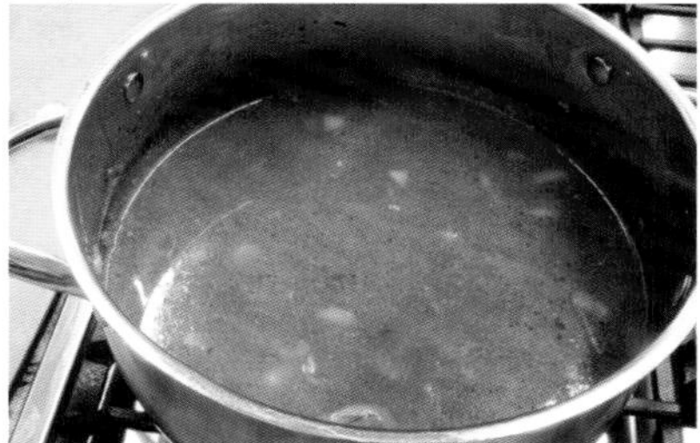

Step 3

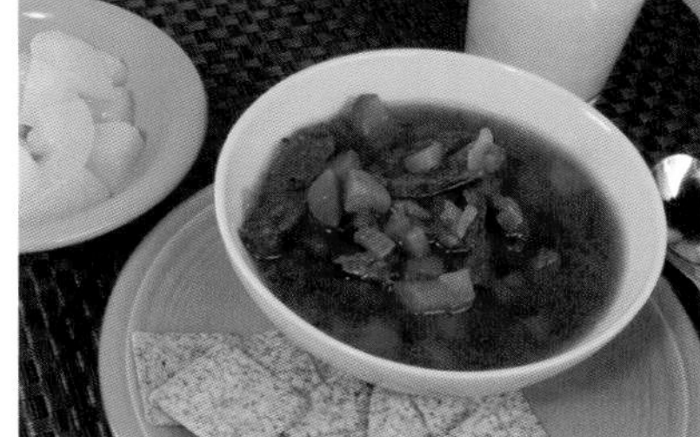

Creditable lunch/supper

Ingredients

2 tablespoons butter
1 pound beef stew meat, cut into thin 1-inch strips
2 teaspoons garlic powder
½ teaspoon dried parsley
½ teaspoon salt
¼ teaspoon black pepper
1 cup onions, chopped
½ cup celery, chopped
½ cup carrots, peeled and chopped
3 cups beef or chicken broth

Directions

1. Heat butter in a large soup pot over medium heat. Add beef and thoroughly brown on all sides, about 10 minutes. Stir in the garlic powder, parsley, salt and pepper, then remove the seasoned meat from the pot and set aside.

2. To the same pot, add the onions, celery and carrots. Cook vegetables until just tender, stirring periodically, 5 minutes.

3. Return browned meat and broth to the pot. Bring to a boil, reduce heat to low, cover and simmer until beef is tender, about 30 minutes.

Vegetable Beef Soup
provides M/MA and VEG at lunch/supper

	Toddler	Pre-School	School Age
Beef Soup	2/3 cup	1 cup	1-1/3 cups
Crackers	1/2 ounce	1/2 ounce	3/4 ounce
Pears	1/8 cup	1/4 cup	1/4 cup
Milk	1/2 cup	3/4 cup	1 cup

Vegetable Minestrone

Prep time - 15 minutes
Cook time - 10 minutes
Total time - 25 minutes

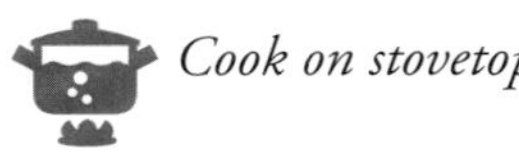

Cook on stovetop

Yield - 9 cups

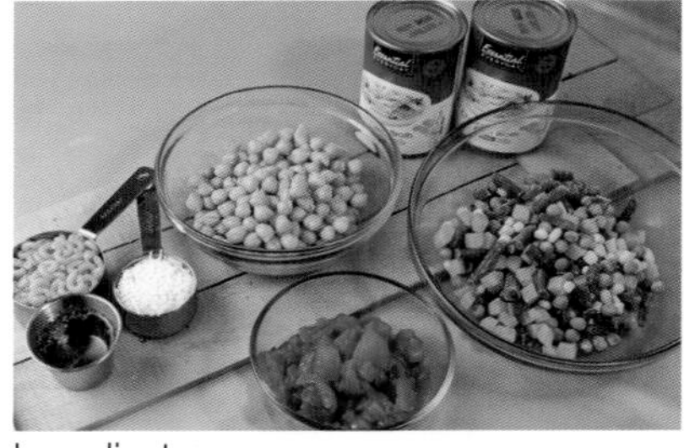

Ingredients

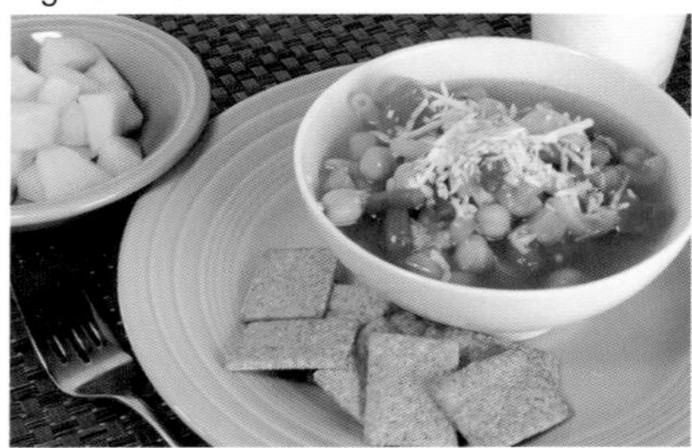

Creditable lunch/supper

Ingredients

3 cups chicken broth
2 ounces (½ cup) dry whole grain elbow macaroni
2¼ cups garbanzo beans, rinsed and drained
1 cup diced tomatoes, with juice
1½ cups frozen Italian vegetables blend
¼ cup Italian dressing
¼ cup shredded Parmesan cheese

Directions

1. In a large saucepan, bring the broth to a boil, add the macaroni and cook for 5 minutes.
2. Add remaining ingredients, except for the cheese, and return to a boil. Reduce heat and simmer, uncovered, over medium-low heat until macaroni is tender, 5-10 minutes.
3. To serve, pour soup into bowls and sprinkle each with ½ tablespoon Parmesan cheese.

Vegetable Minestrone
provides M/MA and VEG at lunch/supper

	Toddler	Pre-School	School Age
Minestrone	1 cup	1-1/2 cups	2 cups
Crackers	1/2 ounce	1/2 ounce	3/4 ounce
Melon	1/8 cup	1/4 cup	1/4 cup
Milk	1/2 cup	3/4 cup	1 cup

White Chicken Chili

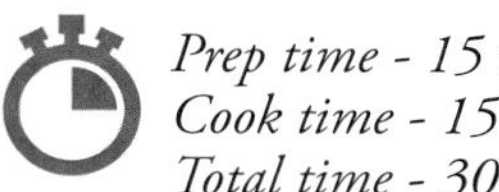
Prep time - 15 minutes
Cook time - 15 minutes
Total time - 30 minutes

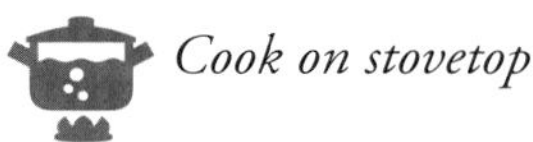
Cook on stovetop

Yield - 8 cups

Ingredients

2 tablespoons vegetable oil
1 pound boneless, skinless chicken breast, finely diced
2 teaspoons ground cumin
½ teaspoon dried oregano
½ cup onions, chopped, optional
4 cups chicken broth
2 cups garbanzo beans, rinsed and drained, divided
⅜ cup (1½ ounces) shredded mozzarella cheese

Directions

1. Heat the oil in a large soup pot over medium heat, then cook the chicken with the onions, cumin and oregano until lightly browned, about 5 minutes. Stir in the broth.
2. Mash half of the beans. Add them and the remaining whole beans to the pot.
3. Bring to a boil. Reduce heat to low and simmer until chicken is tender, with an internal temperature of 165 degrees, about 10 minutes.
4. To serve, pour soup into bowls and sprinkle each with 1 tablespoon cheese.

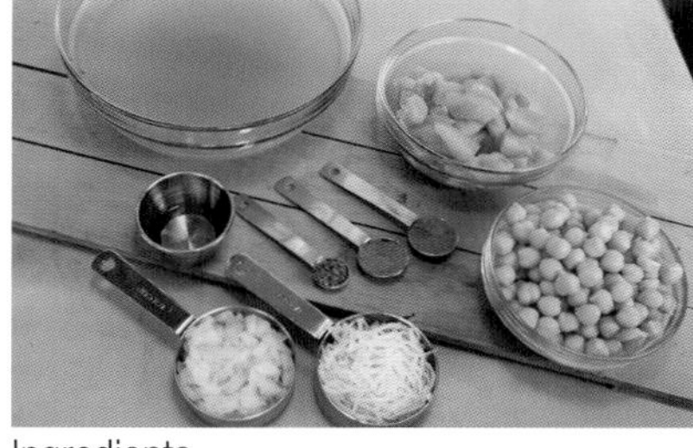
Ingredients

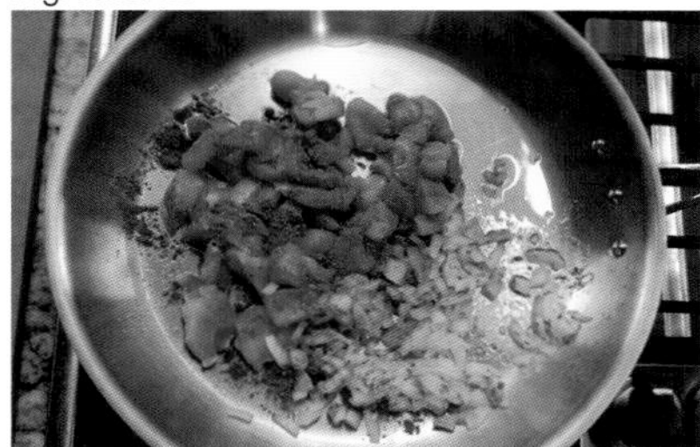
Step 1

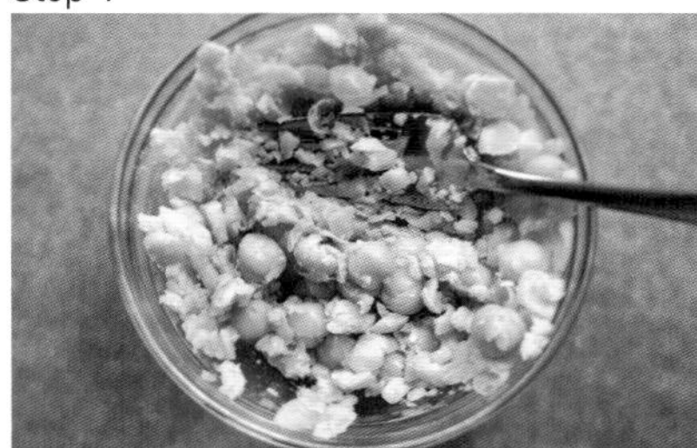
Step 2

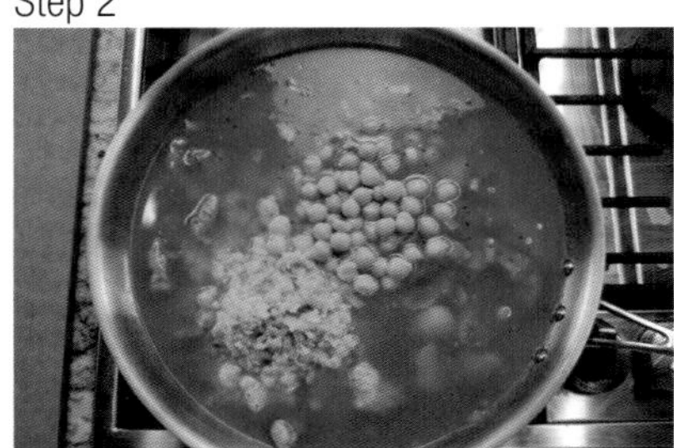
Step 3

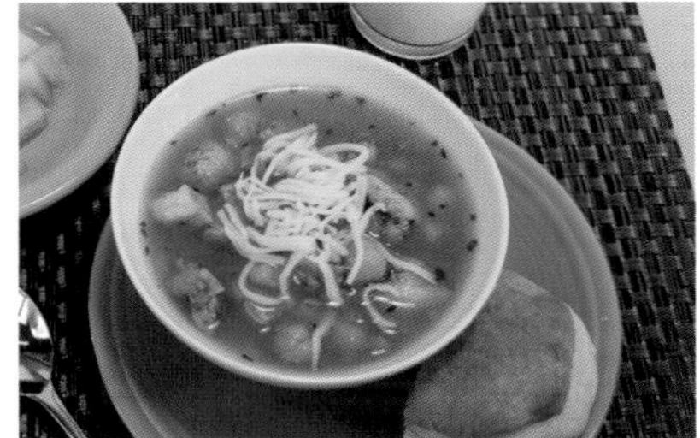
Creditable lunch/supper

White Chicken Chili
provides M/MA and VEG at lunch/supper

	Toddler	Pre-School	School Age
Chicken Chili	2/3 cup	1 cup	1-1/3 cup
Biscuits	1/2 ounce	1/2 ounce	1 ounce
Melon	1/8 cup	1/4 cup	1/4 cup
Milk	1/2 cup	3/4 cup	1 cup

Barbeque Sandwich

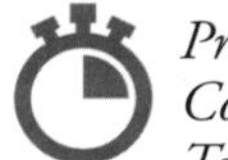

Prep time - 15 minutes
Cook time - 10 minutes
Total time - 25 minutes

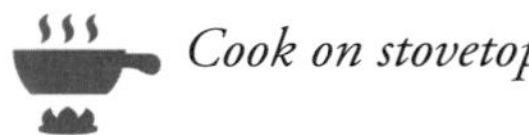

Cook on stovetop

Yield - 3 sandwiches

Ingredients

1 pound ground beef, at least 80% lean
¼ cup tomato paste
1 tablespoon mustard
2 teaspoons brown sugar
3 whole wheat hamburger buns, at least 1½ ounces each

Directions

1. In a skillet, brown ground beef until it reaches an internal temperature of 160 degrees and is no longer pink, about 10 minutes.
2. Stir in the tomato paste, mustard and brown sugar and mix well.
3. Fill each bun with one-third of the barbeque beef.

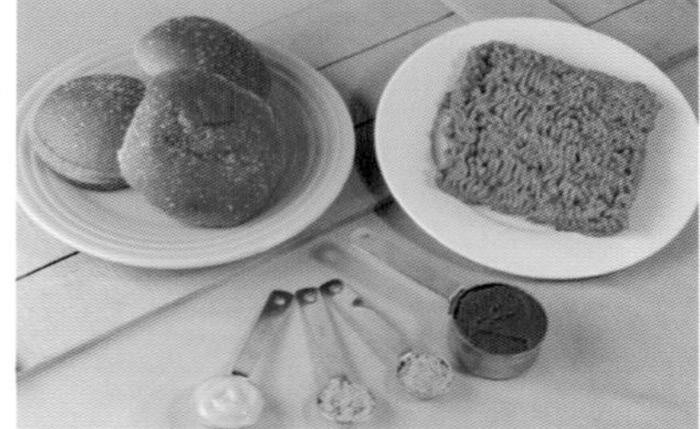

Ingredients

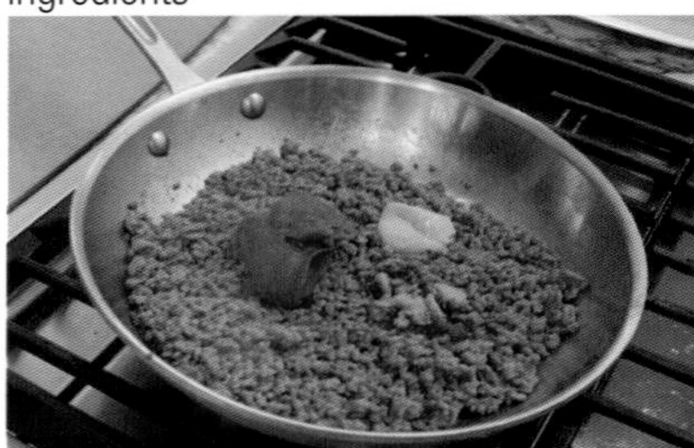

Step 2

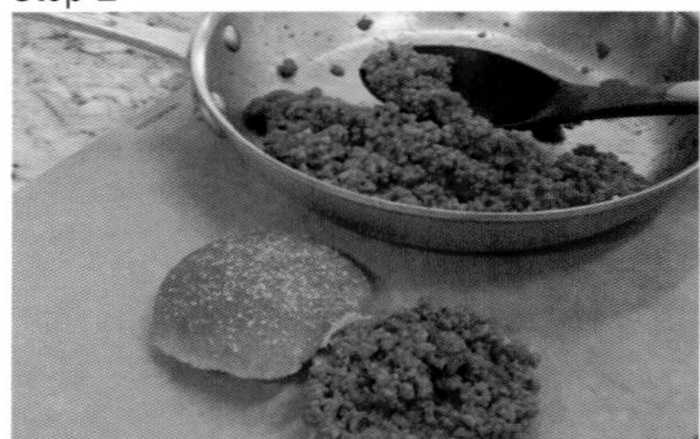

Step 3

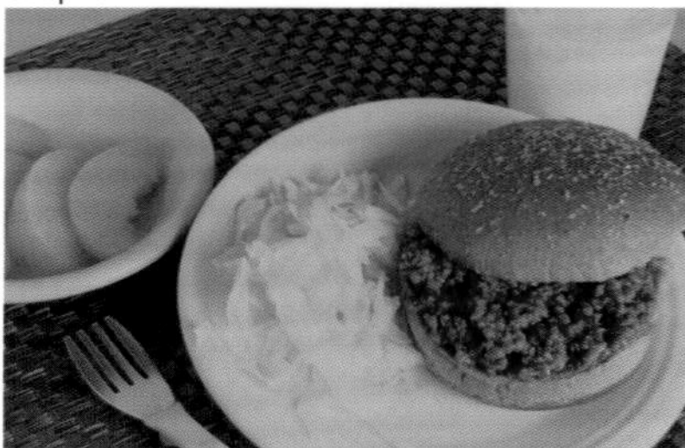

Creditable lunch/supper

Barbeque Sandwich provides G/B and M/MA at lunch/supper			
	Toddler	Pre-School	School Age
BBQ Sandwich	1/2 sandwich	1/2 sandwich	1 sandwich
Lettuce Salad	1/8 cup	1/4 cup	1/2 cup
Peaches	1/8 cup	1/4 cup	1/4 cup
Milk	1/2 cup	3/4 cup	1 cup

Black Bean Burger

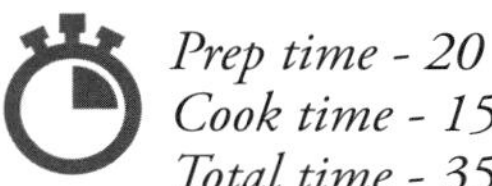

Prep time - 20 minutes
Cook time - 15 minutes
Total time - 35 minutes

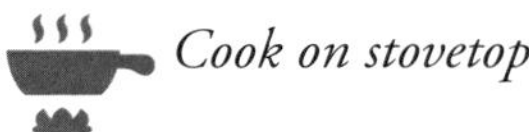

Cook on stovetop

Yield - 3 burgers

Ingredients

2¼ cups black beans, rinsed and drained
1 teaspoon vegetable oil
½ cup green peppers, diced
½ cup onions, diced
2 teaspoons garlic powder
2 teaspoons ground cumin
½ cup bread crumbs
2 eggs, beaten
3 whole wheat hamburger buns, at least 1½ ounces each

Directions

1. Preheat oven to 375 degrees. Line a baking sheet with foil or parchment paper, or coat with cooking spray.
2. In a small skillet, sauté green peppers and onions over medium heat until peppers are tender, about 5 minutes.
3. In a medium bowl, mash black beans with a fork until thick and pasty.
4. Add the sautéed vegetables, garlic powder, cumin, bread crumbs and the eggs to the beans and mix thoroughly.
5. Form 3 patties and place on baking sheet. Bake until lightly golden and firm, about 10-15 minutes. Flip burgers over once, about halfway through cooking. Serve on buns.

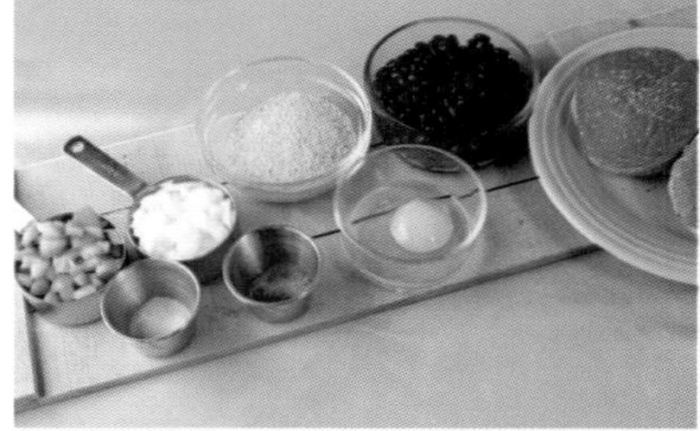

Ingredients

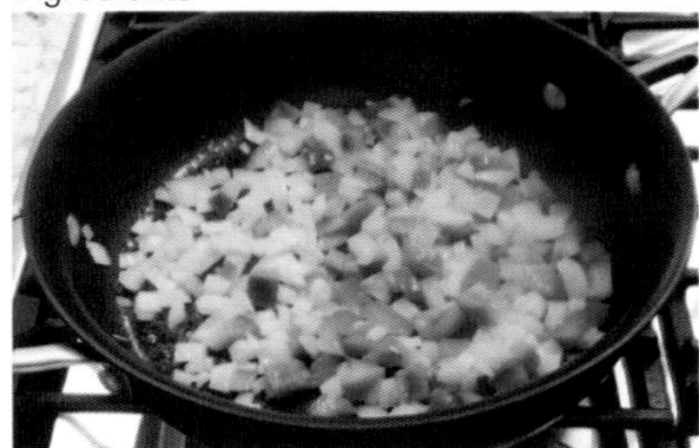

Step 2

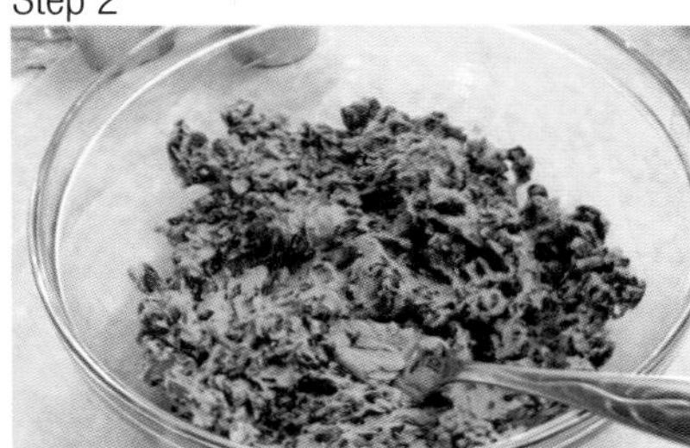

Step 3

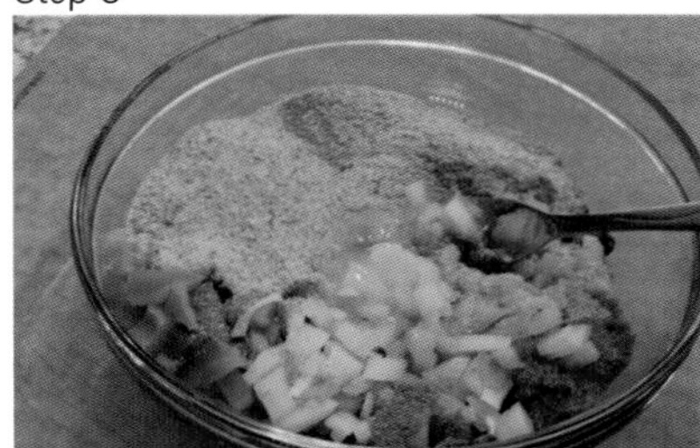

Step 4

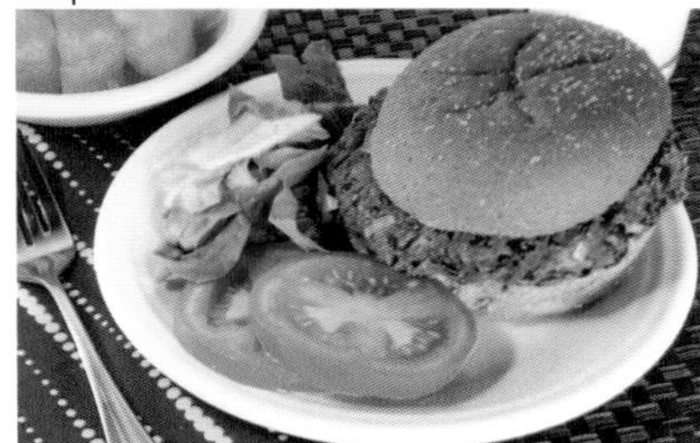

Creditable lunch/supper

Black Bean Burger
provides G/B and M/MA at lunch/supper

	Toddler	Pre-School	School Age
Bean Burger	1/2 burger	1/2 burger	1 burger
Lettuce & Tomato	1/8 cup	1/4 cup	1/2 cup
Watermelon	1/8 cup	1/4 cup	1/4 cup
Milk	1/2 cup	3/4 cup	1 cup

California Burger

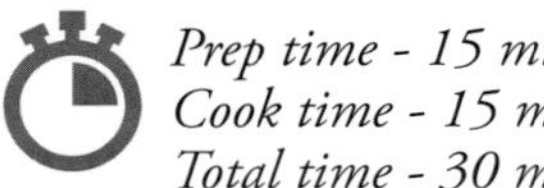
Prep time - 15 minutes
Cook time - 15 minutes
Total time - 30 minutes

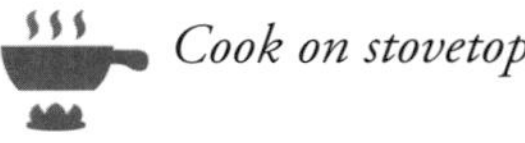
Cook on stovetop

Yield - 3 burgers

Ingredients

1 pound ground beef, at least 80% lean
1 cup sliced tomatoes
1½ cups lettuce leaves
3 1-ounce slices cheddar cheese
3 whole wheat hamburger buns, at least 1½ ounces each

Directions

1. Preheat oven to 400 degrees. Line a baking sheet with foil or parchment paper, or coat with cooking spray.
2. Make 3 burger patties, about 5 ounces each, and place on baking sheet.
3. Bake until patties are brown and firm to the touch, with an internal temperature of 160 degrees, about 15-20 minutes. Remove from oven.
4. Serve burgers on buns and top with cheese, lettuce and tomatoes.

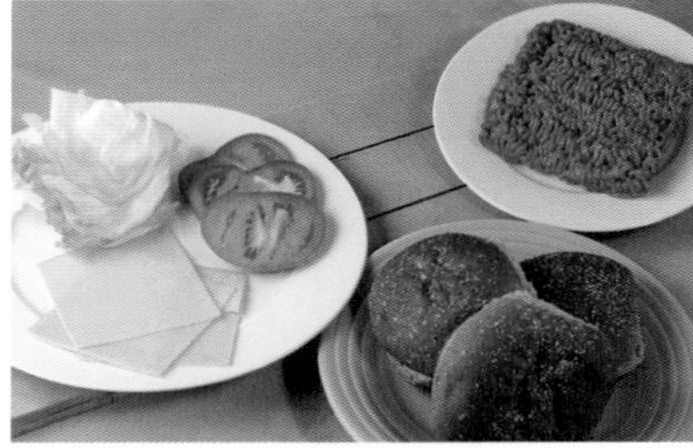
Ingredients

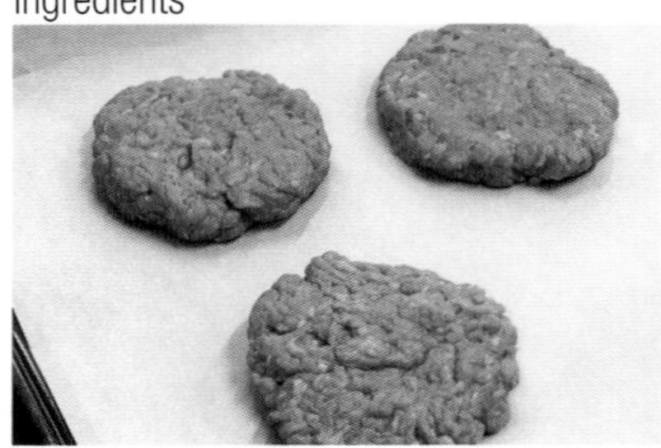
Step 2

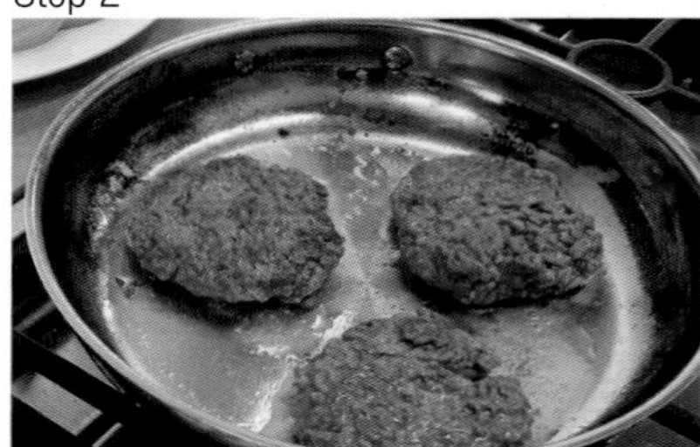
Step 3

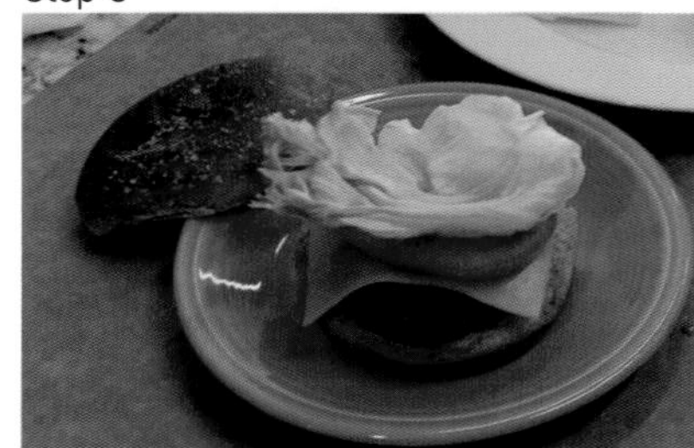
Step 4

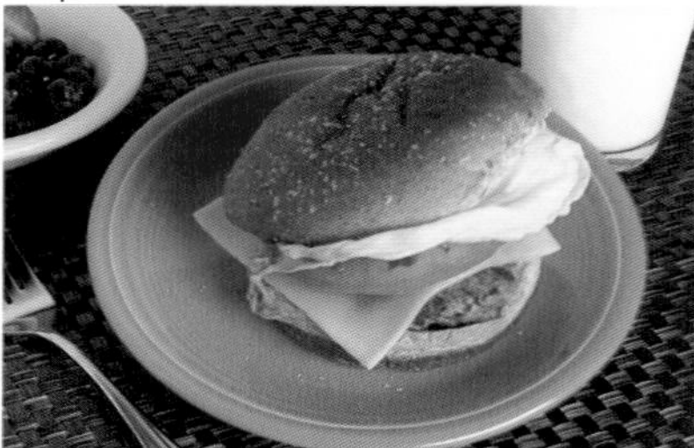
Creditable lunch/supper

California Burger provides G/B, M/MA and VEG at lunch/supper			
	Toddler	Pre-School	School Age
California Burger	1/2 burger	1/2 burger	1 burger
Mixed Berries	1/8 cup	1/4 cup	1/4 cup
Milk	1/2 cup	3/4 cup	1 cup

Chicken Caesar Pita Sandwich

Prep time - 20 minutes
Cook time - 0 minutes
Total time - 20 minutes

No cook, no bake

Yield - 6 sandwiches

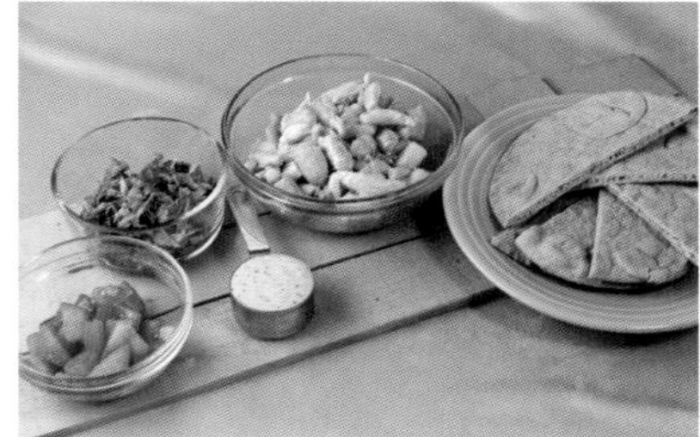

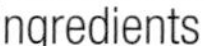
Ingredients

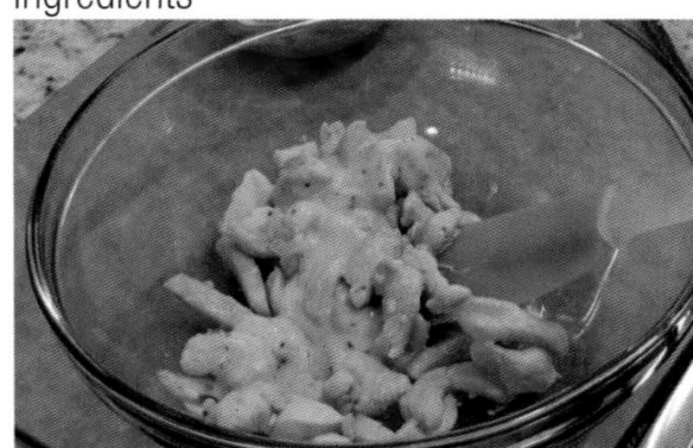

Step 1

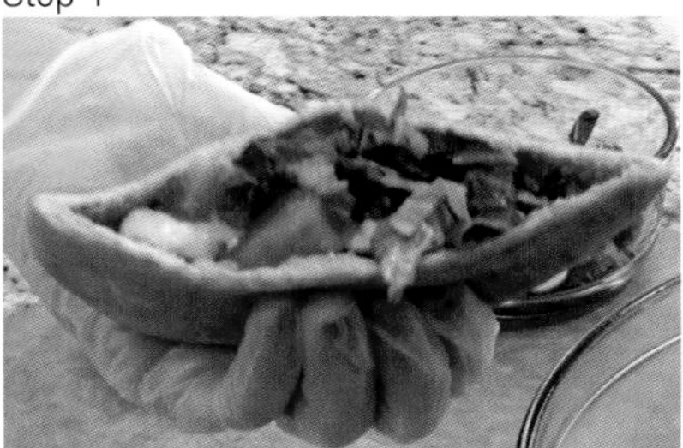

Step 3

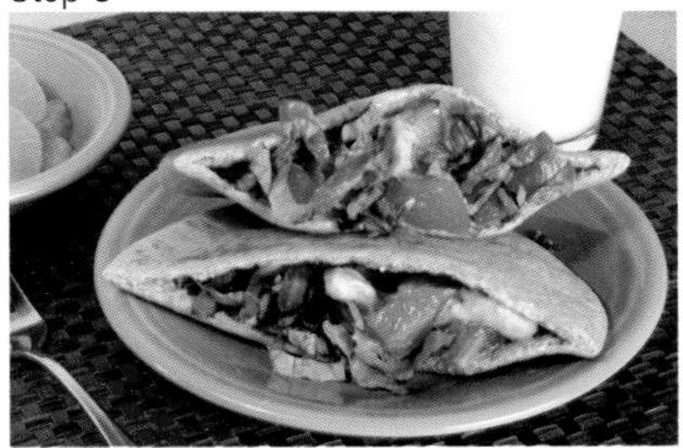

Creditable lunch/supper

Ingredients

9 ounces cooked chicken, diced
¼ cup caesar salad dressing
¾ cup lettuce, shredded
¾ cup fresh tomatoes, diced
3 whole wheat pita bread rounds, at least 1½ ounces each

Directions

1. In a mixing bowl, toss chicken with the salad dressing.
2. Slice each pita round in half and open the pockets.
3. Stuff each pita pocket with 1½ ounces chicken and ⅛ cup each of tomato and lettuce.

Chicken Caesar Pita Sandwich provides G/B, M/MA and VEG at lunch/supper			
	Toddler	Pre-School	School Age
Pita Sandwich	1/2 round	1/2 round	1 round
Mandarin Oranges	1/8 cup	1/4 cup	1/4 cup
Milk	1/2 cup	3/4 cup	1 cup

Chicken Mozzarella Melt

Prep time - 15 minutes
Cook time - 10 minutes
Total time - 25 minutes

Bake in oven

Yield - 3 sandwiches

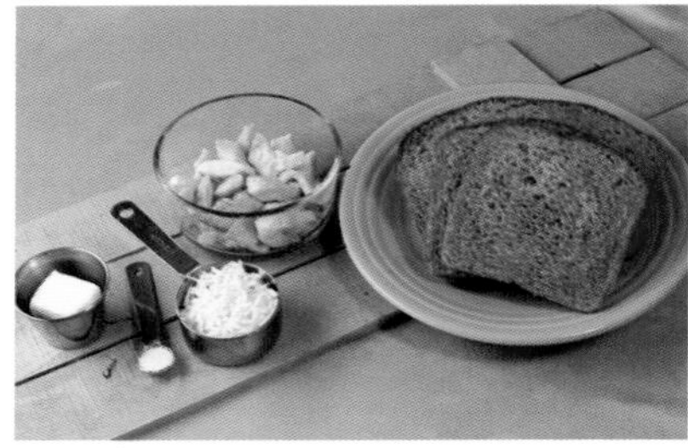

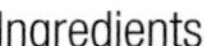

Ingredients

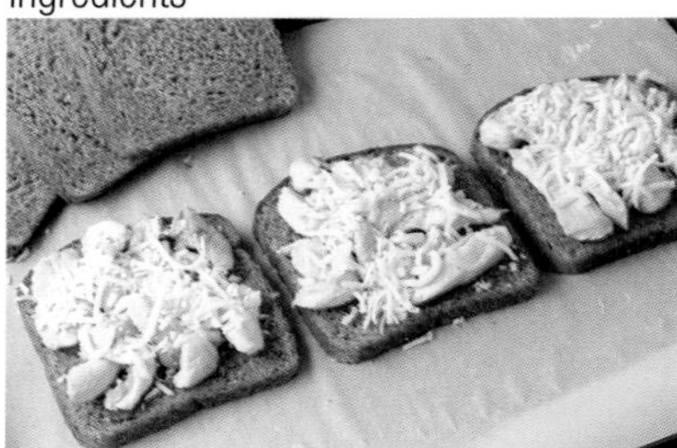

Step 3

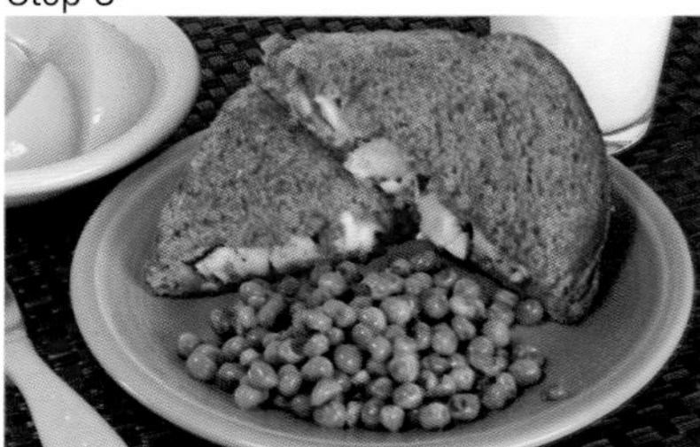

Creditable lunch/supper

Ingredients

6 slices whole grain bread, at least 1½ ounces each
2 tablespoons butter
6 ounces cooked chicken, sliced
¾ cup (3 ounces) shredded mozzarella cheese
⅛ teaspoon salt per sandwich, or to taste

Directions

1. Preheat oven to 350 degrees. Line a baking sheet with foil or parchment paper, or coat with cooking spray.
2. Butter one side of each bread slice. Place 3 slices on baking sheet, buttered side down.
3. Place 2 ounces of chicken and 1 ounce (¼ cup) of cheese on each slice of bread. Top with remaining slices of bread, buttered sides up.
4. Bake until golden brown, chicken is warmed through and cheese is melted, about 10 minutes. Flip sandwiches halfway through baking.

Chicken Mozzarella Melt Sandwich provides G/B and M/MA at lunch/supper			
	Toddler	Pre-School	School Age
Chicken Melt	1/2 sandwich	1/2 sandwich	1 sandwich
Peas	1/8 cup	1/4 cup	1/2 cup
Peaches	1/8 cup	1/4 cup	1/4 cup
Milk	1/2 cup	3/4 cup	1 cup

Chicken Sandwich

Prep time - 15 minutes
Cook time - 25 minutes
Total time - 40 minutes

Bake in oven

Yield - 3 sandwiches

Ingredients

1 pound boneless, skinless chicken breast,
—cut into 6-ounce portions
¼ teaspoon salt
¼ teaspoon Italian seasoning
3 lettuce leaves
3 tomato slices
3 1-ounce slices mozzarella cheese
3 whole wheat hamburger buns, at least 1½ ounces each

Directions

1. Preheat oven to 450 degrees. Line a baking sheet with foil or coat with cooking spray.
2. Season chicken with salt and Italian seasoning and place on baking pan.
3. Bake until chicken reaches an internal temperature of 165 degrees, about 25 minutes.
4. Remove from oven and cut into slices. Serve on buns topped with 1 ounce mozzarella cheese, tomato and lettuce.

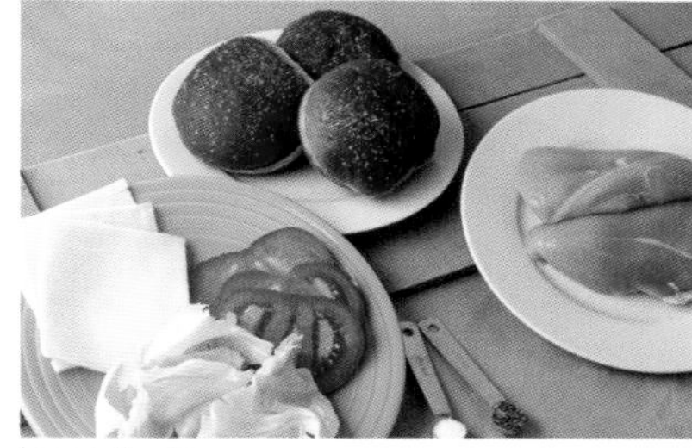

Ingredients

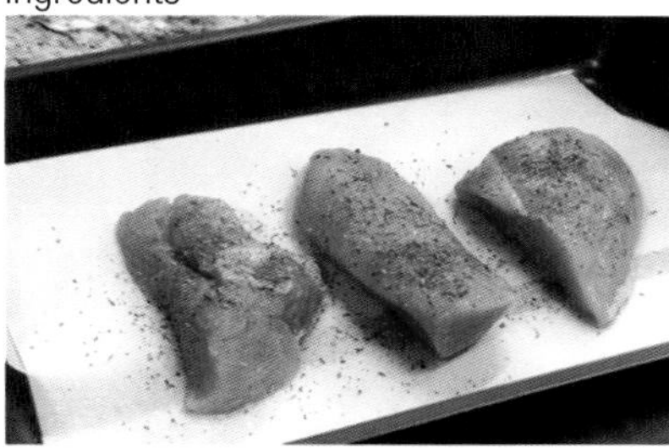

Step 2

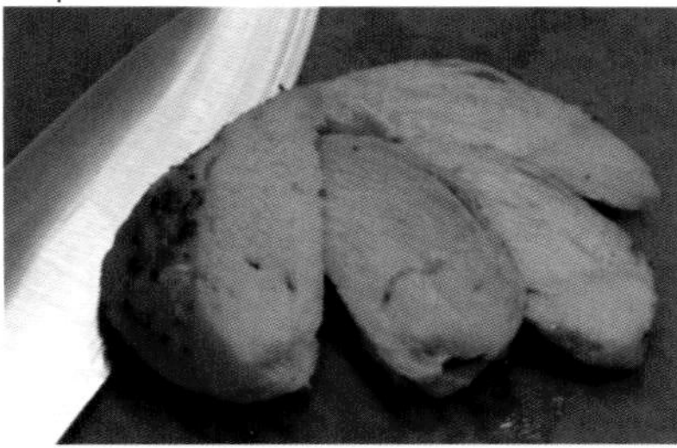

Step 4

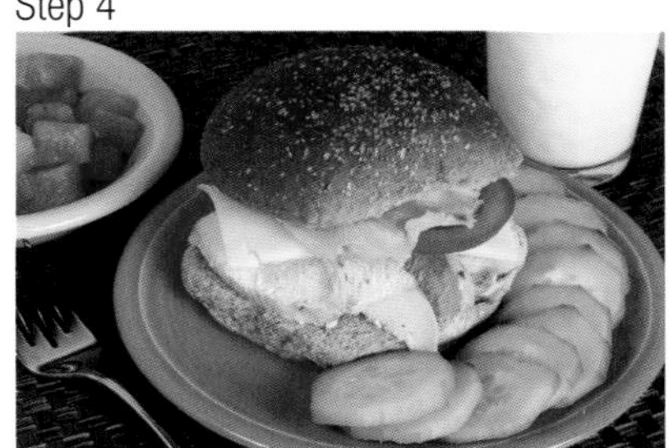

Creditable lunch/supper

Chicken Sandwich provides G/B and M/MA at lunch/supper			
	Toddler	Pre-School	School Age
Chicken Sandwich	1/2 sandwich	1/2 sandwich	1 sandwich
Cucumber	1/8 cup	1/4 cup	1/2 cup
Watermelon	1/8 cup	1/4 cup	1/4 cup
Milk	1/2 cup	3/4 cup	1 cup

Club Sandwich

Prep time - 15 minutes
Cook time - 0 minutes
Total time - 15 minutes

No cook, no bake

Yield - 3 sandwiches

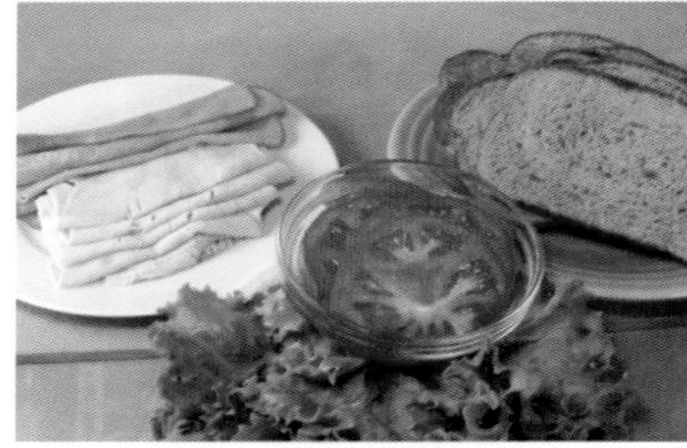
Ingredients

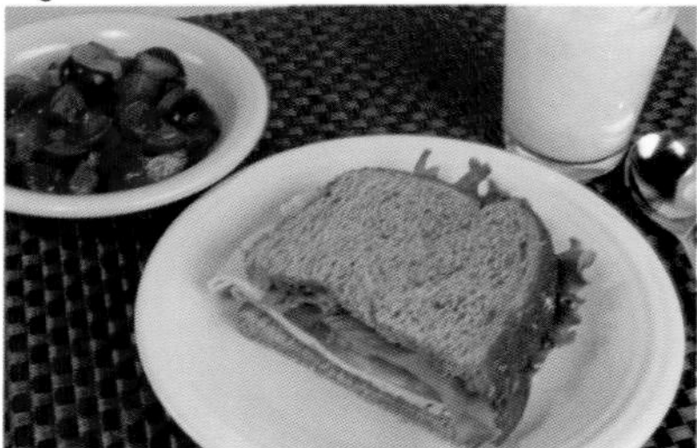
Creditable lunch/supper

Ingredients

6 slices whole grain bread, at least 1½ ounces each
3 tablespoons mayonnaise
6 ounces turkey, thinly sliced
6 ounces turkey ham, thinly sliced
3 lettuce leaves
3 tomato slices
⅛ teaspoon salt per sandwich, or to taste

Directions

1. Spread ½ tablespoon of mayonnaise on each slice of bread.
2. Place 2 ounces of turkey and 2 ounces of turkey ham on each of 3 slices bread. Season with salt, if desired.
3. Top each with a tomato slice, lettuce leaf and the remaining slice of bread.

Club Sandwich
provides G/B, M/MA and VEG at lunch/supper

	Toddler	Pre-School	School Age
Club Sandwich	1/2 sandwich	1/2 sandwich	1 sandwich
Carrots	1/8 cup	1/4 cup	1/2 cup
Grapes	1/8 cup	1/4 cup	1/4 cup
Milk	1/2 cup	3/4 cup	1 cup

Grilled Ham & Cheese

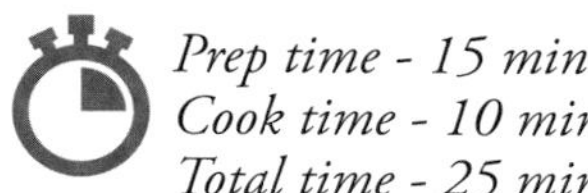
Prep time - 15 minutes
Cook time - 10 minutes
Total time - 25 minutes

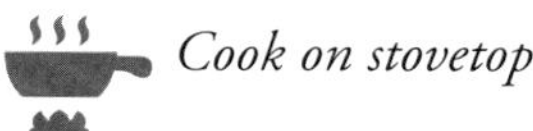
Cook on stovetop

Yield - 3 sandwiches

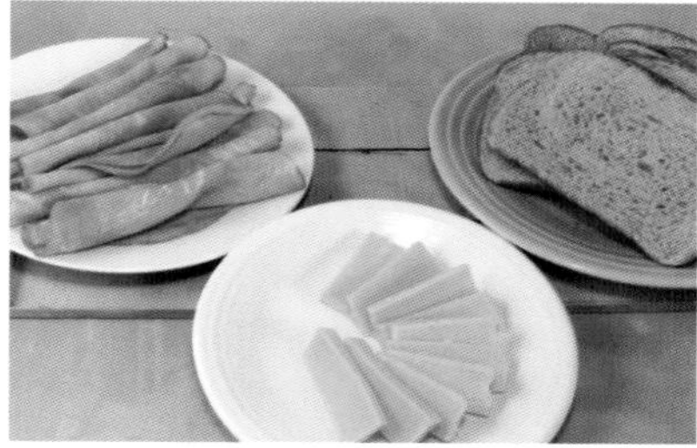
Ingredients

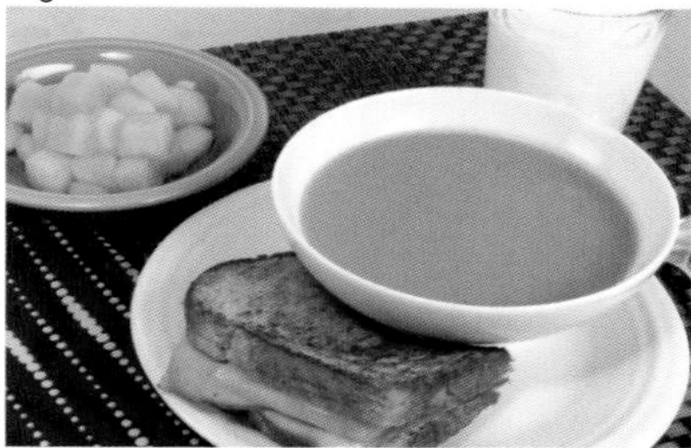
Creditable lunch/supper

Ingredients

6 slices whole grain bread, at least 1½ ounces each
6 ounces turkey ham, thinly sliced
3 1-ounce slices cheddar cheese
2 tablespoons butter

Directions

1. Butter both sides of the bread slices and place 3 slices on work surface.
2. Place 2 ounces of turkey ham and 1 ounce of cheese on each slice. Top with the remaining slices of bread.
3. Heat griddle or grill pan over medium heat. Place sandwiches on the grill/griddle. Heat first side until bread is toasted. Flip sandwiches and continue grilling until ham is hot and cheese is melted, about 10 minutes total.

Grilled Ham & Cheese Sandwich
provides G/B and M/MA at lunch/supper

	Toddler	Pre-School	School Age
Ham Sandwich	1/2 sandwich	1/2 sandwich	1 sandwich
Tomato Soup	1/4 cup	1/2 cup	1 cup
Melon	1/8 cup	1/4 cup	1/4 cup
Milk	1/2 cup	3/4 cup	1 cup

Grilled Tuna Salad Sandwich

Prep time - 15 minutes
Cook time - 10 minutes
Total time - 25 minutes

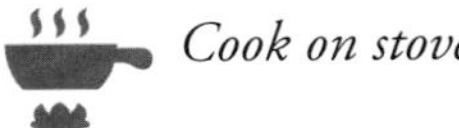

Cook on stovetop

Yield - 3 sandwiches

Ingredients

10 ounces water-packed tuna, drained
3 tablespoons plain yogurt
1 rib celery, finely diced
2 tablespoons onions, minced, optional
1 tablespoon pickle relish, optional
1 tablespoon lemon juice
Salt and pepper to taste
6 slices whole grain bread, at least 1½ ounces each
Butter for spreading

Directions

1. Place tuna in a mixing bowl. Add yogurt, celery, lemon juice, onions and pickle relish, salt and pepper. Mix well.
2. Butter both sides of the bread and lay 3 slices on a work surface. Spread ½ cup of tuna salad on each slice and top with the remaining 3 slices.
3. Place sandwiches on the grill/griddle over medium heat. Grill sandwiches until golden brown, about 10-15 minutes. Flip sandwiches about halfway through grilling.

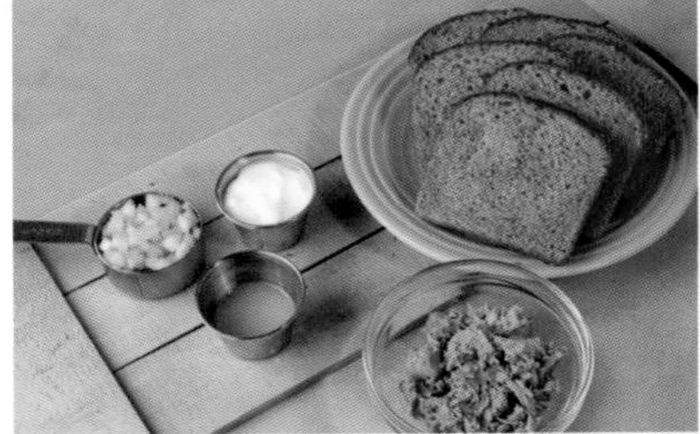

Ingredients

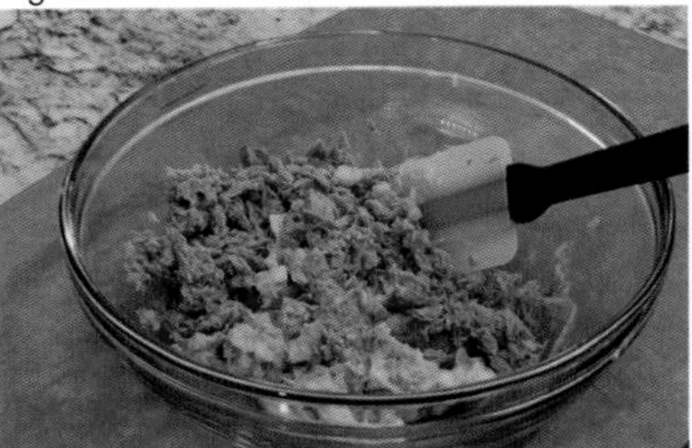

Step 1

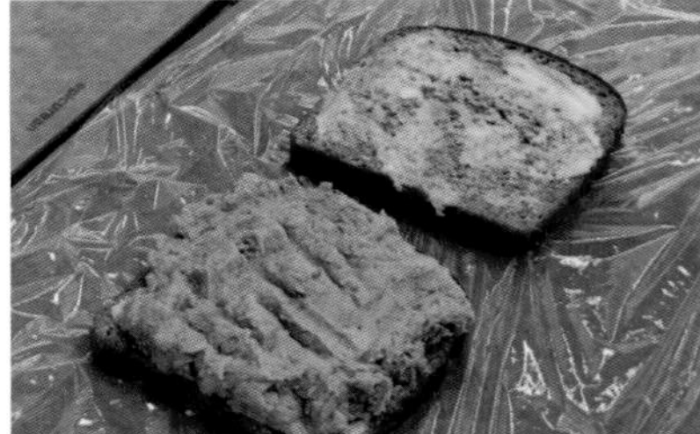

Step 3

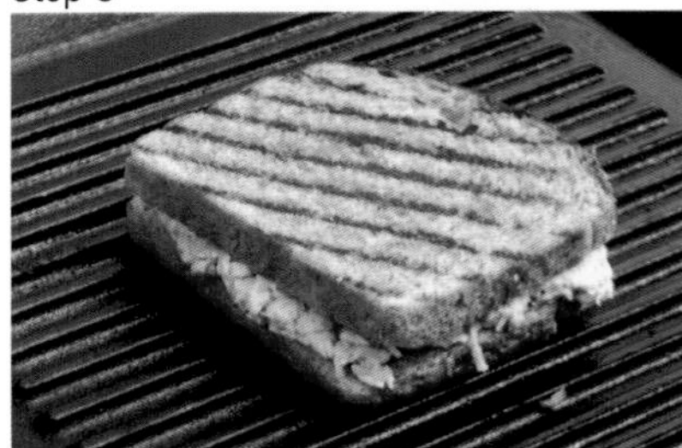

Step 4

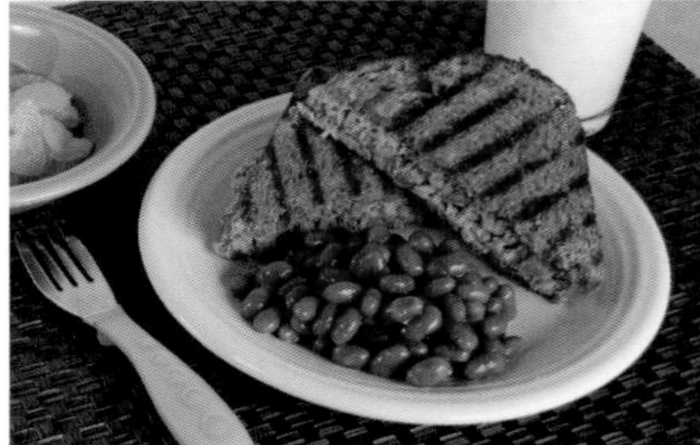

Creditable lunch/supper

Grilled Tuna Salad Sandwich
provides G/B and M/MA at lunch/supper

	Toddler	Pre-School	School Age
Tuna Sandwich	1/2 sandwich	1/2 sandwich	1 sandwich
Baked Beans	1/4 cup	1/4 cup	1/2 cup
Mandarin Oranges	1/8 cup	1/4 cup	1/4 cup
Milk	1/2 cup	3/4 cup	1 cup

Hot Chicken Pita Sandwich

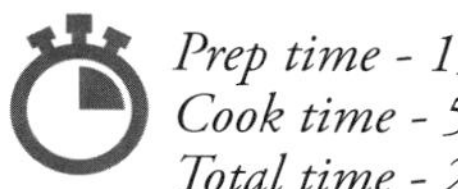

Prep time - 15 minutes
Cook time - 5 minutes
Total time - 20 minutes

Bake in oven

Yield - 6 sandwiches

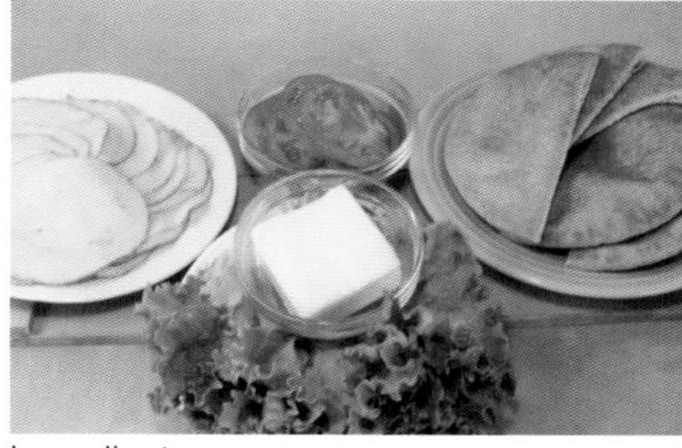

Ingredients

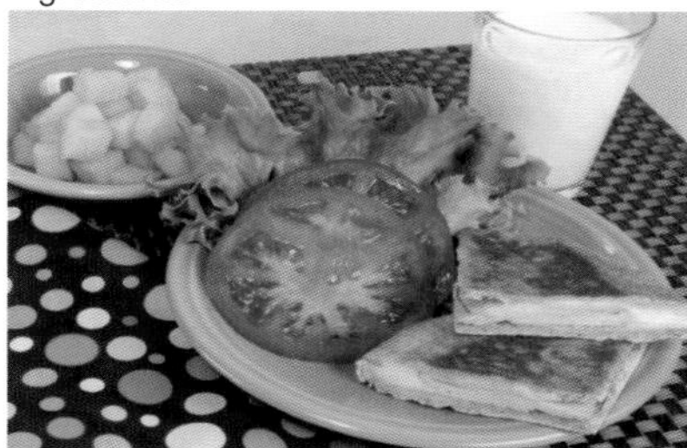

Creditable lunch/supper

Ingredients

3 whole wheat pita bread rounds, at least 1½ ounces each
9 ounces cooked chicken breast, thinly sliced
6 ½-ounce slices mozzarella cheese

Directions

1. Preheat oven to 350 degrees. Line a baking sheet with foil or parchment paper, or coat with cooking spray.
2. Slice each pita round in half and open the pocket.
3. Stuff each pocket with 1½ ounces chicken and ½ ounce cheese.
4. Place on baking sheet and heat until cheese melts, about 5 minutes.

Hot Chicken Pita Sandwich provides G/B and M/MA at lunch/supper			
	Toddler	Pre-School	School Age
Chicken Sandwich	1/2 round	1/2 round	1 round
Lettuce, Tomato	1/8 cup	1/4 cup	1/2 cup
Melon	1/8 cup	1/4 cup	1/4 cup
Milk	1/2 cup	3/4 cup	1 cup

Honey Mustard Turkey Melt

Prep time - 15 minutes
Cook time - 10 minutes
Total time - 25 minutes

Bake in oven

Yield - 3 sandwiches

Ingredients

6 slices whole grain bread, at least 1½ ounces each
Butter for spreading
12 ounces cooked turkey, thinly sliced
2 tablespoons honey mustard
2 tablespoons mayonnaise, optional

Directions

1. Preheat oven to 350 degrees. Line a baking sheet with foil or parchment paper, or coat with cooking spray.
2. Butter both sides of bread and place 3 slices on the baking sheet.
3. In a small bowl, mix honey mustard and mayonnaise.
4. Spread honey mustard on the 3 slices and top each with 4 ounces of turkey and the second slice of bread. Place on baking sheet.
5. Bake until bread is golden brown and turkey is warmed through, about 10 minutes. Flip sandwiches halfway through baking.

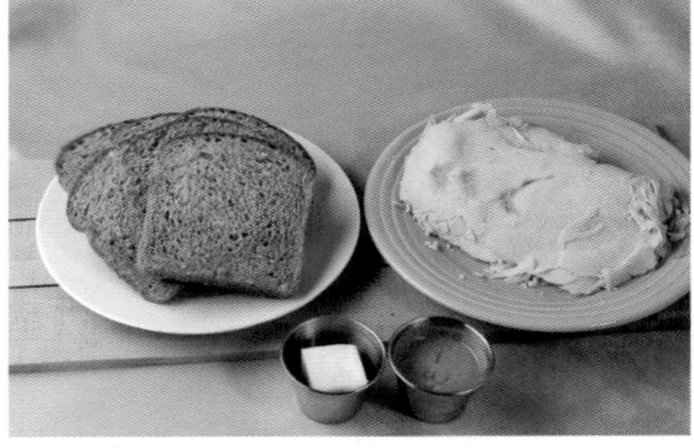

Ingredients

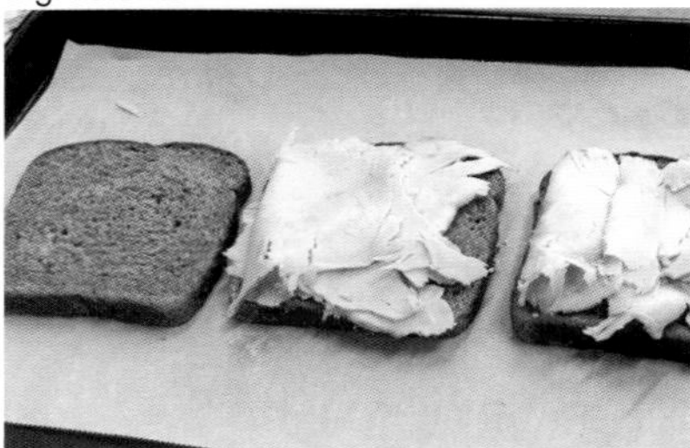

Step 2

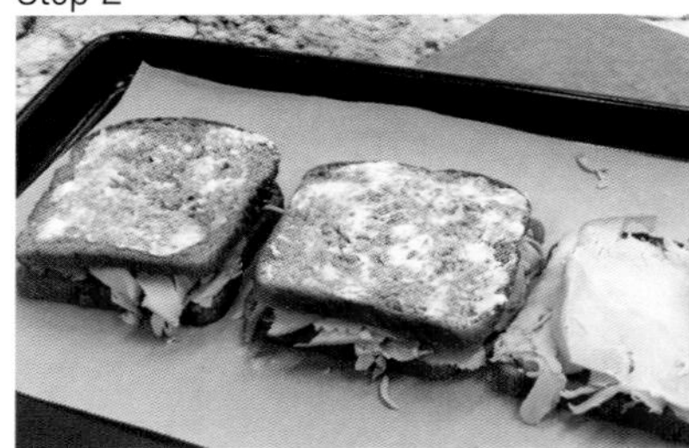

Step 4

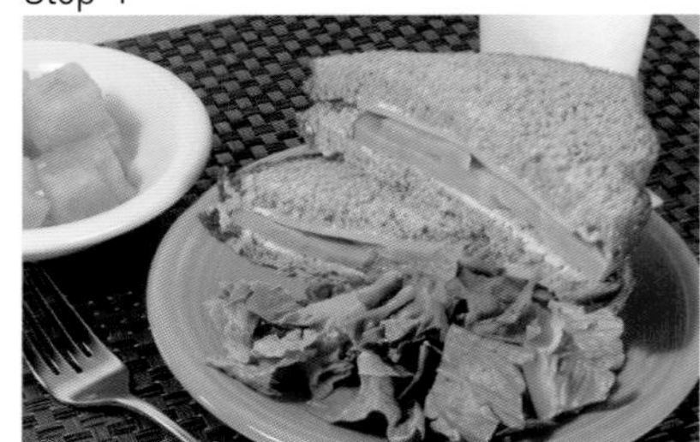

Creditable lunch/supper

Honey-Mustard Turkey Melt provides G/B and M/MA at lunch/supper			
	Toddler	Pre-School	School Age
Turkey Sandwich	1/2 sandwich	1/2 sandwich	1 sandwich
Romaine Lettuce	1/8 cup	1/4 cup	1/2 cup
Watermelon	1/8 cup	1/4 cup	1/4 cup
Milk	1/2 cup	3/4 cup	1 cup

Hot Ham & Cheese Sandwich

Prep time - 15 minutes
Cook time - 10 minutes
Total time - 25 minutes

Bake in oven

Yield - 3 sandwiches

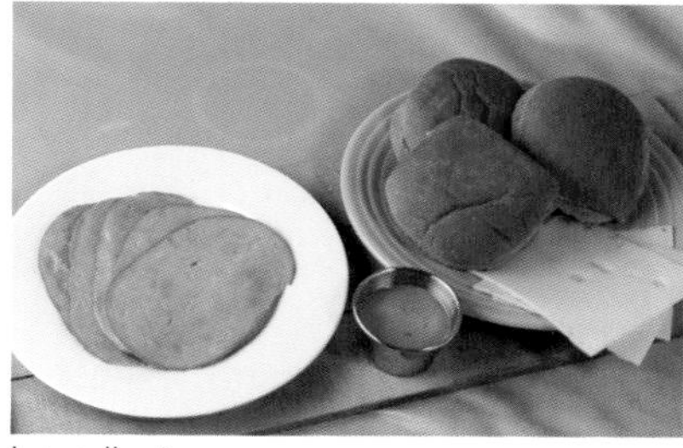

Ingredients

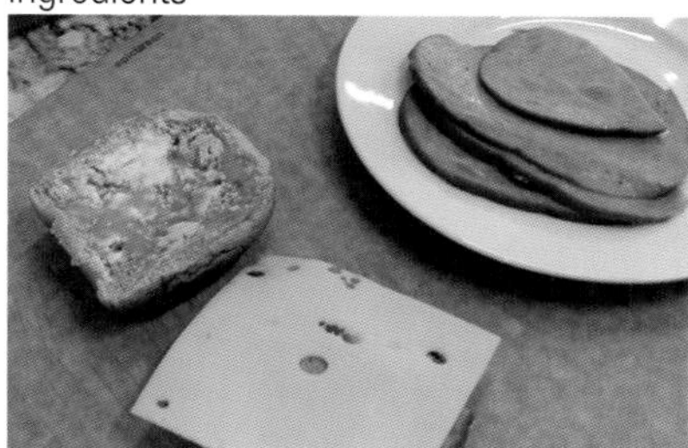

Step 3

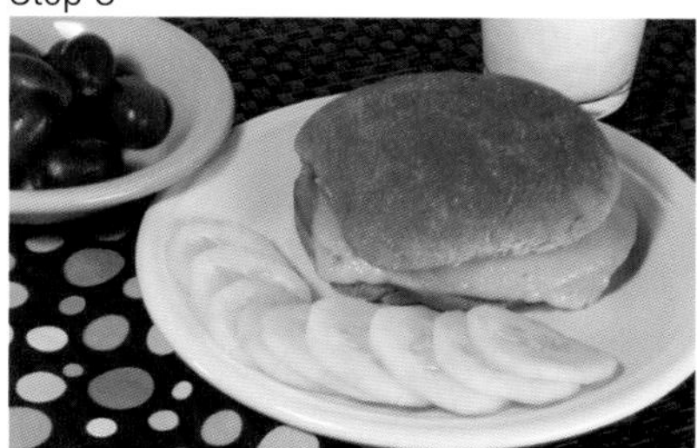

Creditable lunch/supper

Ingredients

3 whole wheat hamburger buns, at least 1½ ounces each
Butter for spreading
6 ounces turkey ham, thinly sliced
3 1-ounce slices Swiss cheese
2 tablespoons honey mustard
2 tablespoons mayonnaise, optional

Directions

1. Preheat oven to 350 degrees. Line a baking sheet with foil or parchment paper, or coat with cooking spray.
2. Butter the buns and spread with honey mustard and mayonnaise. Place on the baking sheet.
3. Fill each bun with 2 ounces of turkey ham and 1 ounce of Swiss cheese.
4. Bake until the ham is hot and the cheese is melted, about 10 minutes.

Hot Ham & Cheese Sandwich
provides G/B and M/MA at lunch/supper

	Toddler	Pre-School	School Age
Ham Sandwich	1/2 sandwich	1/2 sandwich	1 sandwich
Cucumber	1/8 cup	1/4 cup	1/2 cup
Grapes	1/8 cup	1/4 cup	1/4 cup
Milk	1/2 cup	3/4 cup	1 cup

Hummus Wrap

Prep time - 20 minutes
Cook time - 0 minutes
Total time - 20 minutes

No cook, no bake

Yield - 3 wrap sandwiches

Ingredients

3 8-inch whole wheat tortillas
½ cup hummus
9 1-ounce slices cheddar, mozzarella or Swiss cheese
½ cup salsa
1 cup lettuce, shredded

Directions

1. Lay tortillas on a work surface. Spread each tortilla with bout 2½ tablespoons hummus and 3 1-ounce cheese slices.
2. Spread 2½ tablespoons salsa over the cheese and sprinkle with ⅓ cup lettuce.
3. Roll up and slice in half.

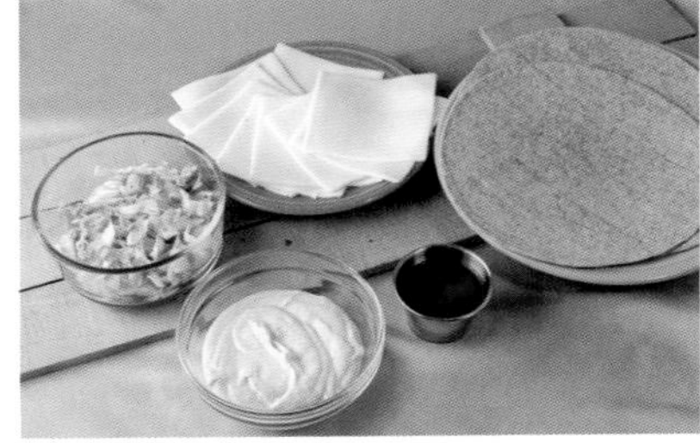

Ingredients

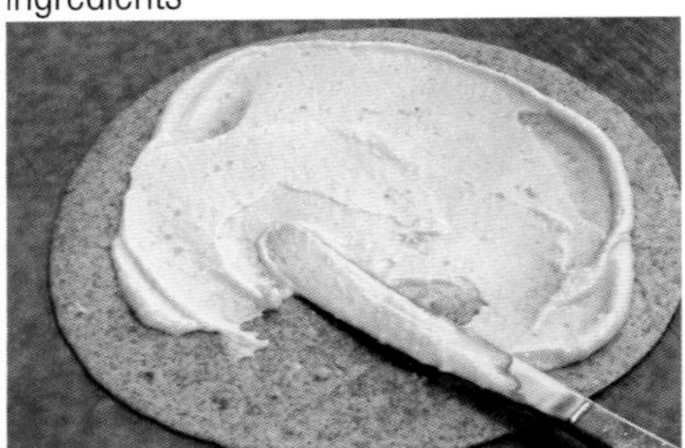

Step 1

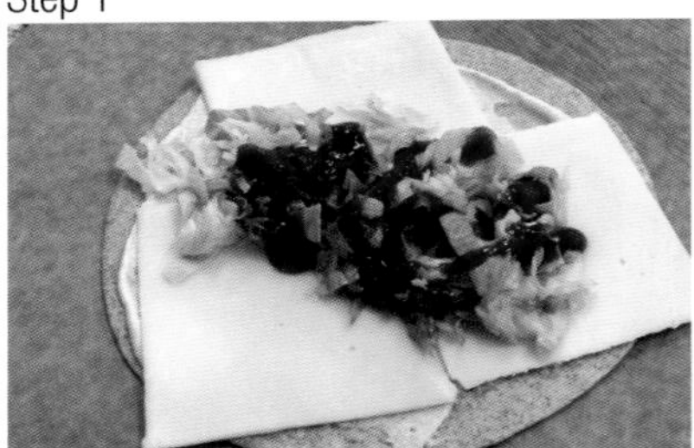

Step 2

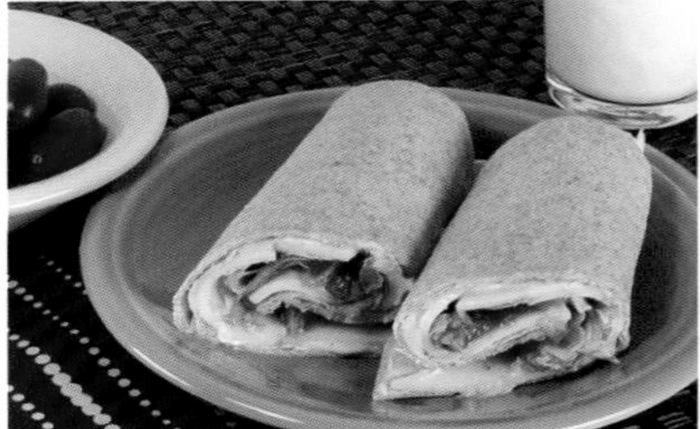

Creditable lunch/supper

Hummus Wrap
provides G/B, M/MA and VEG at lunch/supper

	Toddler	Pre-School	School Age
Hummus Wrap	1/2 wrap	1/2 wrap	1 wrap
Grapes	1/8 cup	1/4 cup	1/4 cup
Milk	1/2 cup	3/4 cup	1 cup

Humpty Dumpty Sandwich

Prep time - 20 minutes
Cook time - 0 minutes
Total time - 20 minutes

No cook, no bake

Yield - 3 sandwiches

Ingredients

3 hard-cooked eggs, chopped
¼ cup celery, finely diced
½ cup cottage cheese
¼ cup (1 ounce) shredded cheddar cheese
2 teaspoons yellow mustard
¼ teaspoon salt
⅛ teaspoon black pepper
6 slices whole grain bread, at least 1½ ounces each
Butter for spreading
3 lettuce leaves

Directions

1. Chop the hard-cooked eggs.
2. Combine all ingredients in a bowl, except for the bread, butter and lettuce. Mix thoroughly.
3. Butter one side of each bread slice.
4. Place one-third of the egg salad on each of 3 bread slices. Top each with 1 lettuce leaf and the remaining bread slice.

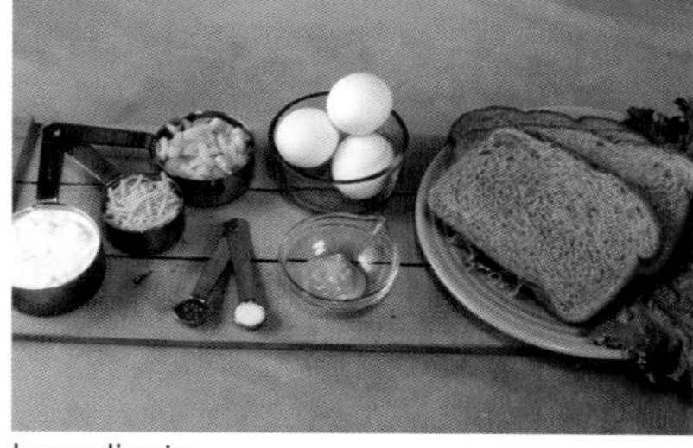

Ingredients

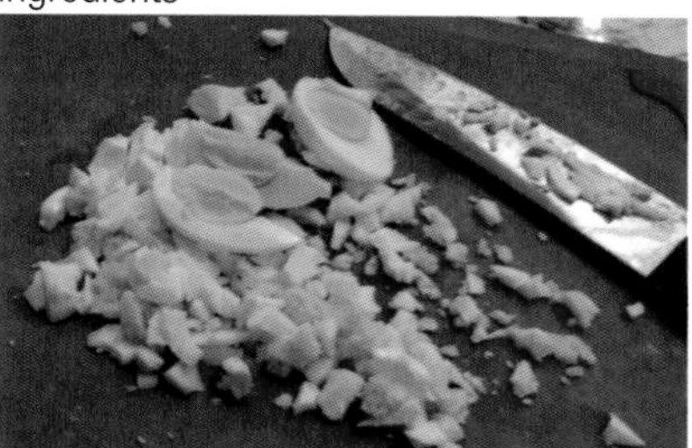

Step 1

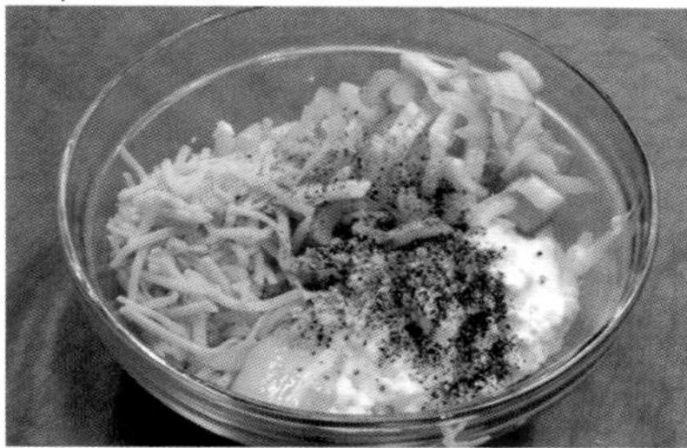

Step 2

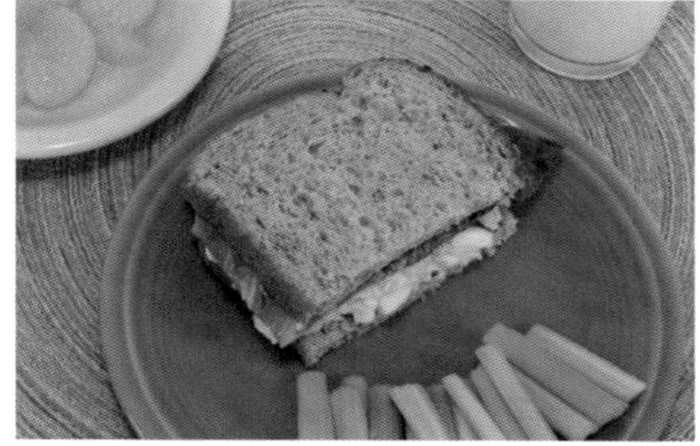

Creditable lunch/supper

Humpty Dumpty Sandwich
provides G/B and M/MA at lunch/supper

	Toddler	Pre-School	School Age
Egg Salad Sandwich	1/2 sandwich	1/2 sandwich	1 sandwich
Celery	1/8 cup	1/4 cup	1/2 cup
Mandarin Oranges	1/8 cup	1/4 cup	1/4 cup
Milk	1/2 cup	3/4 cup	1 cup

Meatball Sub

Prep time - 15 minutes
Cook time - 10 minutes
Total time - 25 minutes

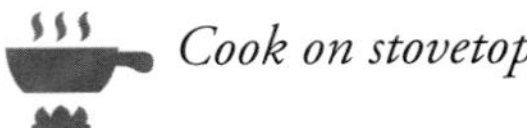
Cook on stovetop

Yield - 3 sandwiches

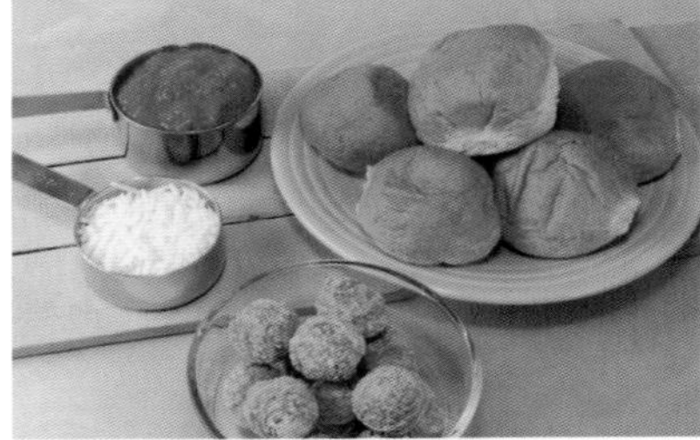
Ingredients

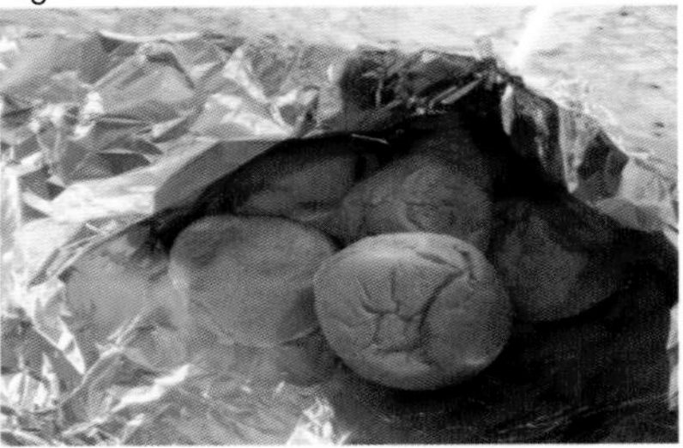
Step 1

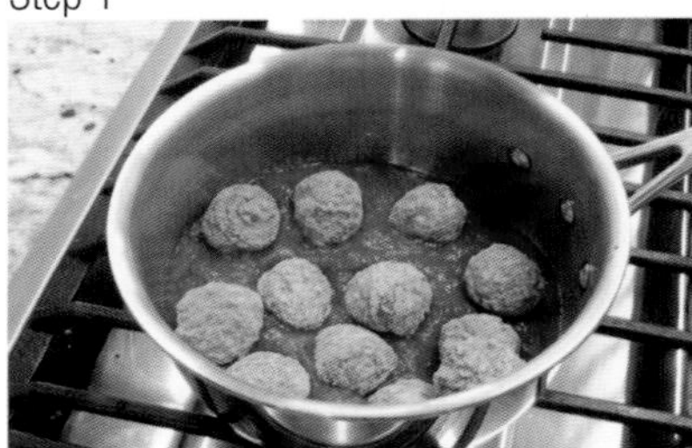
Step 2a

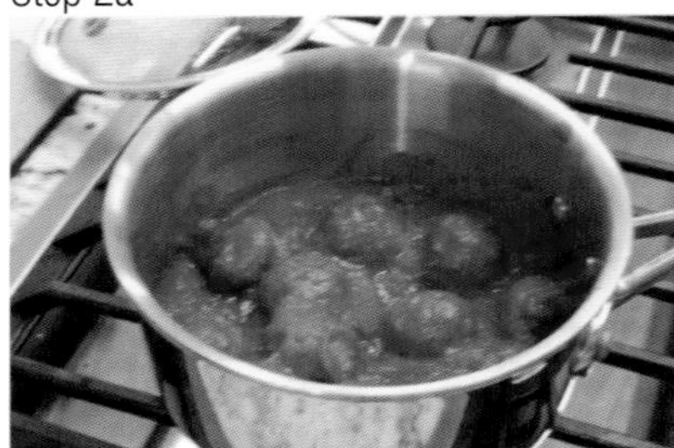
Step 2b

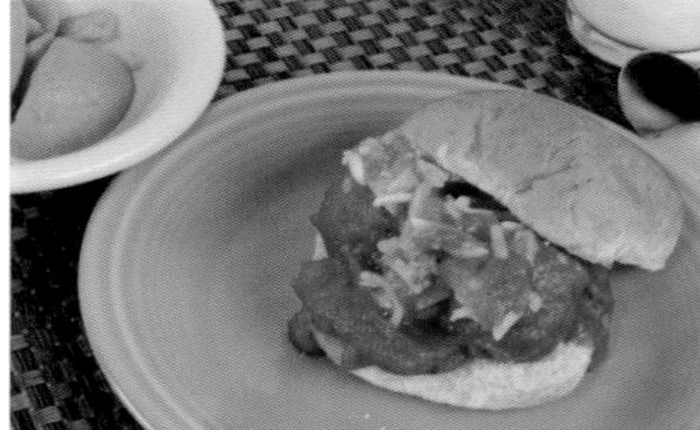
Creditable lunch/supper

Ingredients

3 whole grain hoagie buns, at least 1½ ounces each
12 1-ounce meatballs*
1½ cups marinara sauce
½ cup (2 ounces) shredded mozzarella cheese

Directions

1. Preheat oven to 300 degrees. Wrap buns in foil and place in oven to warm, about 10 minutes.
2. In a partially-covered saucepan, heat the meatballs in the marinara sauce over low heat, about 10 minutes.
3. When meatballs and buns are warm, place four meatballs on the bottom of each bun. Top with ½ cup marinara sauce, 2½ tablespoons cheese and cover with top of bun.

**CN labeled*

Meatball Sub
provides G/B, M/MA and VEG at lunch/supper

	Toddler	Pre-School	School Age
Meatball Sandwich	1/2 sandwich	1/2 sandwich	1 sandwich
Sweet Potatoes	1/8 cup	1/4 cup	1/2 cup
Milk	1/2 cup	3/4 cup	1 cup

Pizza Sandwich

Prep time - 20 minutes
Cook time - 10 minutes
Total time - 20 minutes

Cook on stovetop and in oven

Yield - 3 sandwiches

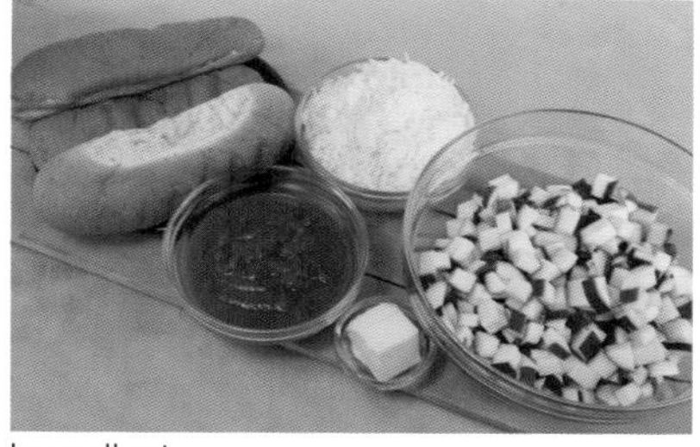
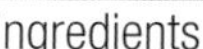
Ingredients

Ingredients

2 tablespoons butter
3 cups zucchini, diced
¾ cup marinara sauce
3 whole wheat hoagie buns, at least 1½ ounces each
2¼ cups (9 ounces) shredded mozzarella cheese

Directions

1. Preheat oven to 400 degrees. Line a baking pan with foil or coat with cooking spray.
2. Melt butter in a large skillet over medium heat. Add zucchini and sauté until tender, about 5 minutes.
3. Add marinara sauce and cook until sauce is heated through, about 2 minutes.
4. Lay the opened buns in the baking pan. Fill each bun with one-third of the zucchini sauce and top with a heaping ¾ cup (3 ounces) of mozzarella cheese.
5. Heat sandwiches in oven until cheese melts, about 3 minutes.

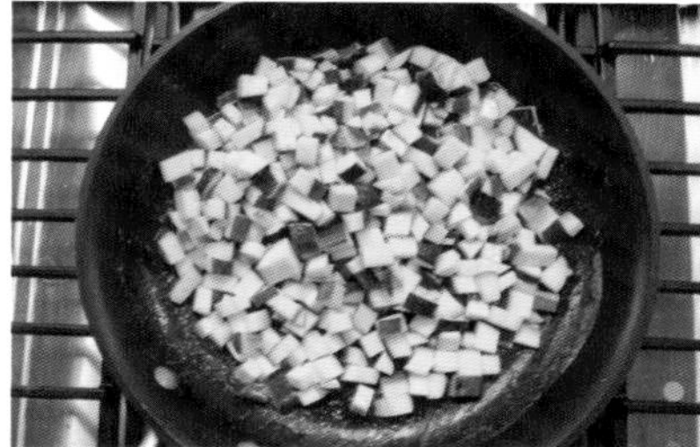
Step 2

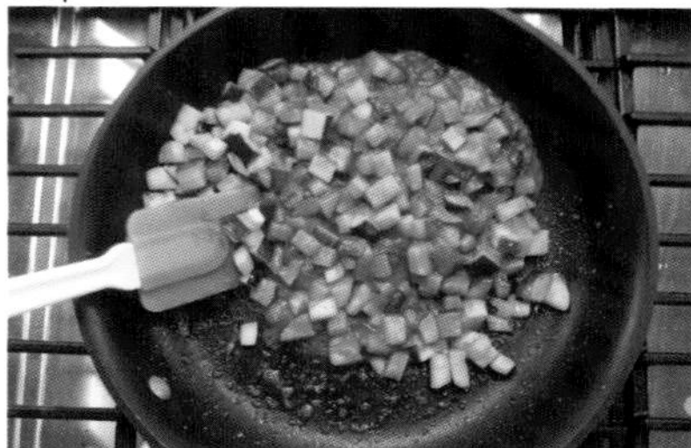
Step 3

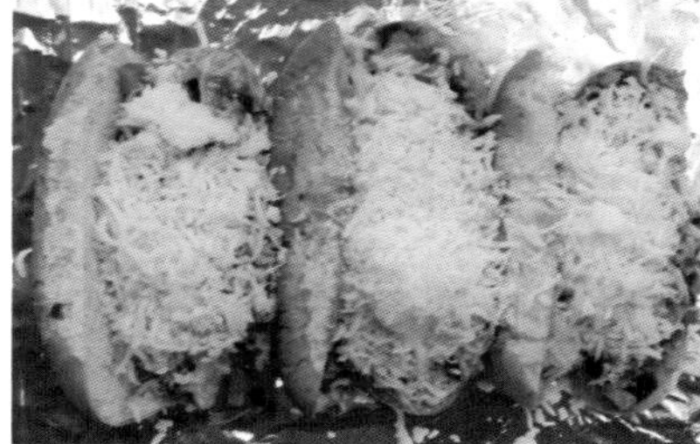
Step 4

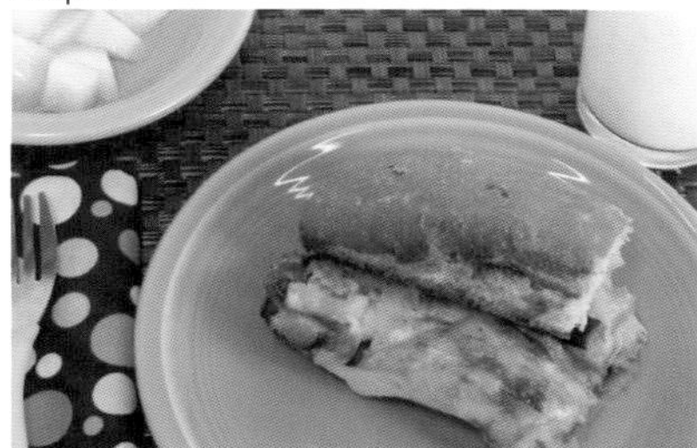
Creditable lunch/supper

Pizza Sandwich
provides G/B, M/MA and VEG at lunch/supper

	Toddler	Pre-School	School Age
Pizza Sandwich	1/2 sandwich	1/2 sandwich	1 sandwich
Honeydew Melon	1/8 cup	1/4 cup	1/4 cup
Milk	1/2 cup	3/4 cup	1 cup

Pork Lettuce Wrap

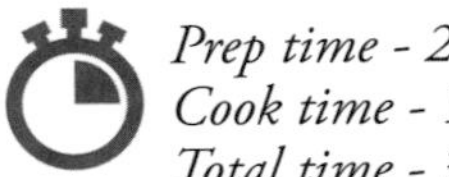

Prep time - 20 minutes
Cook time - 10 minutes
Total time - 30 minutes

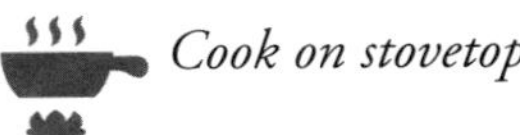

Cook on stovetop

Yield - 6 wraps

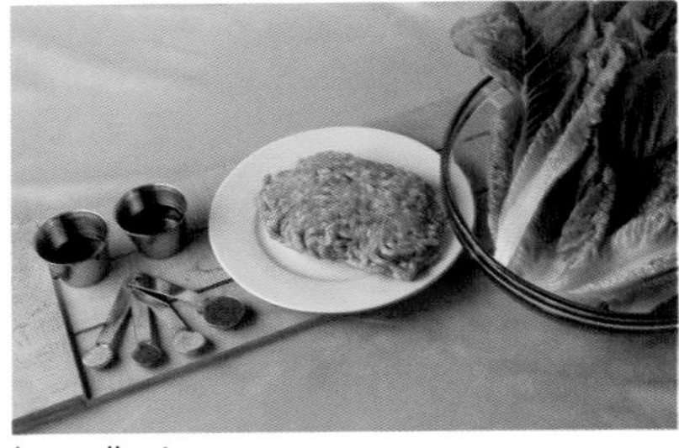

Ingredients

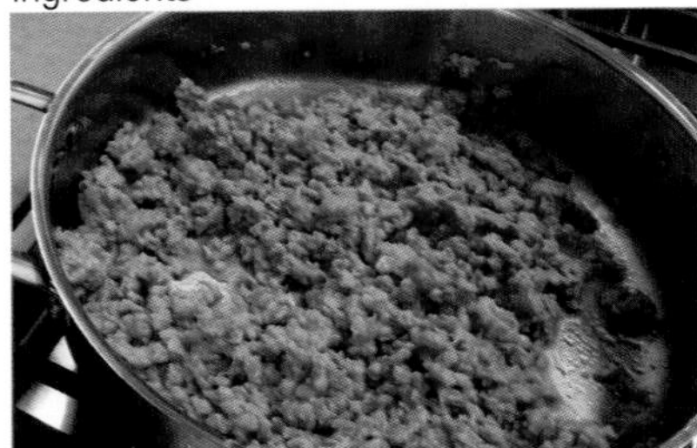

Step 1

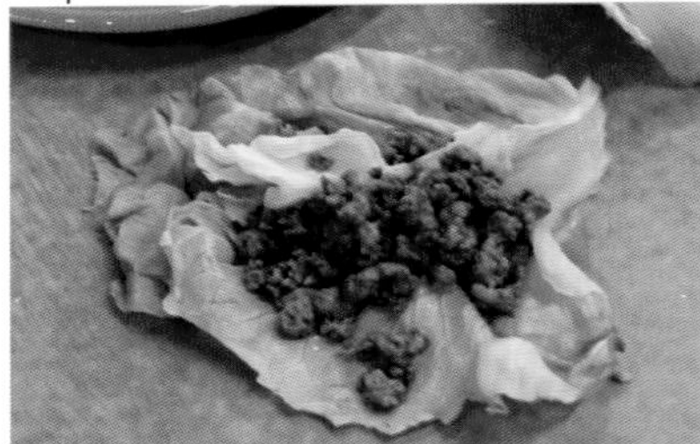

Step 3

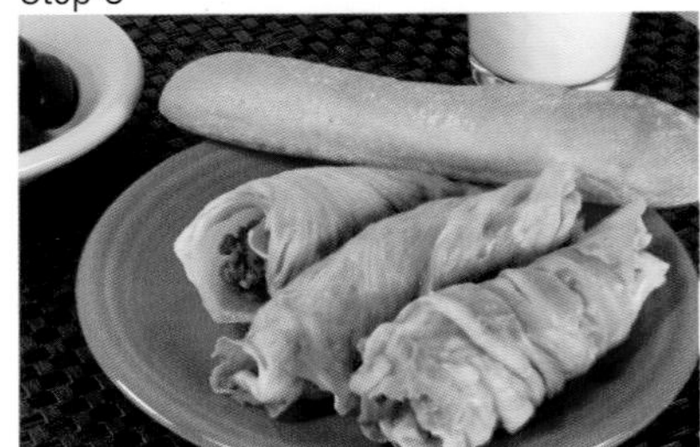

Creditable lunch/supper

Ingredients

2 teaspoons vegetable oil
1 pound ground pork, at least 80% lean
1¼ teaspoons ground allspice
¾ teaspoon ground ginger
2 tablespoons soy sauce
12 romaine lettuce leaves

Directions

1. Heat oil in a large sauté pan over medium-high heat. Add pork and cook, stirring frequently, until pork begins to brown, about 5 minutes; drain excess fat.
2. Stir in allspice, ginger and soy sauce and cook until pork is cooked through, with an internal temperature of 160 degrees, another 5 minutes.
3. To make the lettuce wraps, place 2 lettuce leaves on each plate. Fill each with 1½ ounces spiced pork and roll up.

Pork Lettuce Wrap
provides M/MA and VEG at lunch/supper

	Toddler	Pre-School	School Age
Lettuce Wrap	1 wrap	1 wrap	1-1/2 wrapss
Breadsticks	1/2 ounce	1/2 ounce	1 ounce
Grapes	1/8 cup	1/4 cup	1/4 cup
Milk	1/2 cup	3/4 cup	1 cup

Roast Beef Sandwich

Prep time - 15 minutes
Cook time - 0 minutes
Total time - 15 minutes

No cook, no bake

Yield - 3 sandwiches

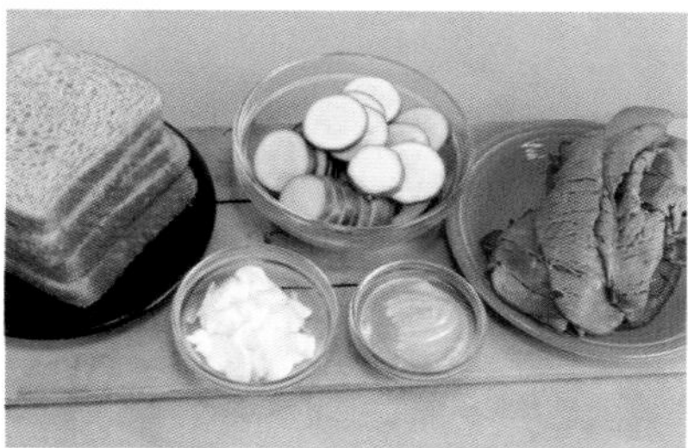
Ingredients

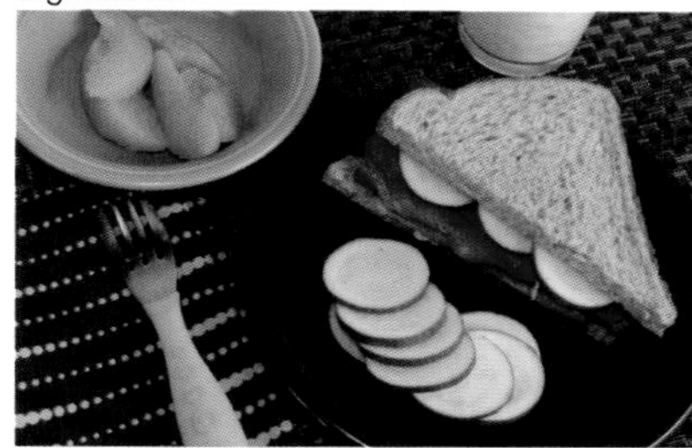
Creditable lunch/supper

Ingredients

3 tablespoons mayonnaise
3 tablespoons mustard
6 slices whole grain bread, at least 1½ ounces each
9 ounces roast beef, thinly sliced
1 large zucchini, thinly sliced

Directions

1. In a small bowl, combine the mayonnaise and mustard.
2. Place bread on work surface and spread each slice with 1 tablespoon of the mayonnaise/mustard.
3. On 3 slices of bread, place 3 ounces of roast beef and 3 zucchini slices. Top with the remaining slices of bread.
4. Slice sandwiches in half and serve remaining zucchini on the side.

Roast Beef Sandwich provides G/B and M/MA at lunch/supper			
	Toddler	Pre-School	School Age
Roast Beef Sandwich	1/2 sandwich	1/2 sandwich	1 sandwich
Extra Zucchini	1/8 cup	1/4 cup	1/2 cup
Peaches	1/8 cup	1/4 cup	1/4 cup
Milk	1/2 cup	3/4 cup	1 cup

Shredded Beef Sandwich

Prep time - 20 minutes
Cook time - 2 hours
Resting time - 15 minutes
Total - 2 hours, 35 minutes

Bake in oven

Yield - 3 sandwiches

Ingredients

½ cup ketchup
1 tablespoon Worcestershire sauce
1 tablespoon Dijon mustard
¼ teaspoon garlic powder
1 pound boneless chuck roast
3 whole wheat hamburger buns, at least 1½ ounces each

Directions

1. Preheat oven to 350 degrees. Line a small baking pan with foil or coat with cooking spray.
2. In a small bowl, mix the ketchup, Worcestershire sauce, mustard and garlic powder. Brush or rub on all sides of the roast.
3. Place roast in baking pan and bake, uncovered, until very tender, about 2 hours. Remove from oven, cut into quarters and allow to cool about 15 minutes.
4. Shred meat with two forks and mix in the pan juices.
5. Fill each bun with 3 ounces of the shredded beef.

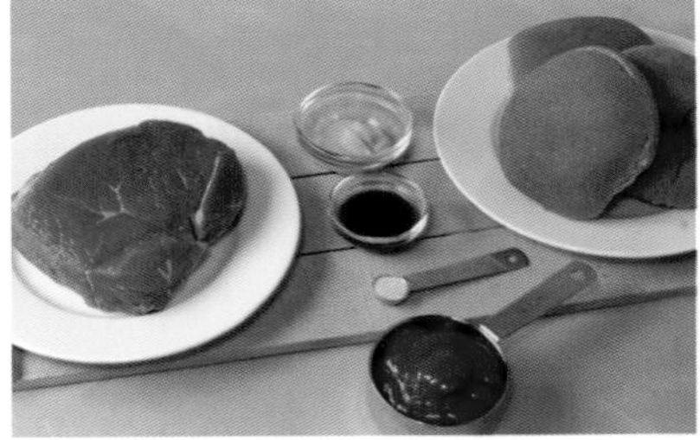

Ingredients

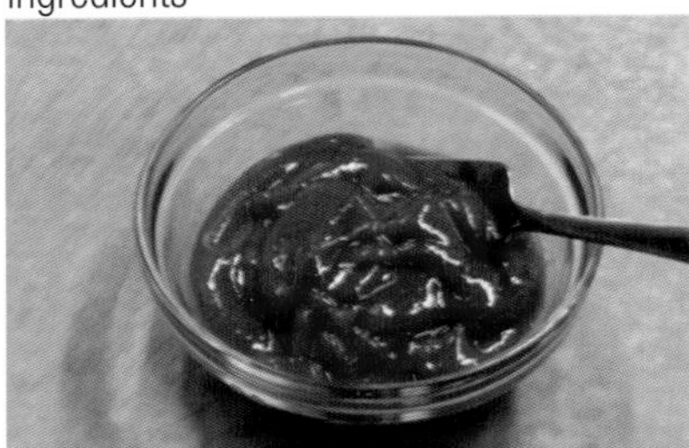

Step 21

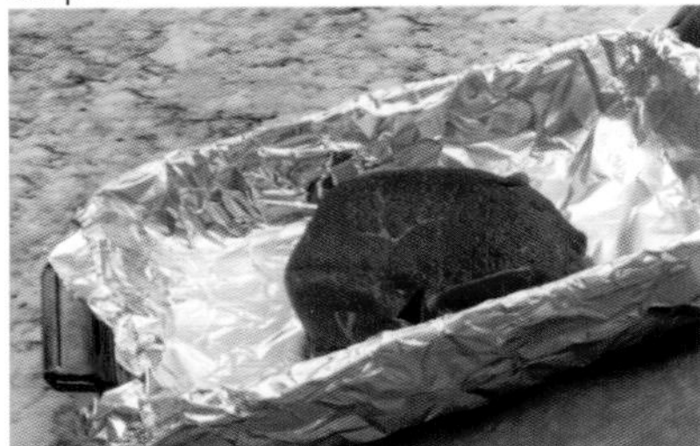

Step 3

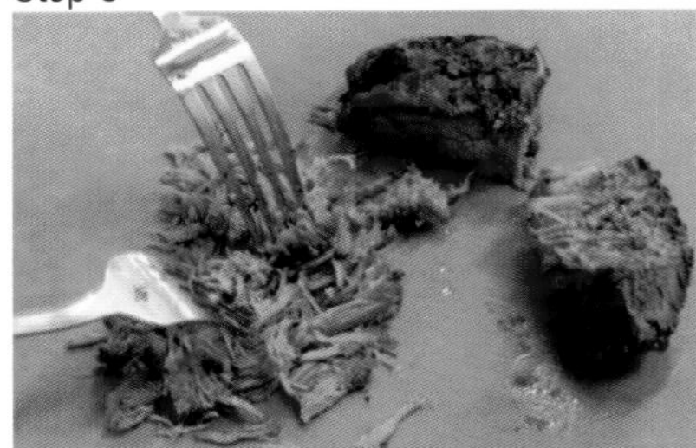

Step 4

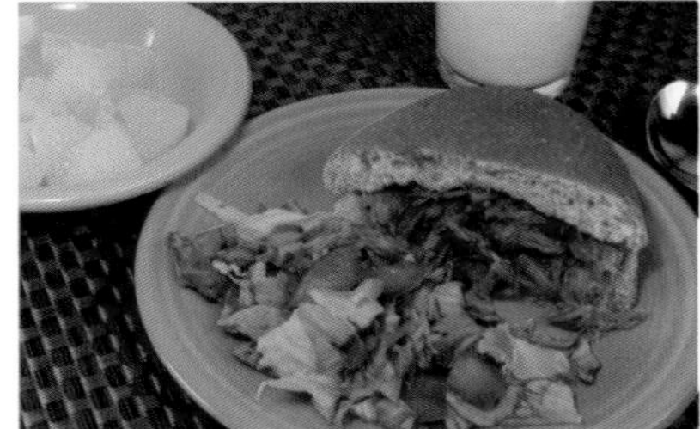

Creditable lunch/supper

Shredded Beef Sandwich
provides G/B and M/MA at lunch/supper

	Toddler	Pre-School	School Age
Beef Sandwich	1/2 sandwich	1/2 sandwich	1 sandwich
Lettuce	1/8 cup	1/4 cup	1/2 cup
Peaches	1/8 cup	1/4 cup	1/4 cup
Milk	1/2 cup	3/4 cup	1 cup

Taco Salad Wraps

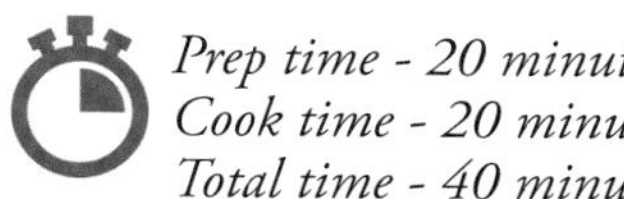

Prep time - 20 minutes
Cook time - 20 minutes
Total time - 40 minutes

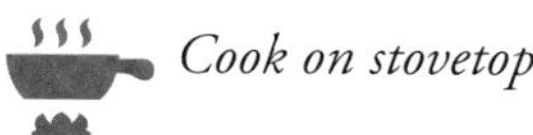

Cook on stovetop

Yield - 3 wraps

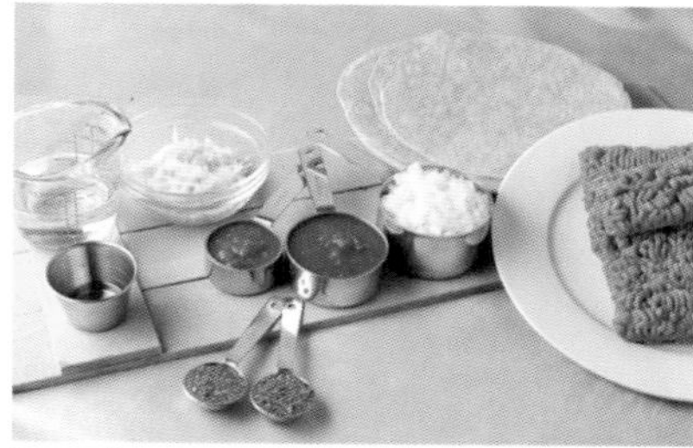

Ingredients

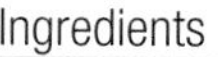

Ingredients

1 tablespoon vegetable oil
1 pound ground beef, at least 80% lean
½ cup onions, chopped
2 tablespoons taco seasoning mix (1 packet)
¾ cup salsa, divided
½ cup water
3 8-inch whole wheat tortillas
¾ cup lettuce, shredded

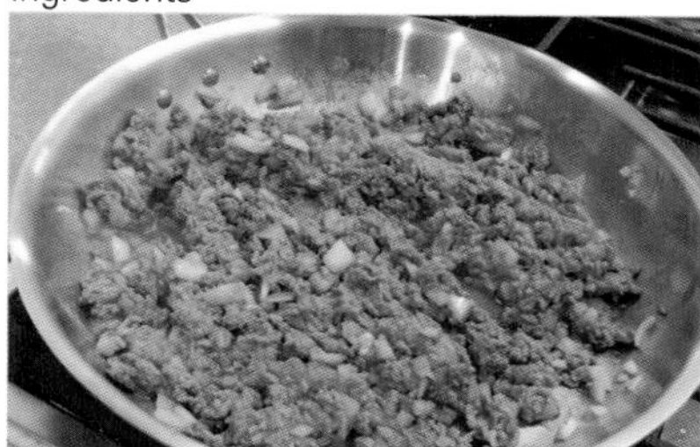

Step 1

Directions

1. Heat oil in skillet over medium heat. Add the onions and ground beef. Cook beef to an internal temperature of 160 degrees, about 10 minutes; drain excess fat.

2. Stir in taco seasoning, ½ cup salsa and water. Reduce heat to low and simmer until most of the liquid is absorbed, about 10 minutes.

3. Lay tortillas on a work surface. Place 3 ounces of seasoned meat, ¼ cup lettuce and 1 tablespoon salsa down the center of each tortilla. Roll up and cut in half.

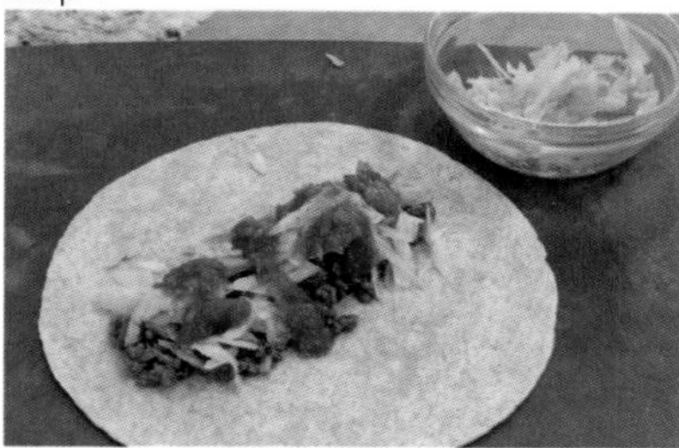

Step 3

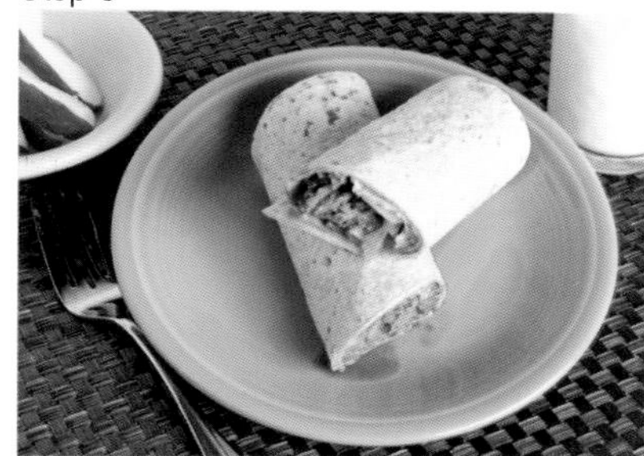

Creditable lunch/supper

Taco Salad Wraps
provides G/B, M/MA and VEG at lunch/supper

	Toddler	Pre-School	School Age
Taco Salad Wrap	1/2 wrap	1/2 wrap	1 wrap
Apple Wedges	1/8 cup	1/4 cup	1/4 cup
Milk	1/2 cup	3/4 cup	1 cup

Under the Sea Burger

Prep time - 20 minutes
Cook time - 10 minutes
Total time - 30 minutes

Bake in oven

Yield - 3 burgers

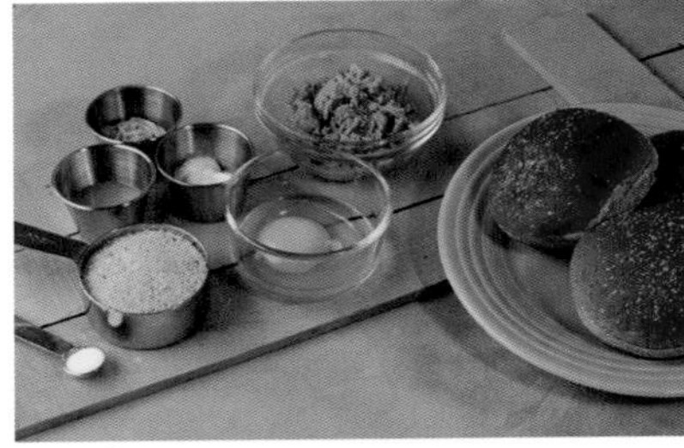

Ingredients

Ingredients

10 ounces water-packed tuna, drained
½ cup bread crumbs
1 egg
2 teaspoons yellow mustard
1 tablespoon mayonnaise
1 teaspoon salt, or to taste
1 tablespoon lemon juice, or to taste
3 whole wheat hamburger buns, at least 1½ ounces each

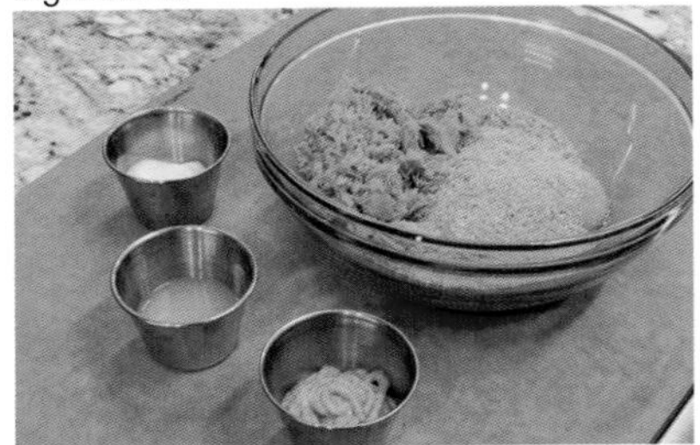

Step 2a

Directions

1. Position oven rack 6 inches from broiler element and preheat broiler. Line a baking sheet with foil or coat with cooking spray.
2. Combine drained tuna, bread crumbs, egg, mustard, mayonnaise, salt, and lemon juice in bowl. Mix well.
3. Form mixture into three patties and place on baking sheet. Bake until patties are lightly golden and firm, about 10 minutes. Serve on a bun.

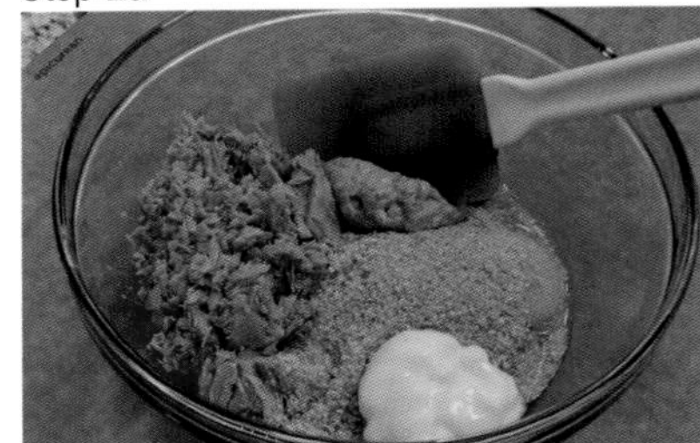

Step 2b

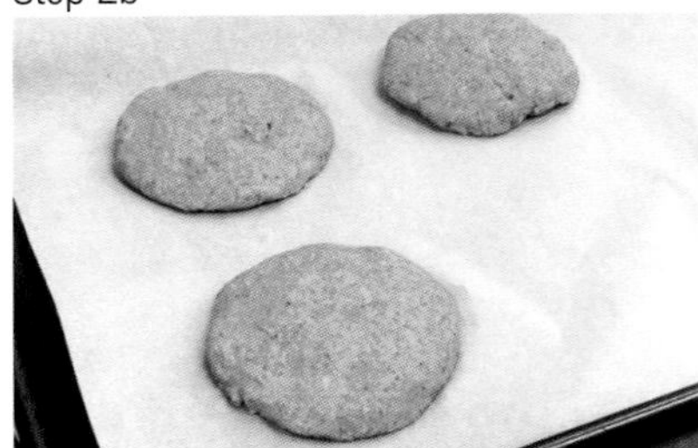

Step 3

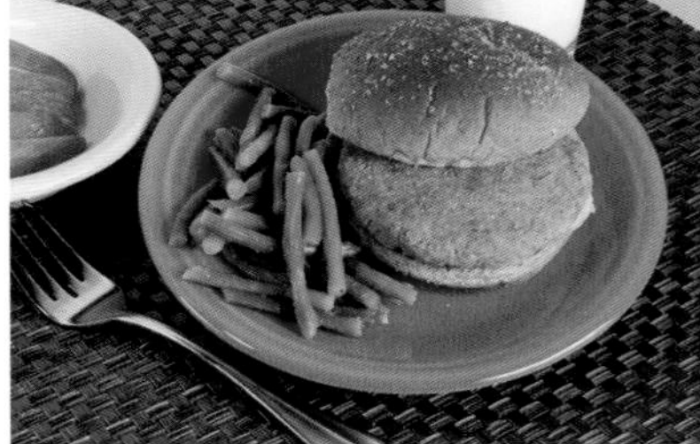

Creditable lunch/supper

Under the Sea Burger
provides G/B and M/MA at lunch/supper

	Toddler	Pre-School	School Age
Tuna Burger	1/2 burger	1/2 burger	1 burger
Green Beans	1/8 cup	1/4 cup	1/2 cup
Apples	1/8 cup	1/4 cup	1/4 cup
Milk	1/2 cup	3/4 cup	1 cup

Very Veggie Bagel Sandwich

Prep time - 15 minutes
Cook time - 0 minutes
Total time - 15 minutes

No cook, no bake

Yield - 6 open-faced sandwiches

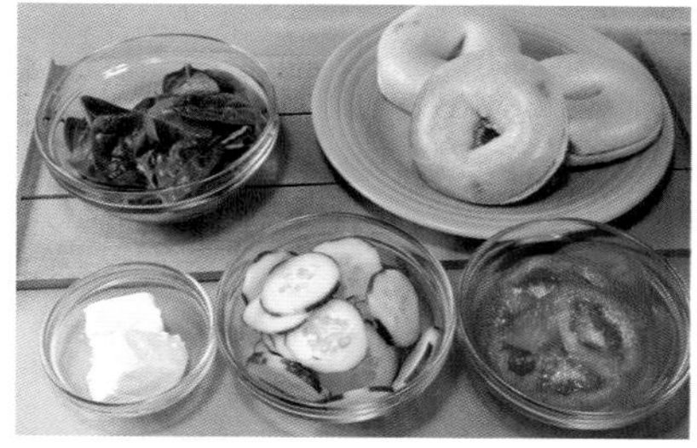

Ingredients

Ingredients

3 whole grain bagels, at least 1½ ounces each
6 tablespoons plain cream cheese
1 cup fresh spinach, washed and dried
1 cup cucumbers, sliced
1 cup tomatoes, sliced

Directions

1. Slice bagels in half and spread each half with 1 tablespoon of cream cheese.

2. Divide the spinach, cucumbers and tomatoes evenly among the 6 half-bagels. Serve open-faced.

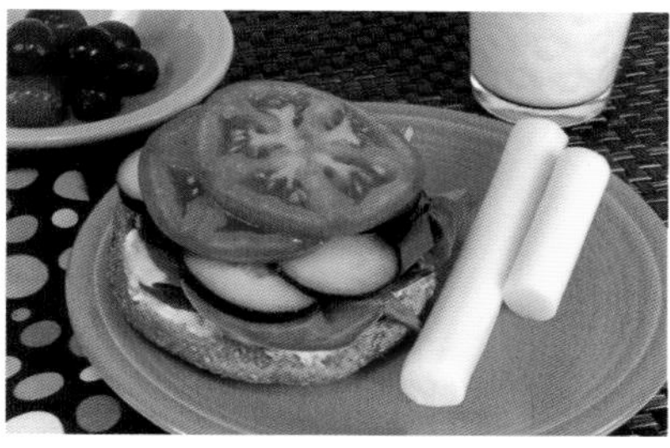

Creditable lunch/supper

Very Veggie Bagel Sandwich provides G/B and VEG at lunch/supper			
	Toddler	Pre-School	School Age
Veggie Sandwich	1/2 bagel	1/2 bagel	1 bagel
String Cheese	1 oz. or 1 stick	1-1/2 oz./sticks	2 oz. or 2 sticks
Grapes	1/8 cup	1/4 cup	1/4 cup
Milk	1/2 cup	3/4 cup	1 cup

Barbeque Chicken Breast

Prep time - 10 minutes
Cook time - 25 minutes
Total time - 35 minutes

Bake in oven

Yield - 12 ounces

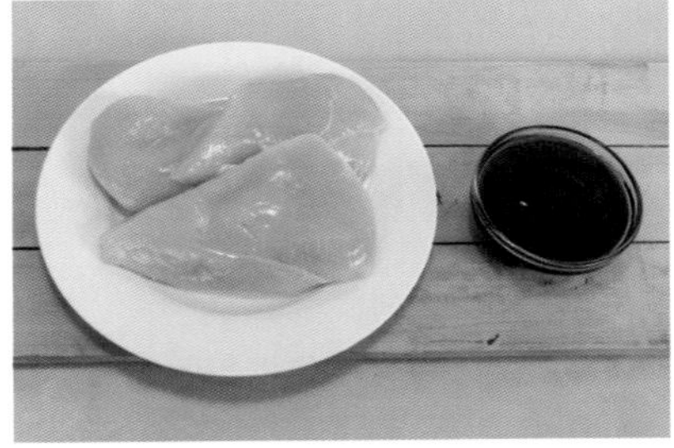
Ingredients

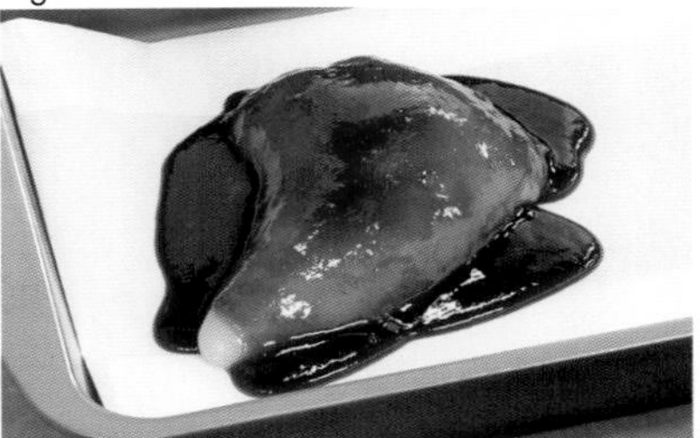
Step 2

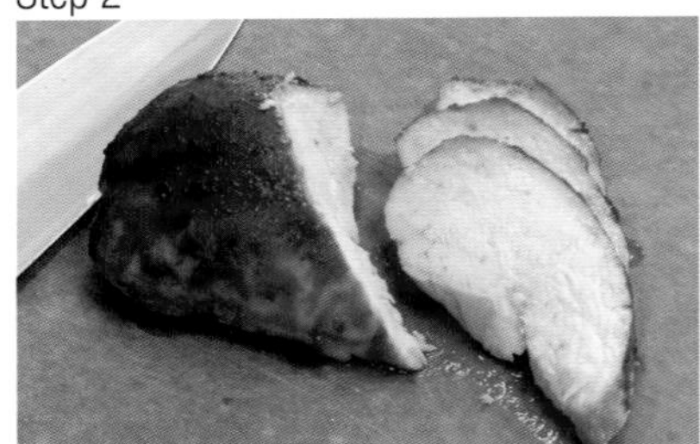
Step 4

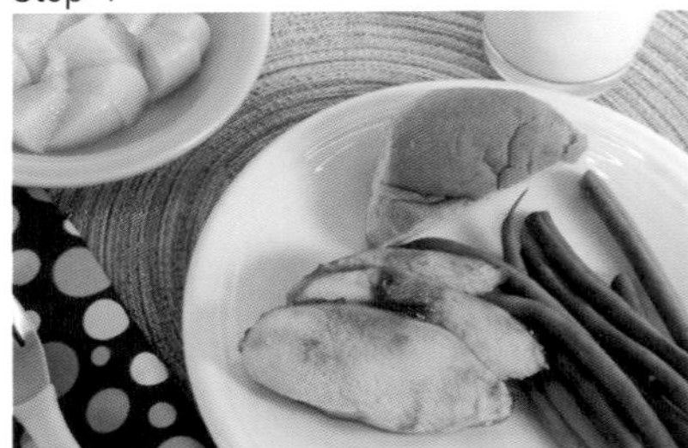
Creditable lunch/supper

Ingredients

½ cup barbeque sauce
1 pound boneless, skinless chicken breasts

Directions

1. Preheat oven to 375 degrees. Line a baking pan with foil or parchment paper, or coat with cooking spray.
2. Pour barbeque sauce over the chicken.
3. Bake until chicken is done, with an internal temperature of 165 degrees, about 25 minutes.
4. To serve, cut into slices.

Barbeque Chicken Breast provides M/MA at lunch/supper			
	Toddler	Pre-School	School Age
BBQ Chicken Breast	1 ounce	1-1/2 ounces	2 ounces
Whole Wheat Roll	1/2 ounce	1/2 ounce	1 ounce
Green Beans	1/8 cup	1/4 cup	1/2 cup
Peaches	1/8 cup	1/4 cup	1/4 cup
Milk	1/2 cup	3/4 cup	1 cup

Beef Stroganoff

Prep time - 15 minutes
Cook time - 30 minutes
Total time - 45 minutes

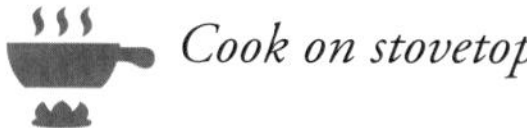
Cook on stovetop

Yield - 5½ cups sauce

Ingredients

4 ounces (3 cups) dry whole grain egg noodles
Water for boiling pasta
1¼ pounds beef chuck, sirloin or round steak
4 tablespoons vegetable oil
2½ cups mushrooms, chopped
1 tablespoon tomato paste
¼ cup water
3 tablespoons cornstarch
3 cups beef broth
¾ cup sour cream

Directions

1. Cook noodles according to package directions; drain.
2. Thinly slice the beef, cutting across the grain.
3. Heat 2 tablespoons of the oil in a large skillet or sauté pan over medium heat. Add beef to pan and brown, about 10 minutes. Set meat aside and discard excess fat.
4. Heat remaining oil in the same pan and cook the mushrooms until lightly browned, about 5 minutes; set aside.
5. Whisk together the water and cornstarch. Combine it with the beef broth and meat juices in the pan. Bring to a boil, then simmer until reduced by a third, about 5 minutes.
6. Add beef and mushrooms to sauce; simmer for 10 minutes.
7. Remove from heat and add sour cream; mix well. Serve over noodles.

Beef Stroganoff
provides G/B and M/MA at lunch/supper

	Toddler	Pre-School	School Age
Beef Stroganoff	1/2 cup	2/3 cup	1 cup
Noodles	1/4 cup	1/4 cup	1/2 cup
Green Beans	1/8 cup	1/4 cup	1/2 cup
Apple Slices	1/8 cup	1/4 cup	1/4 cup
Milk	1/2 cup	3/4 cup	1 cup

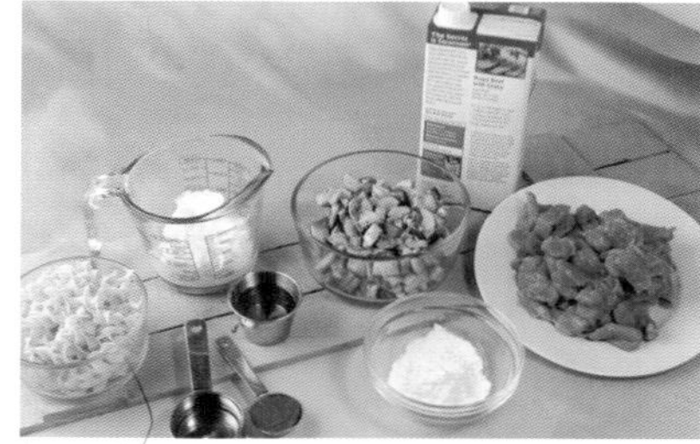
Ingredients

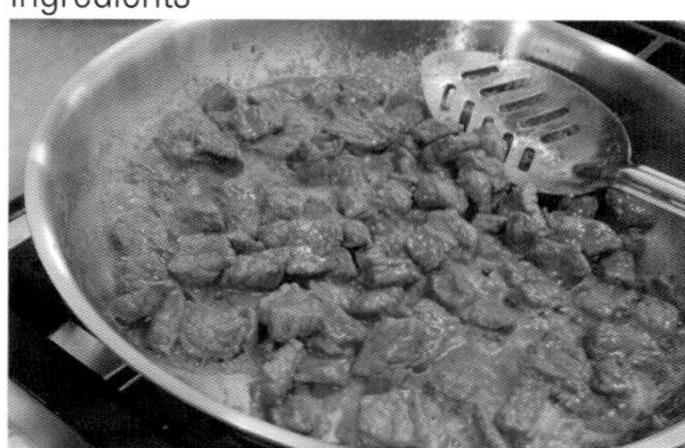
Step 1

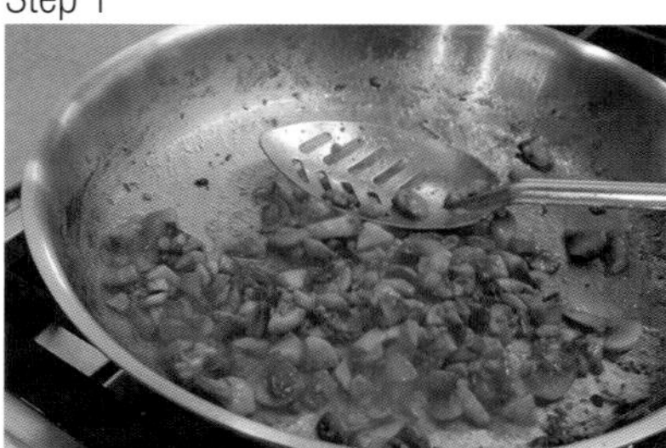
Step 2

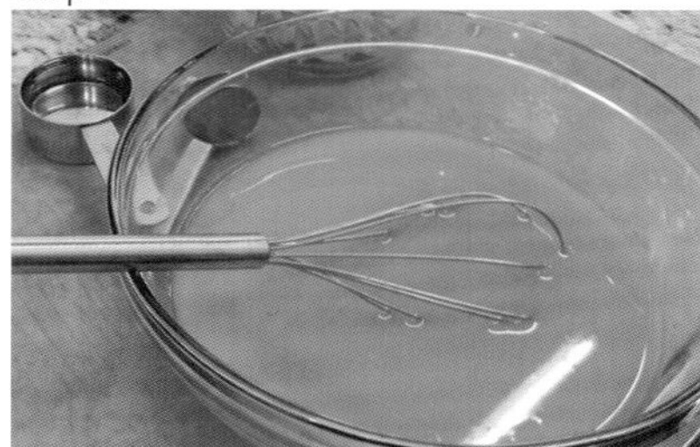
Step 3

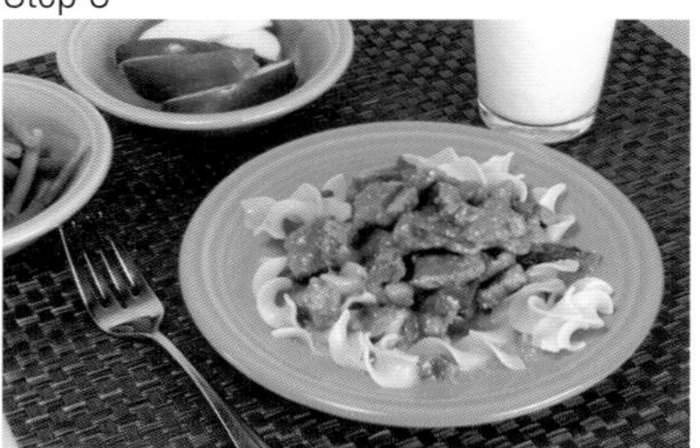
Creditable lunch/supper

Braised Turkey Breast

Prep time - 15 minutes
Cook time - 55 minutes
Total time - 70 minutes

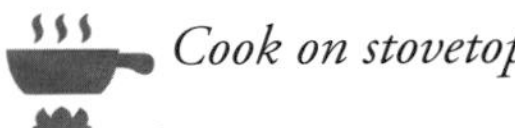

Cook on stovetop

Yield - 16 ounces turkey
1¾ cups gravy

Ingredients

1 tablespoon vegetable oil
¼ teaspoon salt
¼ teaspoon pepper
¼ teaspoon dried thyme
¼ teaspoon paprika
¼ teaspoon garlic powder
1¾ pounds turkey breast
3 cups water
1½ tablespoons cornstarch
1½ tablespoons water

Directions

1. Remove turkey skin. In a small bowl, combine the spices. Sprinkle evenly over all sides of the turkey breast and rub in.
2. Heat a large skillet over medium heat. Add the oil and the turkey breast and brown it on all sides, about 10 minutes.
3. When turkey is browned, add water to the pan carefully, as it will splatter. Cover and simmer for 15 minutes, then turn the turkey breast over. Simmer another 15 minutes until turkey breast is cooked through and tender, with an internal temperature of 165 degrees. Remove turkey from skillet.
4. Simmer pan juices until reduced by half, about 10 minutes.
5. In a small bowl, whisk the cornstarch and water until smooth. Add to the reduced pan juices and, whisking constantly, simmer until thickened, about 5 minutes.

Braised Turkey Breast provides M/MA at lunch/supper			
	Toddler	Pre-School	School Age
Turkey Breast	1 ounce	1-1/2 ounces	2 ounces
Gravy	1 tablespoon	1-1/2 tablespoons	2 tablespoons
Wild Rice	1/4 cup	1/4 cup	1/2 cup
Peas	1/8 cup	1/4 cup	1/2 cup
Apricots	1/8 cup	1/4 cup	1/4 cup
Milk	1/2 cup	3/4 cup	1 cup

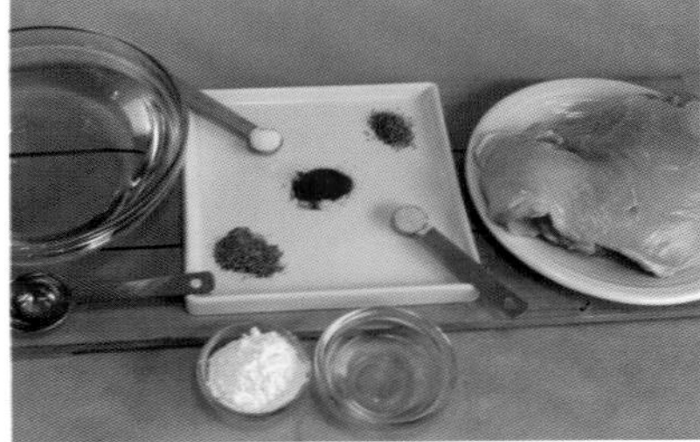

Ingredients

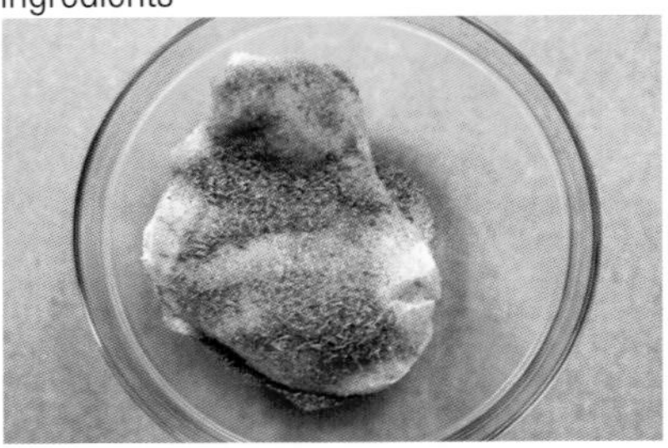

Step 1

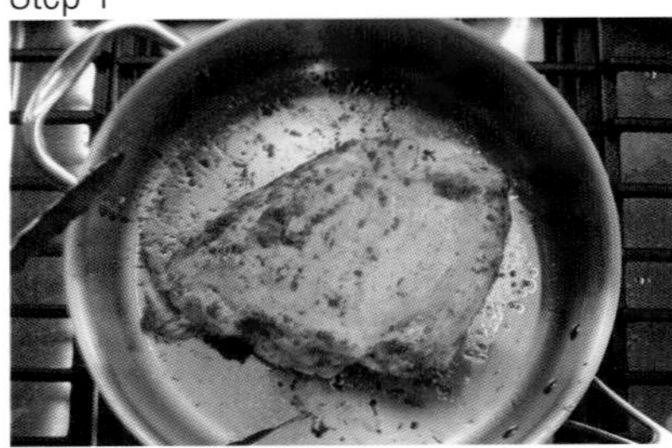

Step 2

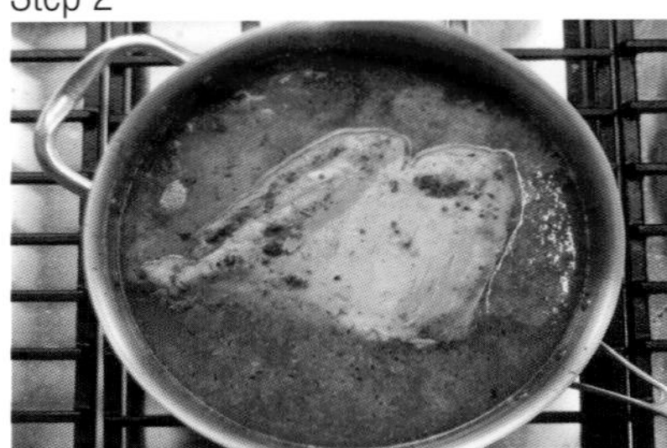

Step 3

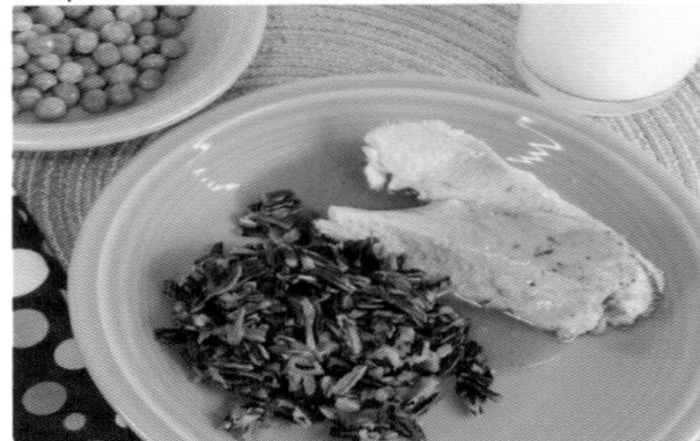

Creditable lunch/supper

Broccoli-Cheddar Baked Potatoes

Prep time - 20 minutes
Cook time - 35 minutes
Total time - 55 minutes

Cook in microwave and in oven

Yield - 6 potatoes

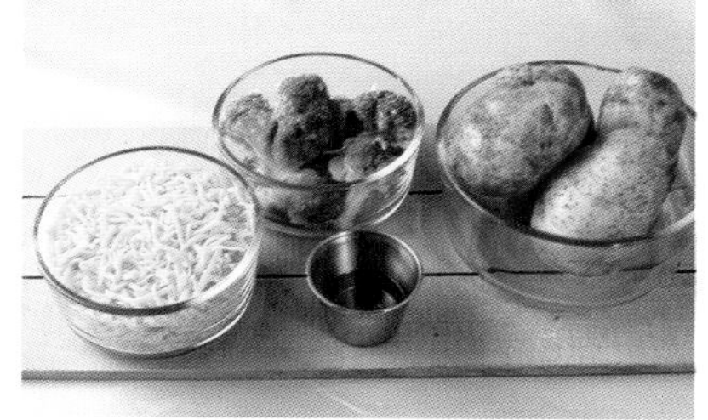
Ingredients

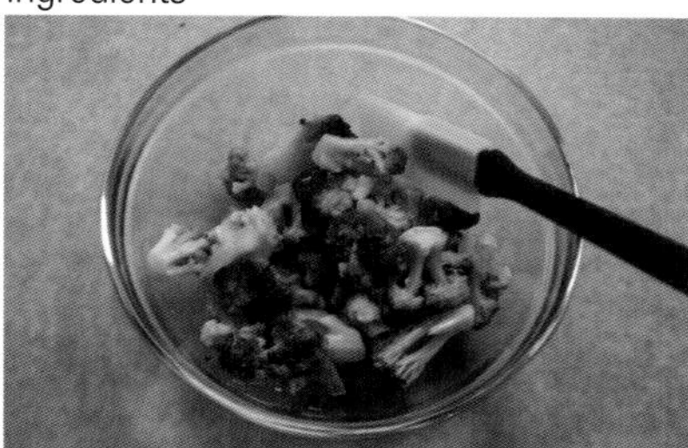
Step 1

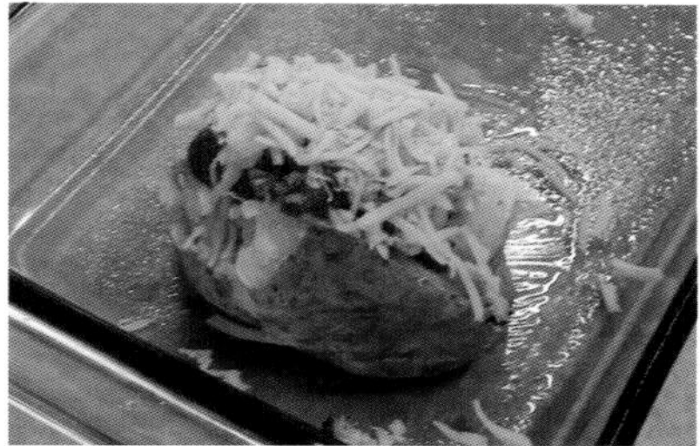
Step 2

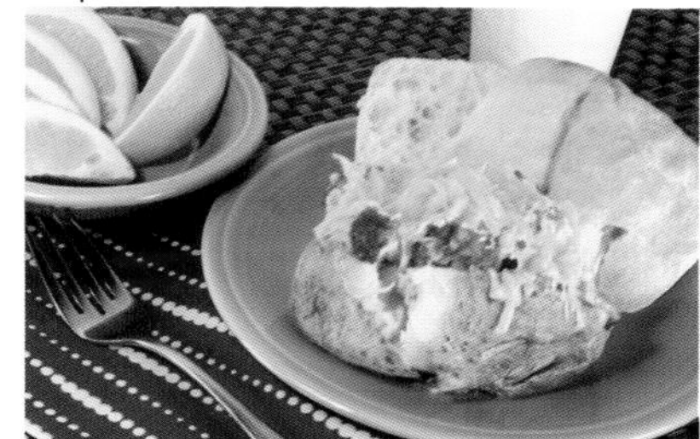
Creditable lunch/supper

Ingredients

2 teaspoons vegetable oil
1½ cups broccoli florets, chopped
2¼ cups (9 ounces) shredded cheddar cheese
6 russet potatoes, washed and dried, about 6 ounces each

Directions

1. Preheat oven to 425 degrees. Line a baking pan with foil or parchment paper, or coat with cooking spray.
2. In small bowl, toss broccoli with oil; set aside.
3. Pierce each potato several times with a fork. Place them in a microwave-safe dish and microwave on high until tender, about 15 minutes. Remove from microwave, cover dish with foil and set aside for 10 minutes to finish cooking.
4. Slit the top of each potato, about 1 inch deep and almost the length of the potato. Squeeze the potato gently to enlarge the opening and place in the baking pan.
5. Stuff each potato with ¼ cup broccoli and top with ⅜ cup cheese.
6. Bake until broccoli is tender, about 20-25 minutes. Cool slightly before serving.

Broccoli-Cheddar Baked Potatoes
provide M/MA and VEG at lunch/supper

	Toddler	Pre-School	School Age
Baked Potato	1 potato	1 potato	1-1/2 potatoes
Whole Wheat Roll	1/2 ounce	1/2 ounce	1 ounce
Oranges	1/8 cup	1/4 cup	1/4 cup
Milk	1/2 cup	3/4 cup	1 cup

Cheddar-Ham Calzone

Prep time - 20 minutes
Cook time - 25 minutes
Total time - 45 minutes

Bake in oven

Yield - 6 calzones

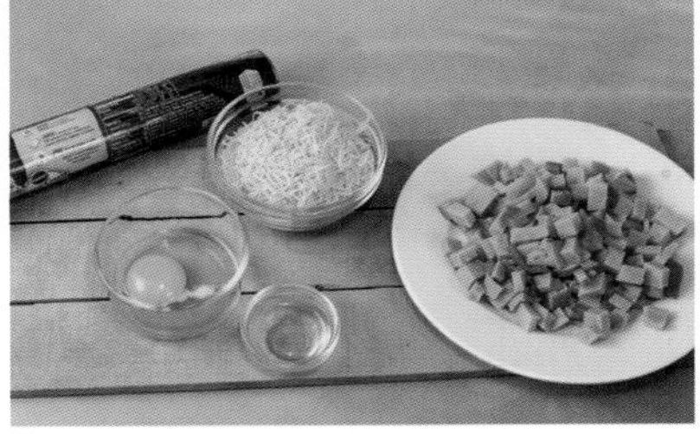
Ingredients

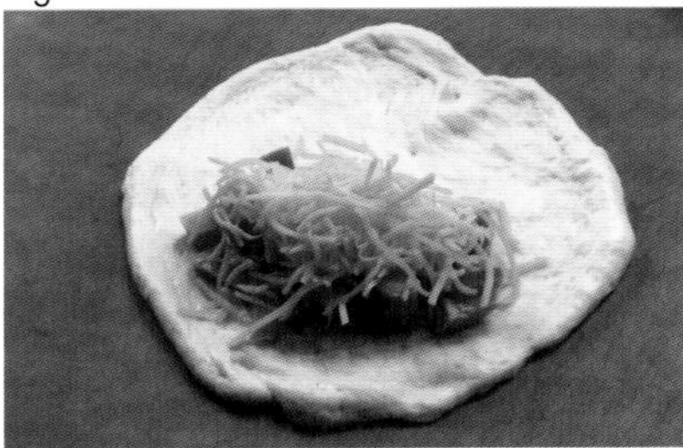
Step 3

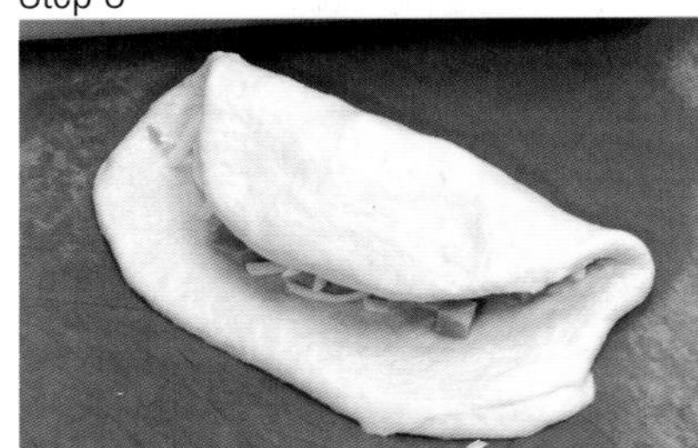
Step 4

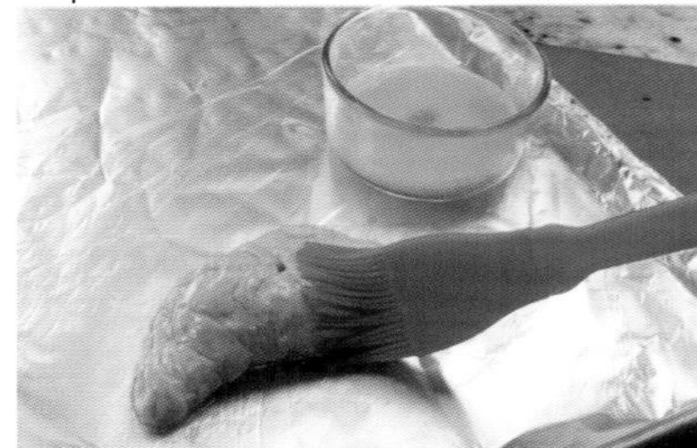
Step 6

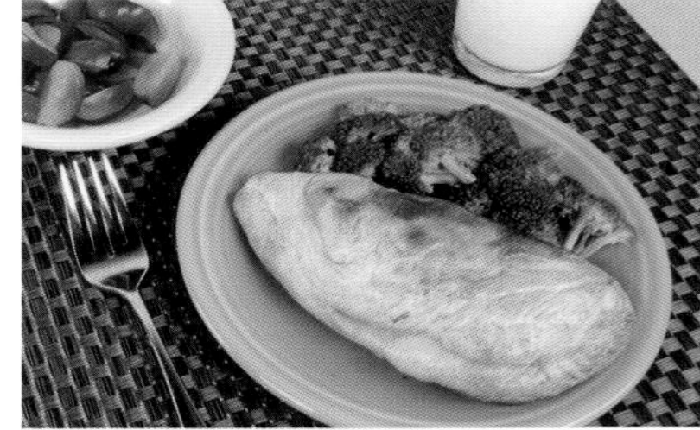
Creditable lunch/supper

Ingredients

1 10-ounce can refrigerated thin crust pizza dough
8 ounces (1½ cups) cooked turkey ham, diced
1½ cups (6 ounces) shredded cheese of your choice
1 egg
1 tablespoon water

Directions

1. Preheat oven to 400 degrees. Line a baking sheet with foil or parchment paper, or coat with cooking spray.
2. Divide dough into 6 portions and roll each into a circle about 7 inches in diameter.
3. Place ¼ cup turkey ham and ¼ cup cheese on one half of the dough circle.
4. Fold dough over to make a half-moon shape, leaving ½ inch of the bottom edge showing.
5. Fold bottom edge over the top edge and press together to seal. Repeat with remaining portions of dough, making 6 calzones.
6. Whisk egg and water together. Brush the top of each calzone with the egg wash.
7. Bake until golden, about 25-30 minutes.

Cheddar-Ham Calzone provides G/B and M/MA at lunch/supper			
	Toddler	Pre-School	School Age
Calzone	1/2 calzone	1/2 calzone	1 calzone
Broccoli	1/8 cup	1/4 cup	1/2 cup
Grapes	1/8 cup	1/4 cup	1/4 cup
Milk	1/2 cup	3/4 cup	1 cup

Chicken Alfredo

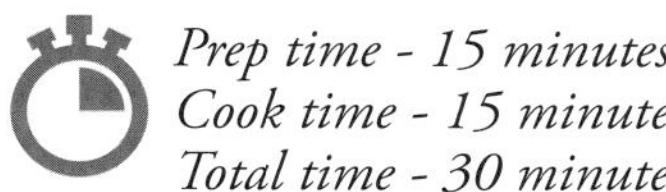

Prep time - 15 minutes
Cook time - 15 minutes
Total time - 30 minutes

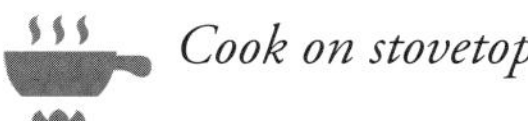

Cook on stovetop

Yield - 3 cups sauce and 1½ cups pasta

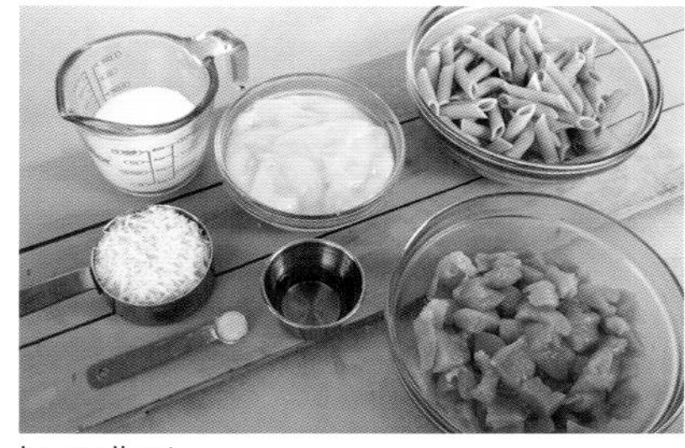

Ingredients

Ingredients

3 ounces (1 cup) dry whole grain rotini (spiral) pasta
Water for boiling pasta
2 tablespoons vegetable oil
1 pound boneless, skinless chicken breast, diced
¼ teaspoon garlic powder
1 14½-ounce can cream of chicken soup
½ cup milk
½ cup grated Parmesan cheese

Directions

1. Cook the pasta according to package directions; drain.
2. Heat large skillet over medium heat. Add oil and chicken and brown, about 5 minutes.
3. Mix in the garlic powder, soup and milk and bring to a simmer, about 2 minutes. Simmer until chicken reaches an internal temperature of 165 degrees, about 8-10 minutes.
4. Stir in Parmesan cheese, then remove from heat. Serve over pasta.

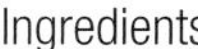

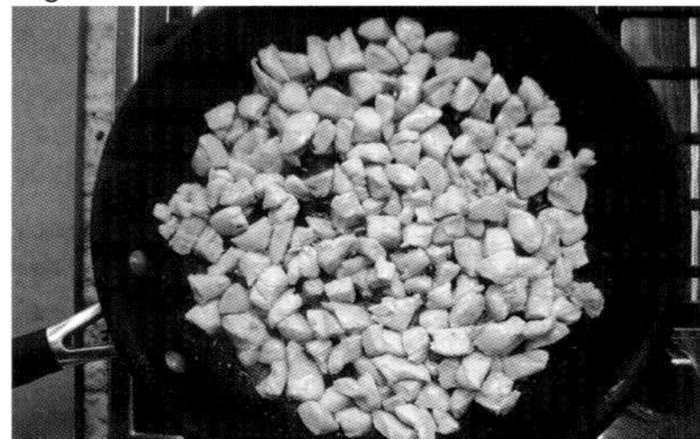

Step 2

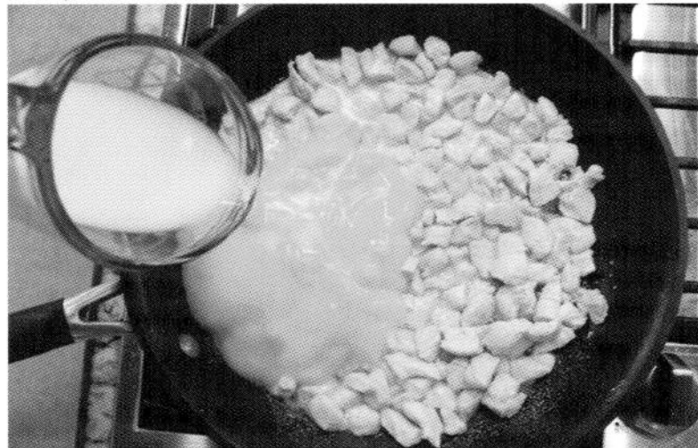

Step 3

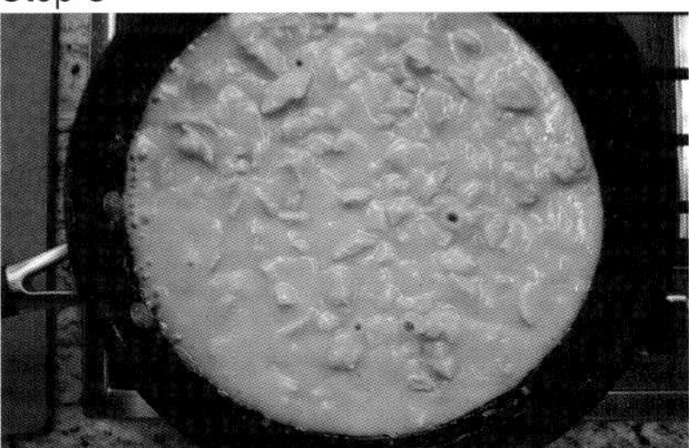

Step 4

Chicken Alfredo
provides M/MA at lunch/supper

	Toddler	Pre-School	School Age
Chicken Alfredo	1/3 cup	1/2 cup	3/4 cup
Rotini Pasta	1/4 cup	1/4 cup	1/2 cup
Green Beans	1/8 cup	1/4 cup	1/2 cup
Mandarin Oranges	1/8 cup	1/4 cup	1/4 cup
Milk	1/2 cup	3/4 cup	1 cup

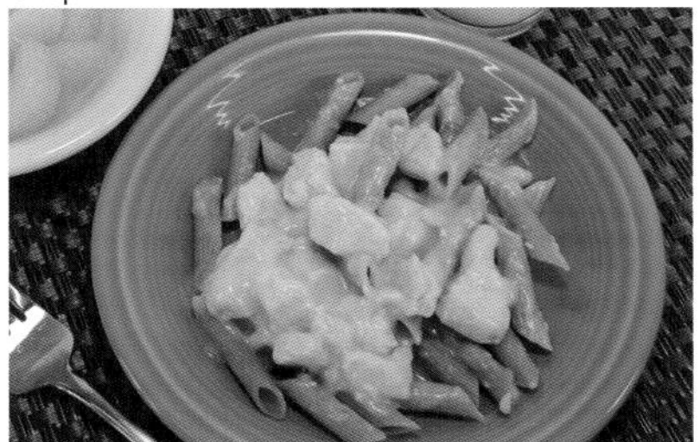

Creditable lunch/supper

Chicken Drumsticks

Prep time - 15 minutes
Cook time - 35 minutes
Total time - 50 minutes

Bake in oven

Yield - 12 drumsticks

Ingredients

1 teaspoon dried basil leaves
1 teaspoon dried thyme leaves
½ teaspoon garlic powder
½ teaspoon salt
1 tablespoon sugar
1 tablespoon vegetable oil
2 pounds bone-in, skinless chicken drumsticks (about 12)

Directions

1. Preheat oven to 350 degrees. Line a baking sheet with foil or parchment paper, or coat with cooking spray.
2. In a large bowl, whisk the spices and sugar together. Stir in the oil.
3. With gloved hands, rub seasoning mix over drumsticks and place on baking sheet.
4. Bake until chicken is golden brown, with an internal temperature of 165 degrees, about 35-45 minutes. Turn chicken halfway through cooking, at about 20 minutes.

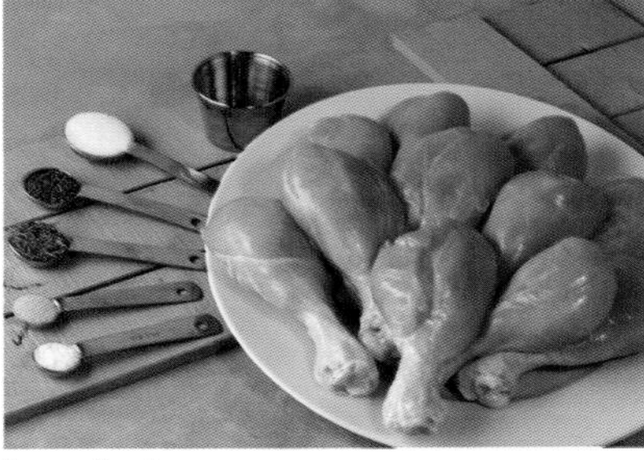
Ingredients

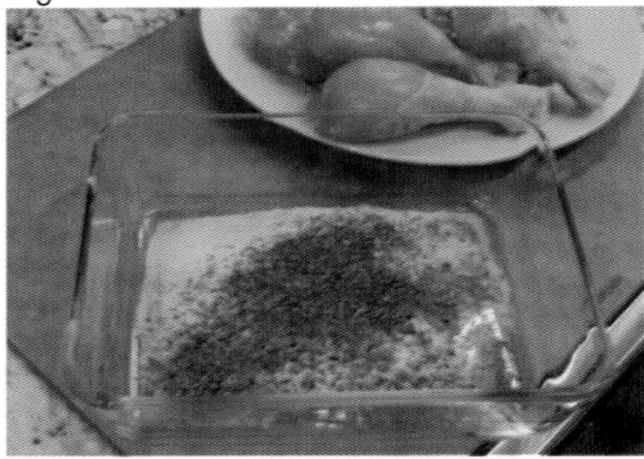
Step 3

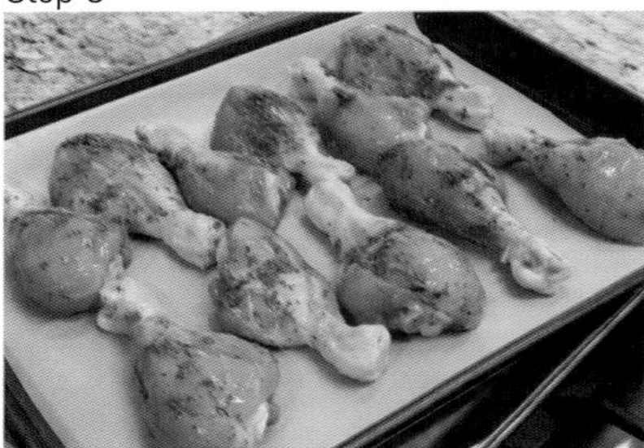
Step 4

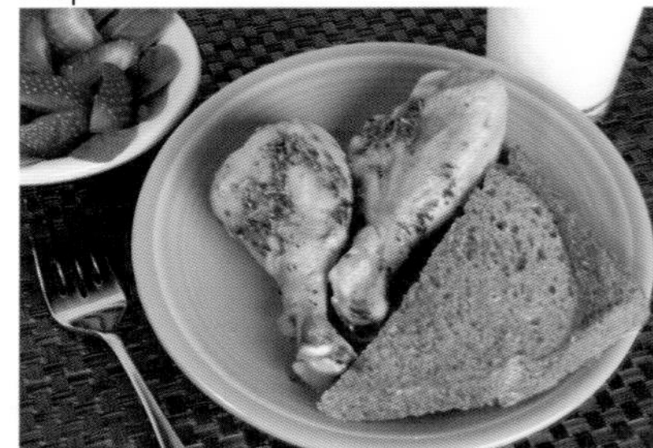
Creditable lunch/supper

Chicken Drumsticks
provide M/MA at lunch/supper

	Toddler	Pre-School	School Age
Chicken Drumstick	1 oz./1 drumstick	1-1/2 oz./2 drums.	2 oz./2 drumsticks
Whole Wheat Bread	1/2 oz. or 1/2 slice	1/2 oz. or 1/2 slice	1 oz. or 1 slice
Spinach	1/8 cup	1/4 cup	1/2 cup
Strawberries	1/8 cup	1/4 cup	1/4 cup
Milk	1/2 cup	3/4 cup	1 cup

Chicken Pasta Primavera

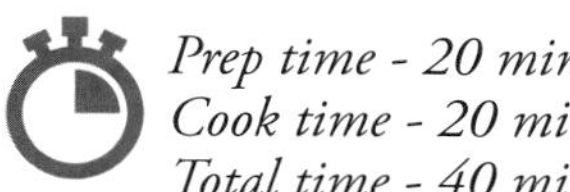
Prep time - 20 minutes
Cook time - 20 minutes
Total time - 40 minutes

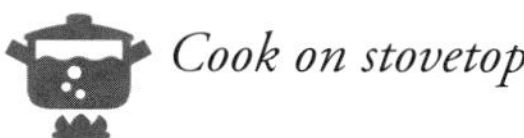
Cook on stovetop

Yield - 6½ cups

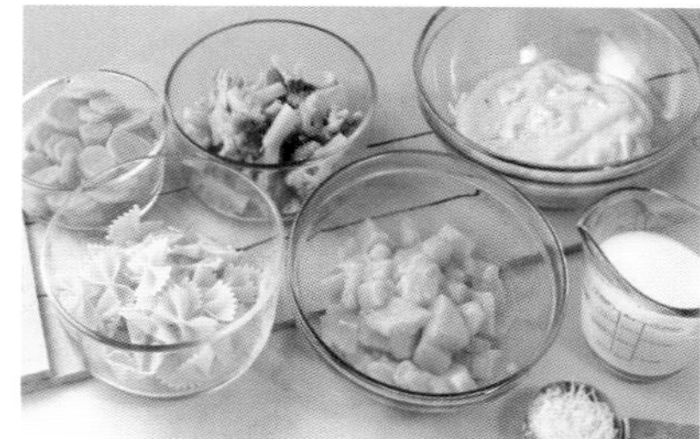
Ingredients

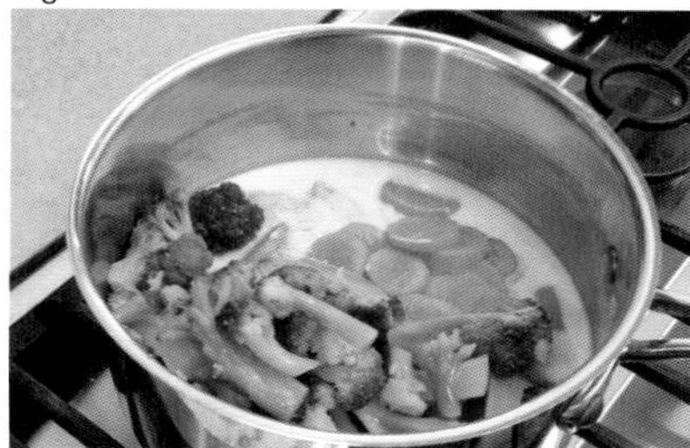
Step 2

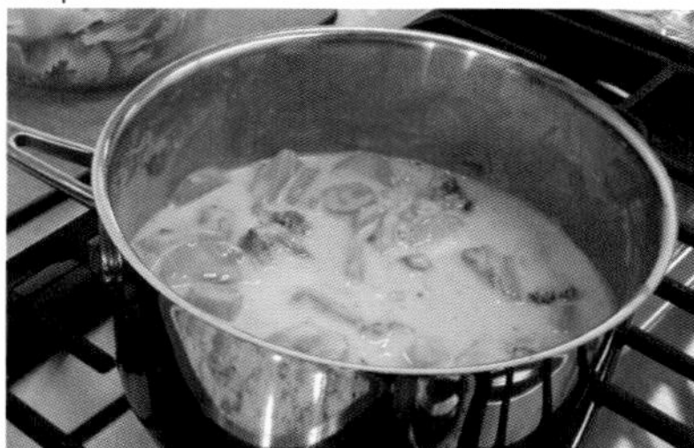
Step 2

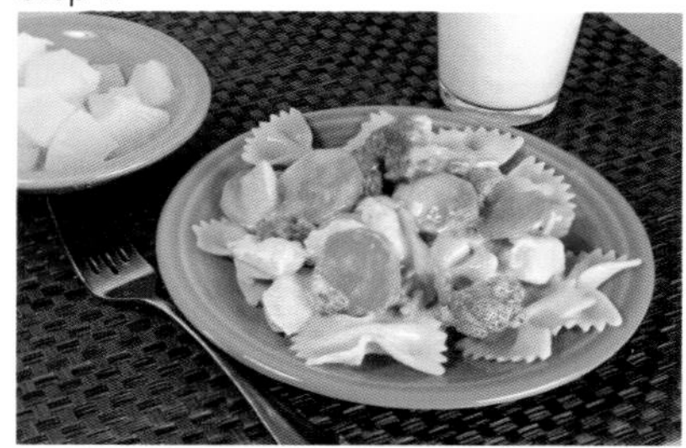
Creditable lunch/supper

Ingredients

4 ounces (2 cups) dry whole grain farfalle (bowtie) pasta
Water for boiling pasta
1 10¾-ounce can cream of mushroom soup
¾ cup milk
¼ cup grated Parmesan cheese
2 cups broccoli florets
1 cup carrots, sliced
9 ounces cooked chicken, chopped

Directions

1. Cook pasta in boiling water until al dente, about 10 minutes. Drain and cover to keep warm.
2. While pasta is cooking, prepare the cream sauce: In a medium saucepan, mix together the mushroom soup, milk, Parmesan cheese, broccoli, and carrots. Bring to a boil over medium heat. Reduce heat to low and cover. Simmer for 10 minutes or until vegetables are tender, stirring occasionally.
3. Pour pasta and chicken into the cream sauce and heat through.

Chicken Pasta Primavera
provides G/B, M/MA and VEG at lunch/supper

	Toddler	Pre-School	School Age
Pasta Primavera	2/3 cup	1 cup	1-1/3 cups
Pineapple	1/8 cup	1/4 cup	1/4 cup
Milk	1/2 cup	3/4 cup	1 cup

Chicken Penne with Broccoli

Prep time - 15 minutes
Cook time - 35 minutes
Total time - 50 minutes

Cook on stovetop and bake in oven

Yield - 10½ cups

Ingredients

7 ounces (2 cups) dry whole grain penne pasta
Water for boiling pasta
4 cups broccoli florets
12 ounces cooked chicken, chopped
1 10¾-ounce can condensed cream of mushroom soup
1½ cups milk
½ teaspoon black pepper
1½ cups (6 ounces) shredded mozzarella cheese, divided
¼ cup shredded Parmesan cheese, divided

Directions

1. Preheat oven to 350 degrees. Grease a shallow 9x13-inch baking pan or coat with cooking spray.
2. Cook the pasta according to the package directions, about 10 minutes. Add the broccoli for the last 4 minutes of cooking time. Drain the pasta mixture well in a colander.
3. In the baking dish, stir together the chicken, soup, milk and pepper. Stir in the cooked pasta and broccoli mixture, ¾ cup mozzarella cheese and 2 tablespoons of the Parmesan cheese; mix well and spread evenly in baking dish.
4. When thoroughly combined, sprinkle the top with the remaining mozzarella and Parmesan cheeses.
5. Bake until hot and bubbling and the cheese is melted, about 25 minutes.

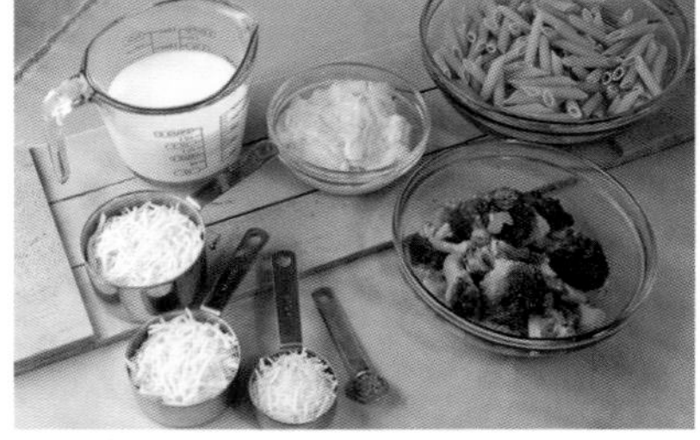

Ingredients

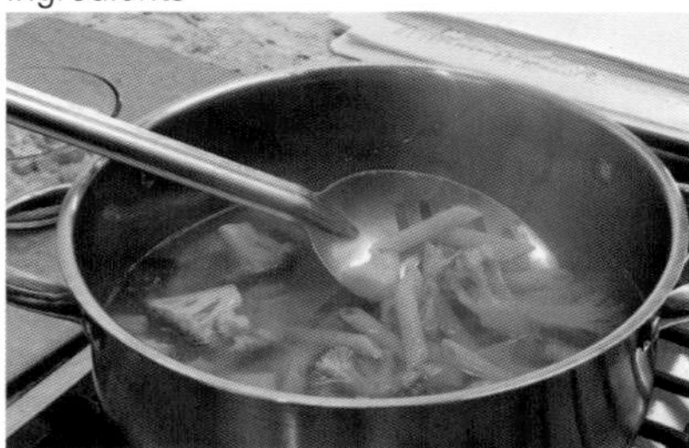

Step 2

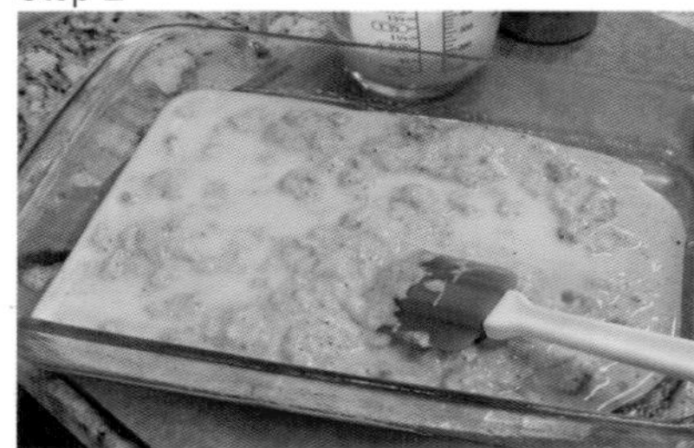

Step 3

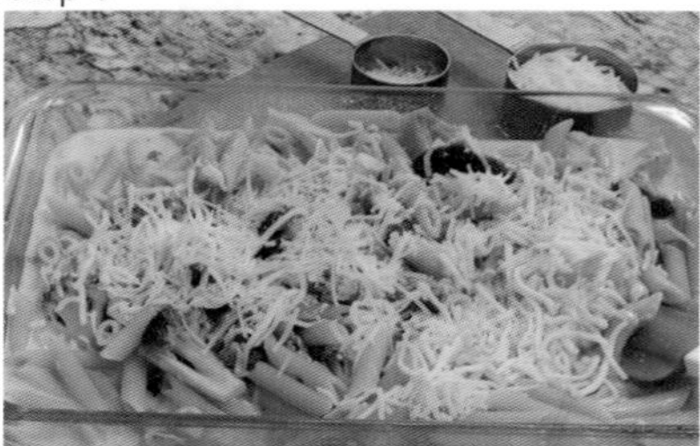

Step 4

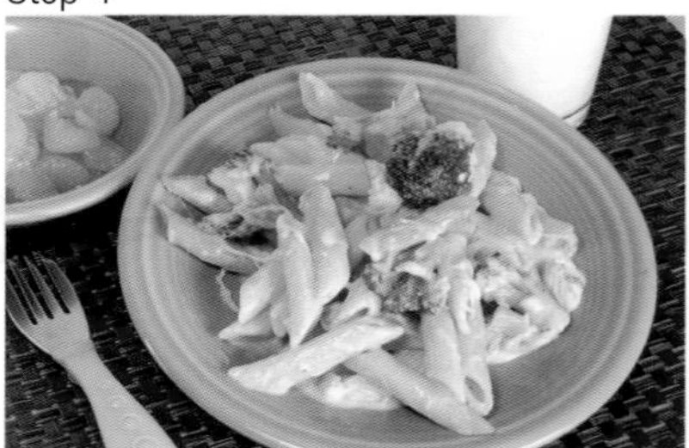

Creditable lunch/supper

Cheesy Penne with Broccoli provides G/B, M/MA and VEG at lunch/supper			
	Toddler	Pre-School	School Age
Chicken Penne	2/3 cup	1 cup	1-1/3 cups
Mandarin Oranges	1/8 cup	1/4 cup	1/4 cup
Milk	1/2 cup	3/4 cup	1 cup

Chicken Pot Pie

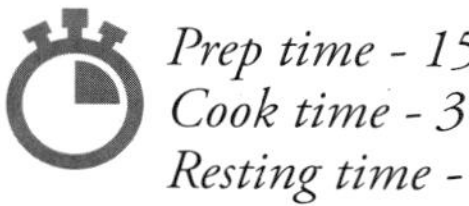

Prep time - 15 minutes
Cook time - 30 minutes
Resting time - 10 minutes
Total time - 55 minutes

Bake in oven

Yield - 12 wedges

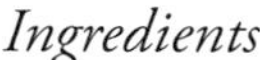

Ingredients

2 sheets pie crust

12 ounces cooked chicken, diced

3 cups frozen vegetable blend, carrots, peas and corn

1 10¾-ounce can condensed cream of mushroom soup

Directions

1. Preheat oven to 400 degrees. Grease a 9-inch deep dish pie plate or coat with cooking spray.
2. Line pie plate with one sheet of pie dough. Pie crust should extend at least 1 inch beyond rim for sealing to top crust.
3. In a large bowl, stir together the chicken, frozen vegetables and the soup.
4. Spoon filling into pastry-lined pie plate.
5. Seal the pie crust together by folding the bottom crust up and over the top crust and crimping with fingers or a fork. Make three slits in the crust to allow steam to escape.
6. Bake until golden brown and heated through, about 30 minutes. Cover the edge with foil to prevent burning.
7. Remove from oven and allow to cool for 10 minutes, if needed to set filling. Cut into 12 wedges.

Chicken Pot Pie
provides G/B and VEG at lunch/supper

	Toddler	Pre-School	School Age
Chicken Pot Pie	1 wedge	1-1/2 wedges	2 wedges
Mandarin Oranges	1/8 cup	1/4 cup	1/4 cup
Milk	1/2 cup	3/4 cup	1 cup

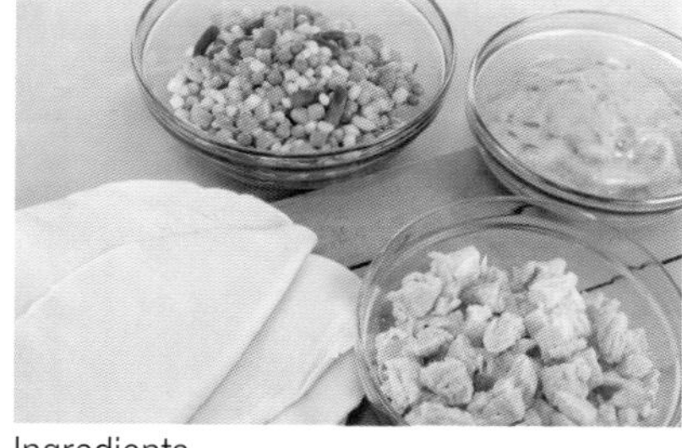

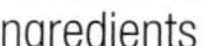

Ingredients

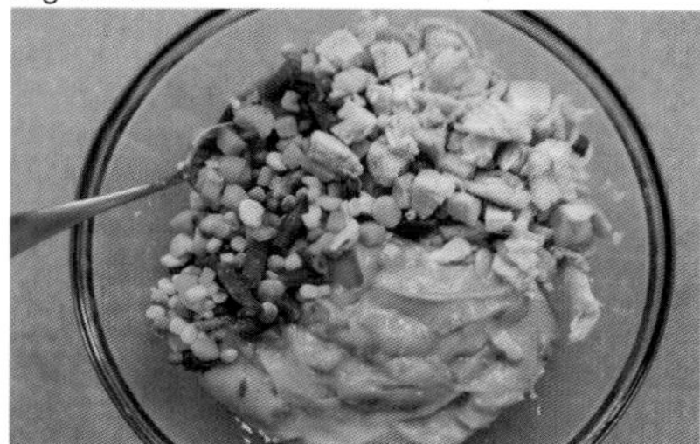

Step 3

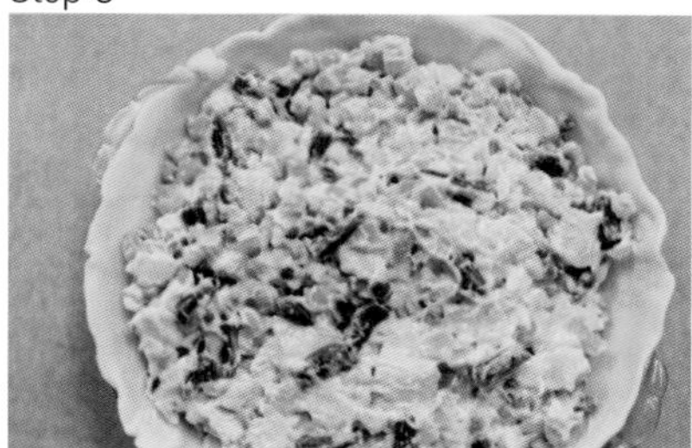

Step 4

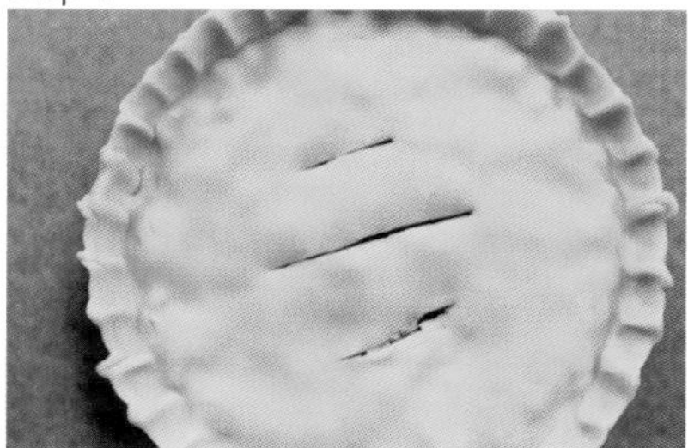

Step 5

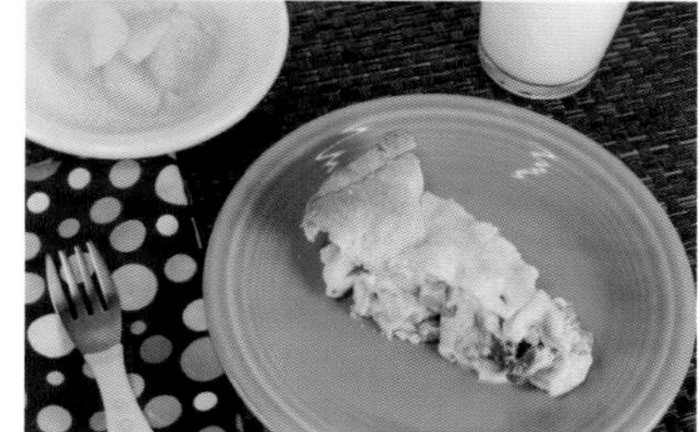

Creditable lunch/supper

Easy Chicken & Rice

Prep time - 15 minutes
Cook time - 35 minutes
Total time - 50 minutes

Cook on stovetop

Yield - 4 cups

Ingredients

1 cup long-grain brown rice
2 cups water for cooking rice
9 ounces cooked chicken, chopped
1 10¾-ounce can condensed cream of chicken soup

Directions

1. Prepare rice according to package directions, about 35 minutes.
2. Heat the cooked chicken in a large saucepan over low heat.
3. When rice is cooked, add it to the chicken and stir to mix. Then add soup and, stirring occasionally, cook until chicken is heated through.

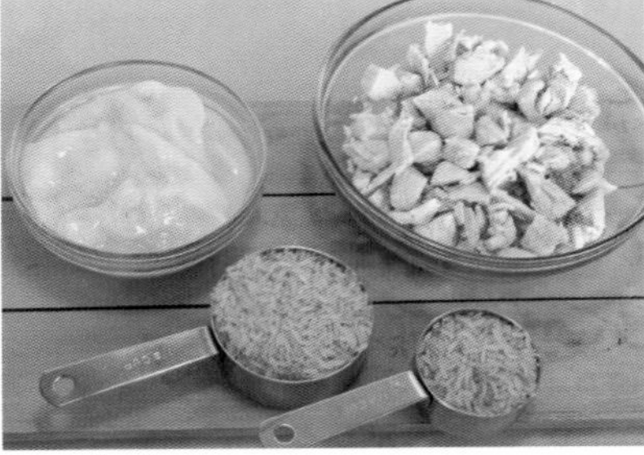

Ingredients

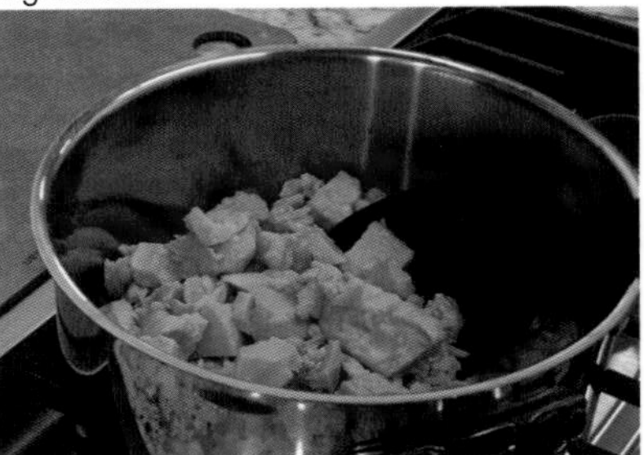

Step 2

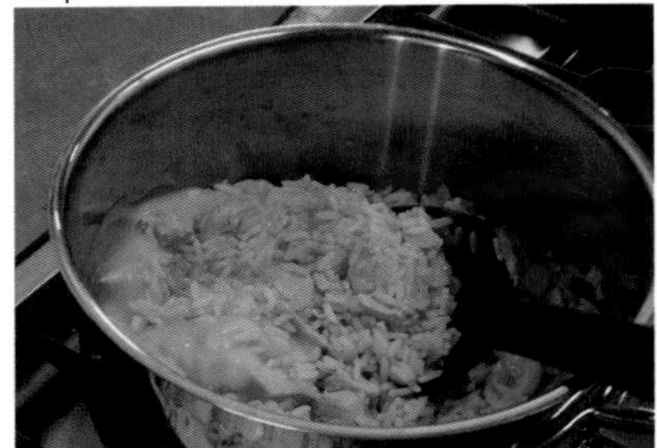

Step 3

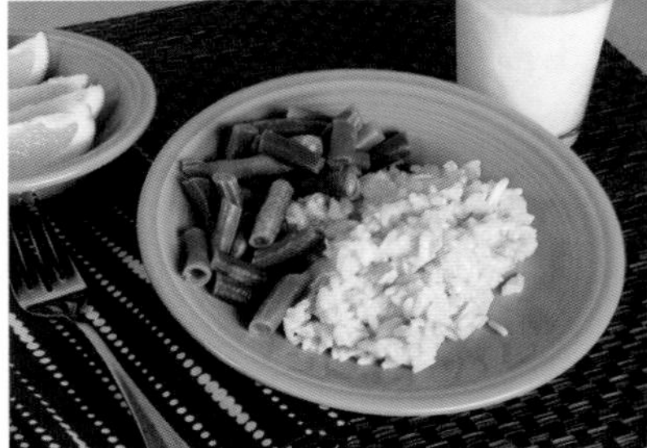

Creditable lunch/supper

Easy Chicken & Rice provides G/B and M/MA at lunch/supper			
	Toddler	Pre-School	School Age
Chicken & Rice	1/2 cup	2/3 cup	1 cup
Green Beans	1/8 cup	1/4 cup	1/2 cup
Oranges	1/8 cup	1/4 cup	1/4 cup
Milk	1/2 cup	3/4 cup	1 cup

Ham & Cheese Pasta Bake

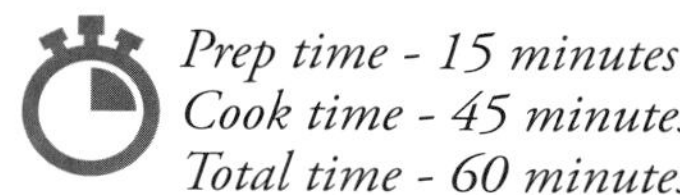

Prep time - 15 minutes
Cook time - 45 minutes
Total time - 60 minutes

Bake in oven

Yield - 6 cups

Ingredients

3 ounces (1¼ cups) dry whole grain rotini (spiral) pasta
3 cups marinara sauce
9 ounces turkey ham, diced
¾ cup (3 ounces) shredded mozzarella cheese

Directions

1. Preheat oven to 350 degrees. Grease a 9x9-inch baking dish or coat with cooking spray.
2. In the baking dish, combine all of the ingredients, including uncooked pasta; mix well. Pasta does not need to be boiled before baking.
3. Bake until hot and bubbling, about 45 minutes.

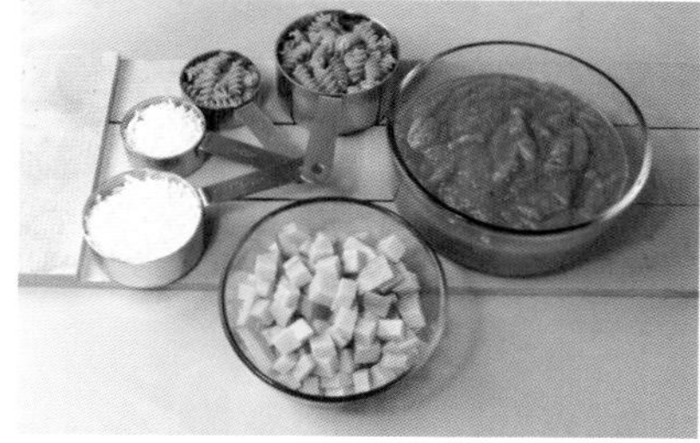

Ingredients

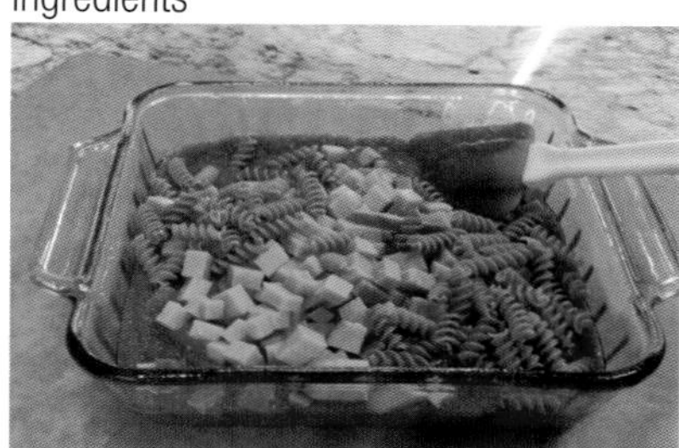

Step 2

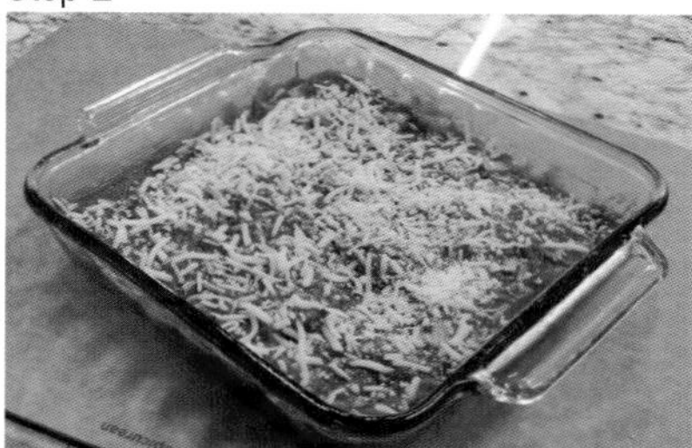

Step 3

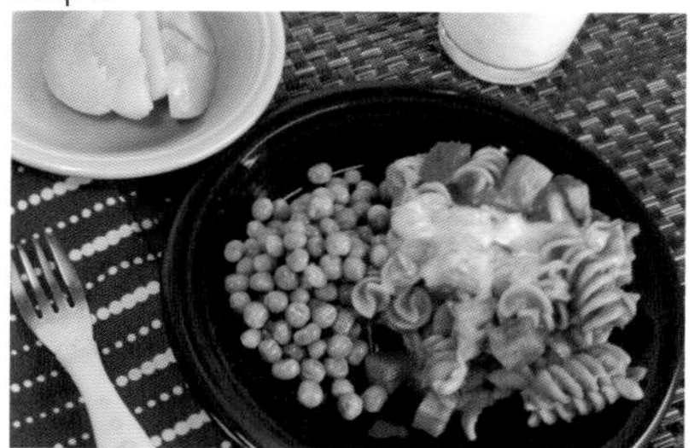

Creditable lunch/supper

Ham & Cheese Pasta Bake provides G/B and M/MA at lunch/supper			
	Toddler	Pre-School	School Age
Pasta Bake	2/3 cup	1 cup	1-1/3 cups
Peas	1/8 cup	1/4 cup	1/2 cup
Peaches	1/8 cup	1/4 cup	1/4 cup
Milk	1/2 cup	3/4 cup	1 cup

Ham & Pea Casserole

Prep time - 15 minutes
Cook time - 40 minutes
Total time - 55 minutes

Cook on stovetop and in oven

Yield - 6 cups

Ingredients

3 ounces (¾ cup) whole grain elbow macaroni
Water for boiling pasta
2 tablespoons butter
2 tablespoons whole wheat flour
1½ cups milk
1 pound turkey ham, diced
1½ cups frozen peas
¼ teaspoon dried basil
¼ cup grated Parmesan cheese

Directions

1. Preheat oven to 350 degrees. Grease a 9x13-inch baking dish or coat with cooking spray.
2. Cook pasta according to package directions, about 10 minutes. Drain.
3. In a large saucepan over medium heat, melt butter. Add flour and stir until well combined. Pour in milk, stirring constantly until it thickens, about 5 minutes.
4. Add the turkey ham, peas, cooked pasta and basil to the thickened sauce. Mix well.
5. Pour into prepared baking dish and sprinkle Parmesan cheese on top.
6. Bake until hot and bubbling, about 25 minutes.

Ham & Pea Casserole provides G/B, M/MA and VEG at lunch/supper			
	Toddler	Pre-School	School Age
Casserole	2/3 cup	1 cup	1-1/3 cups
Pears	1/8 cup	1/4 cup	1/4 cup
Milk	1/2 cup	3/4 cup	1 cup

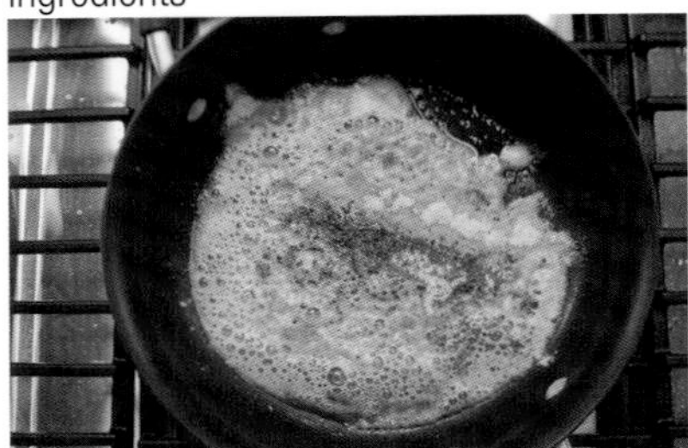

Ingredients

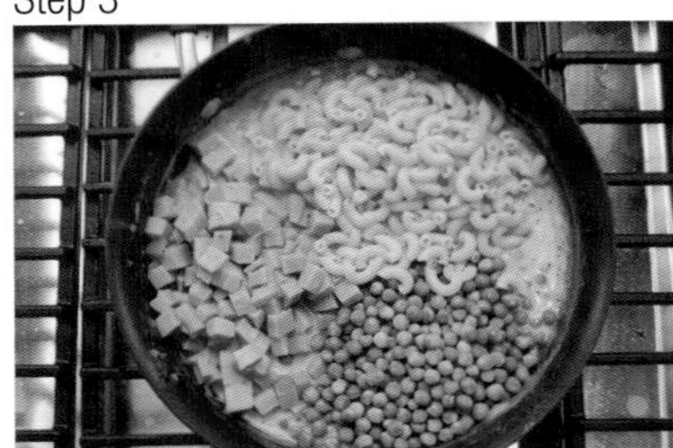

Step 3

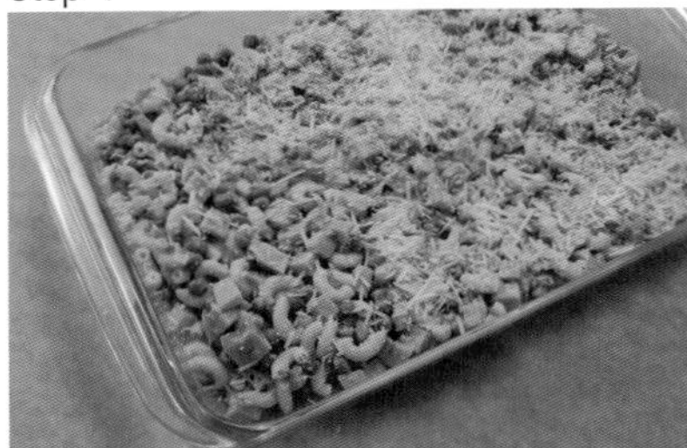

Step 4

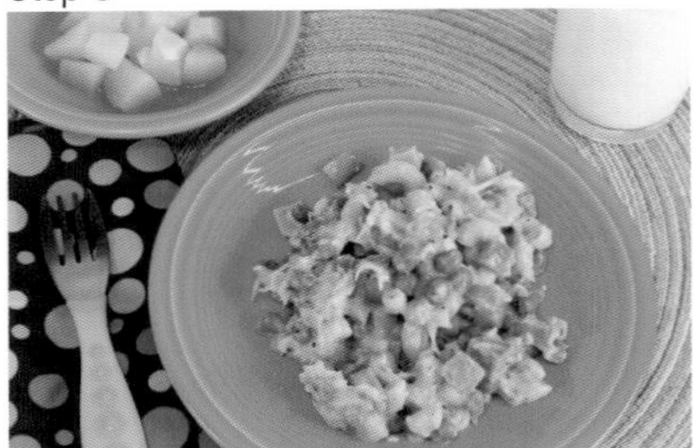

Step 5

Creditable lunch/supper

Lentil-Beef Meatloaf

Prep time - 15 minutes
Cook time - 70 minutes
Total time - 85 minutes

Cook on stovetop and in oven

Yield - 12 slices

Ingredients

1 cup dry lentils
2 cups water
1 tablespoon vegetable oil
1¾ pounds ground beef, at least 80% lean
½ cup onions, finely chopped
1 cup instant oats
2 teaspoons Italian seasoning
¾ teaspoon salt
¼ cup grated Parmesan cheese

Directions

1. Preheat oven to 350 degrees. Grease 9x5-inch loaf pan or coat with cooking spray.
2. In a large saucepan, combine water and lentils. Bring to a boil, reduce heat, cover and simmer until tender, about 45-55 minutes. Set aside to cool.
3. In a large bowl, thoroughly mix the cooked lentils, beef, onions, oats, Italian seasoning and Parmesan cheese.
4. Gently press mixture into loaf pan.
5. Bake until lightly golden and firm to the touch, with an internal temperature of 160 degrees, about 25-35 minutes.
6. Remove from oven, cool slightly and cut into 12 slices.

Batch Cooking Tip *- Make ahead, freeze and reheat.*
This recipe provides 12 1½-ounce servings M/MA

Lentil-Beef Meatloaf provides M/MA and VEG at lunch/supper			
	Toddler	Pre-School	School Age
Meatloaf	2/3 slice	1 slice	1-1/3 slices
Rice	1/4 cup	1/4 cup	1/2 cup
Mixed Fruit	1/8 cup	1/4 cup	1/4 cup
Milk	1/2 cup	3/4 cup	1 cup

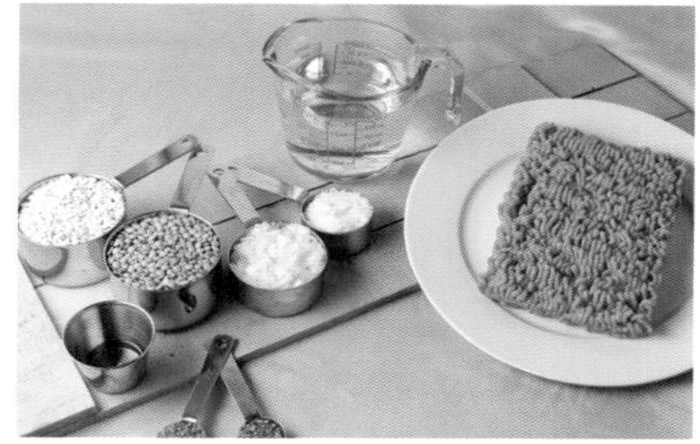

Ingredients

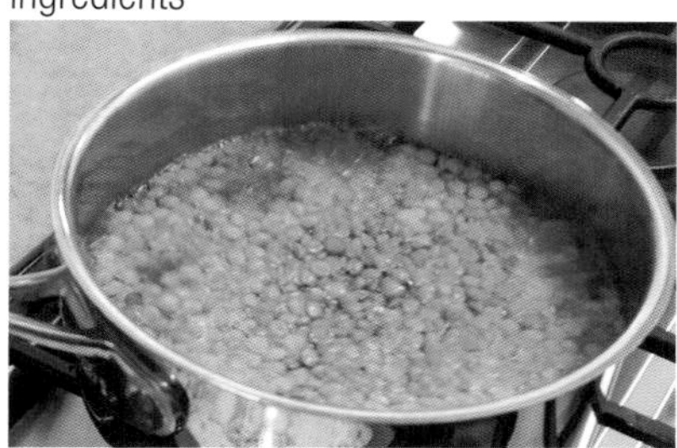

Step 2

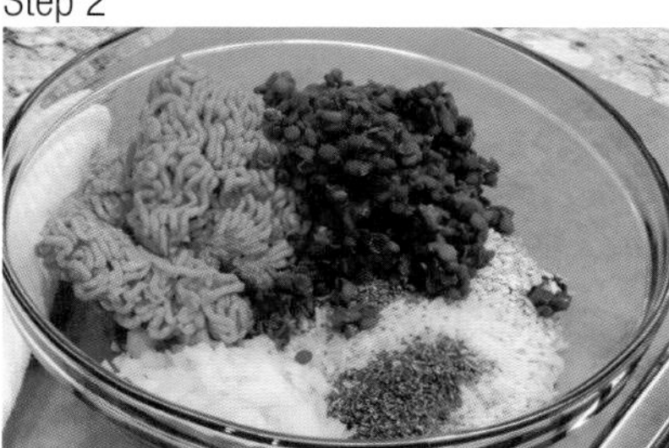

Step 3

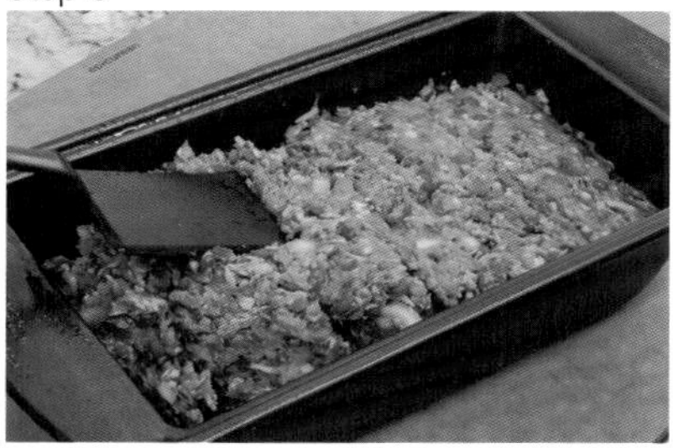

Step 4

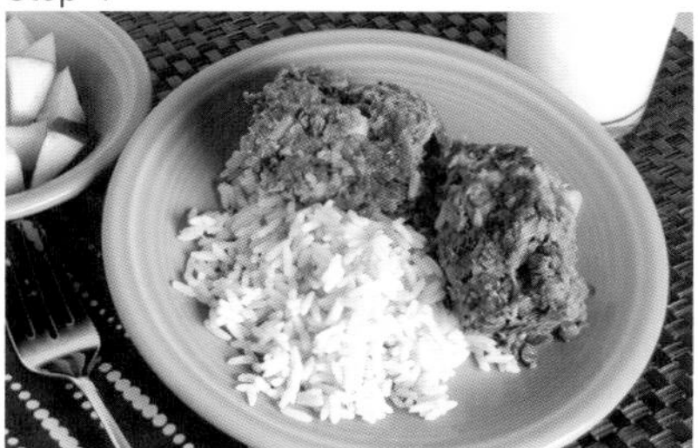

Creditable lunch/supper

On Top of Spaghetti

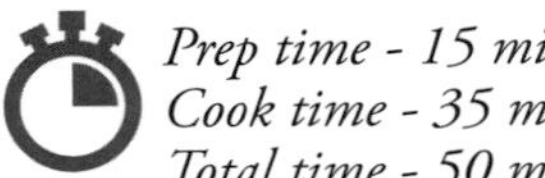

Prep time - 15 minutes
Cook time - 35 minutes
Total time - 50 minutes

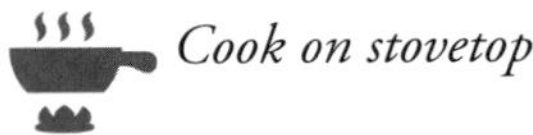

Cook on stovetop

Yield - 4½ cups sauce

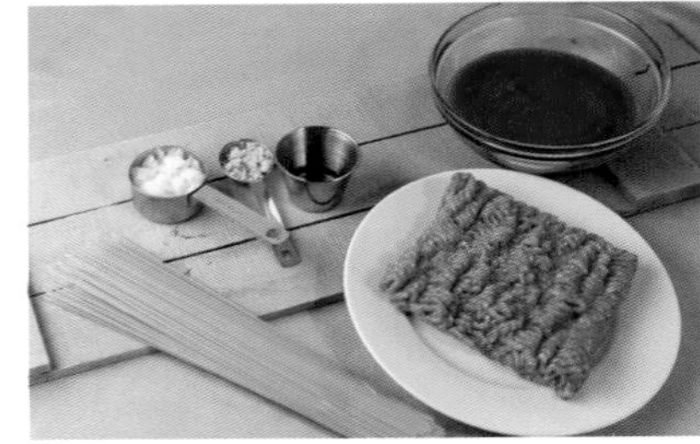

Ingredients

Ingredients

1 teaspoon vegetable oil
¼ cup onions, minced
1 tablespoon fresh garlic, minced
1 pound ground beef, at least 80% lean
3 cups marinara sauce
5 ounces (1 cup) dry whole grain spaghetti
Water for boiling pasta

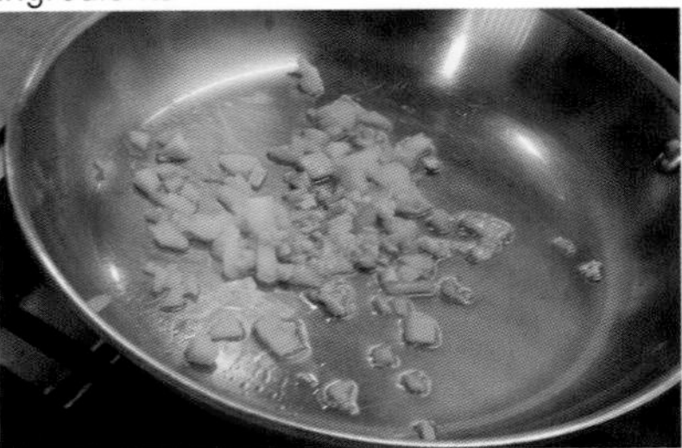

Step 1

Directions

1. In a large skillet, sauté onions and garlic over medium heat until tender, about 5 minutes.
2. Add ground beef and cook until it reaches an internal temperature of 160 degrees and no pink remains, about 10 minutes.
3. Add marinara sauce to the beef and simmer over low heat for 20 minutes.
4. While sauce is cooking, cook spaghetti according to package directions.
5. Serve meat sauce over spaghetti.

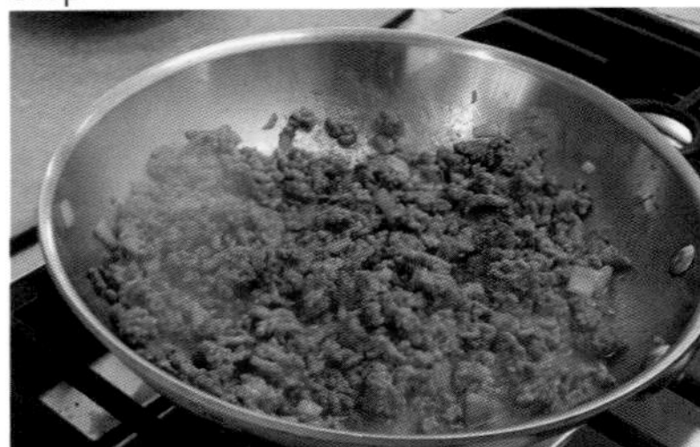

Step 2

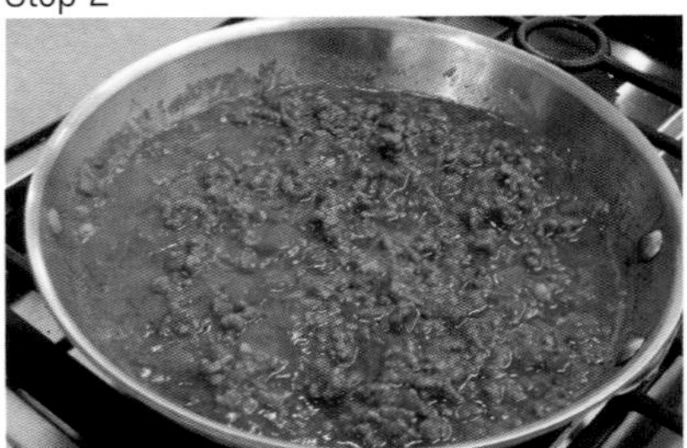

Step 3

On Top of Spaghetti
provides G/B, M/MA and VEG at lunch/supper

	Toddler	Pre-School	School Age
Spaghetti	1/4 cup	1/4 cup	1/2 cup
Marinara Sauce	1/2 cup	3/4 cup	1 cup
Green Beans	1/8 cup	1/4 cup	1/2 cup
Milk	1/2 cup	3/4 cup	1 cup

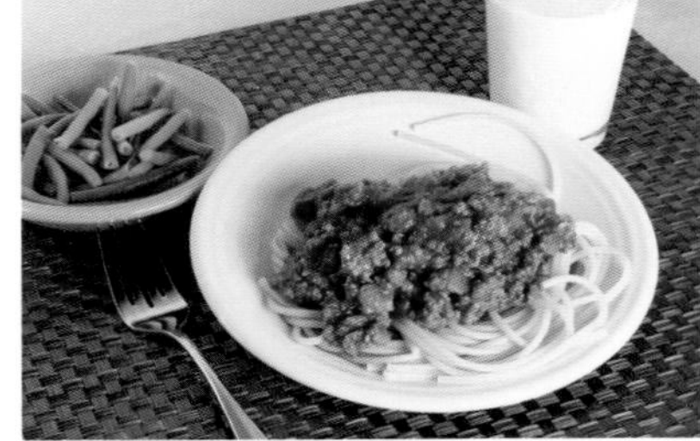

Creditable lunch/supper

Parmesan Chicken

Prep time - 15 minutes
Cook time - 35 minutes
Total time - 50 minutes

Bake in oven

Yield - 12 ounces

Ingredients

2 tablespoons vegetable oil
¼ teaspoon garlic, minced
1 cup dry bread crumbs
⅔ cup grated Parmesan cheese
1 teaspoon dried basil
¼ teaspoon black pepper
1 pound boneless, skinless chicken breast

Directions

1. Preheat oven to 350 degrees. Lightly grease a 9x13-inch baking pan.
2. In a small bowl, blend the oil and garlic. In a separate bowl, mix the bread crumbs, Parmesan cheese, basil, and pepper.
3. Brush each chicken breast with the oil mixture, then roll it in the bread crumbs. Place coated chicken in the baking pan, and sprinkle with any remaining bread crumbs.
4. Bake until chicken reaches an internal temperature of 165 degrees, about 35 minutes.

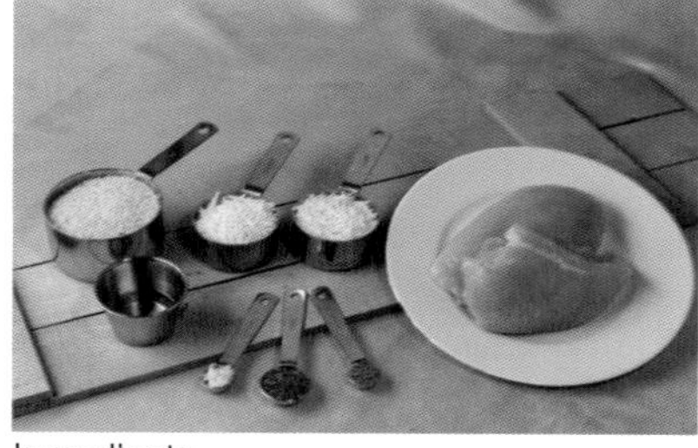
Ingredients

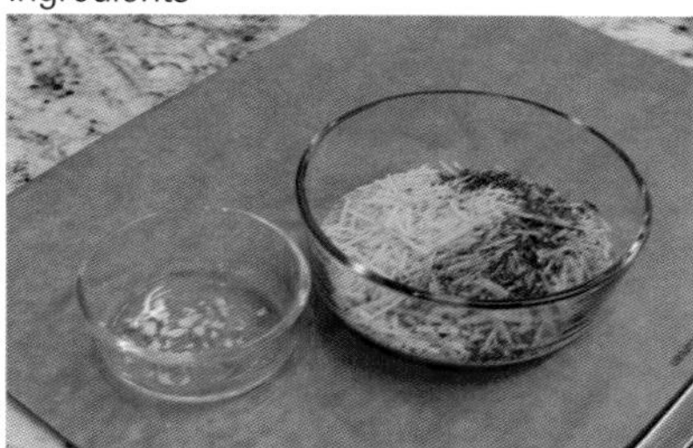
Step 2

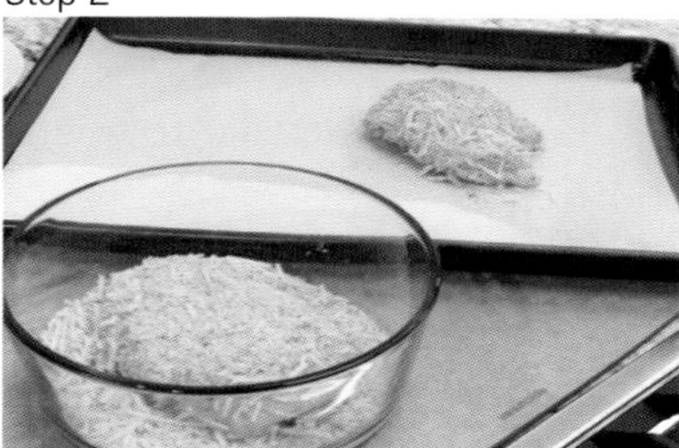
Step 3

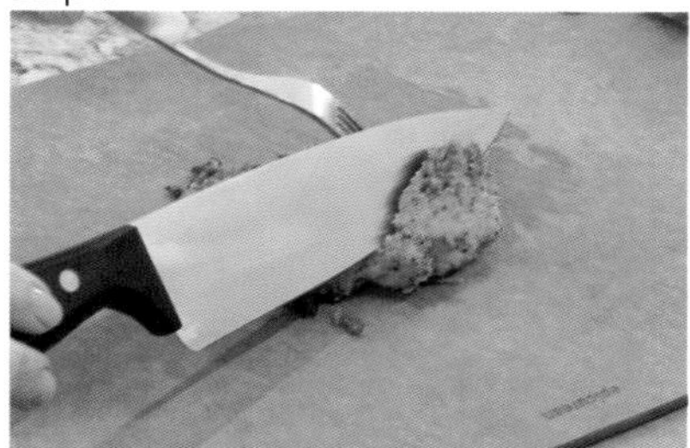
Step 4

Parmesan Chicken provides M/MA at lunch/supper			
	Toddler	Pre-School	School Age
Parmesan Chicken	1 ounce	1-1/2 ounces	2 ounces
Noodles	1/4 cup	1/4 cup	1/2 cup
Peas	1/8 cup	1/4 cup	1/2 cup
Pears	1/8 cup	1/4 cup	1/4 cup
Milk	1/2 cup	3/4 cup	1 cup

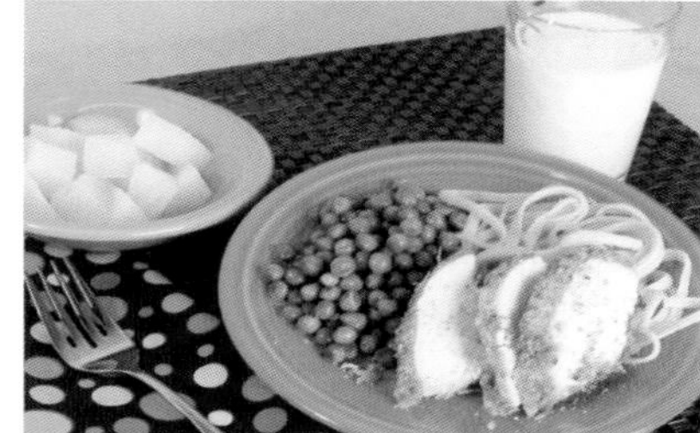
Creditable lunch/supper

Pork Roast

Prep time - 15 minutes
Cook time - 45 minutes
Resting time - 10 minutes
Total time - 70 minutes

Bake in oven

Yield - 10 ounces

Ingredients

1 teaspoon garlic powder
¼ teaspoon paprika
¼ teaspoon salt
1 tablespoon vegetable oil
1 pound pork loin

Directions

1. Preheat oven to 350 degrees. Line a baking pan with foil or parchment paper, or coat with cooking spray.
2. In a small bowl, stir together the spices and the oil.
3. Brush or rub seasoned oil on all sides of the roast.
4. Bake until internal temperature is 160 degrees, about 45-60 minutes.
5. Remove from oven and let rest for 10-15 minutes before slicing.

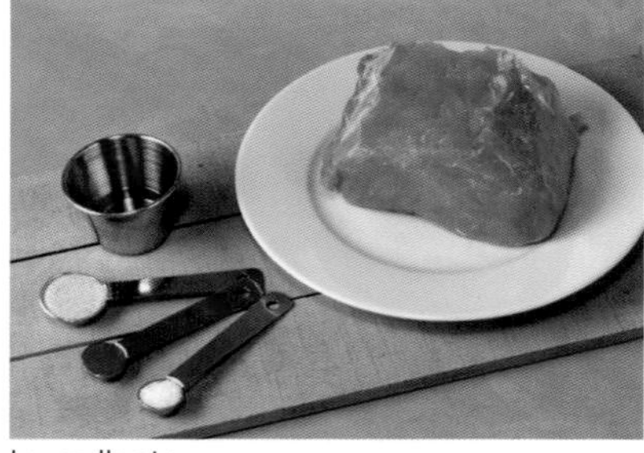

Ingredients

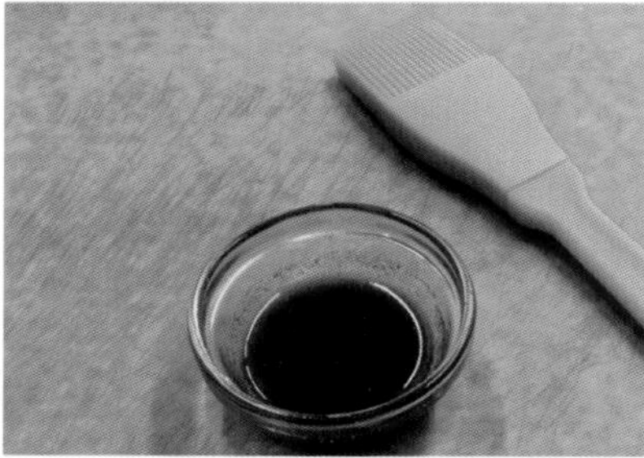

Step 2

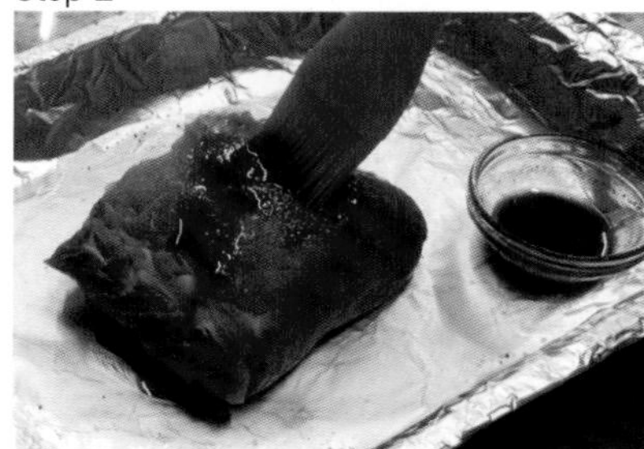

Creditable lunch/supper

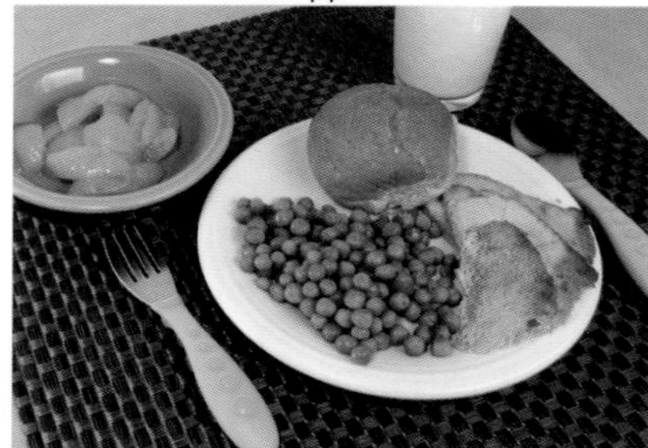

Creditable lunch/supper

Pork Roast provides M/MA at lunch/supper			
	Toddler	Pre-School	School Age
Pork Roast	1 ounce	1-1/2 ounces	2 ounces
Whole Wheat Roll	1/2 ounce	1/2 ounce	1 ounce
Peas	1/8 cup	1/4 cup	1/2 cup
Apricots	1/8 cup	1/4 cup	1/4 cup
Milk	1/2 cup	3/4 cup	1 cup

Quiche

Prep time - 15 minutes
Cook time - 40 minutes
Total time - 55 minutes

Bake in oven

Yield - 6 slices

Ingredients

1 9-inch deep dish pie crust, unbaked
6 tablespoons (1½ ounces) shredded mozzarella cheese
3 cups broccoli, finely chopped
8 ounces cooked turkey ham, finely diced
6 eggs
2 tablespoons whole wheat flour

Directions

1. Preheat oven to 375 degrees.
2. Pierce the bottom and sides of the pie crust several times with a fork, then bake until very lightly golden, about 8 minutes. Set aside to cool.
3. Distribute broccoli, turkey ham and cheese evenly in the baked crust.
4. Whisk eggs and flour together and pour over quiche filling.
5. Place the quiche in the oven on top of a baking sheet. Bake until brown and firm, 32-35 minutes. Quiche is done when a toothpick inserted into the center comes out clean.
6. Remove from oven and cool slightly before serving. Cut into 6 slices.

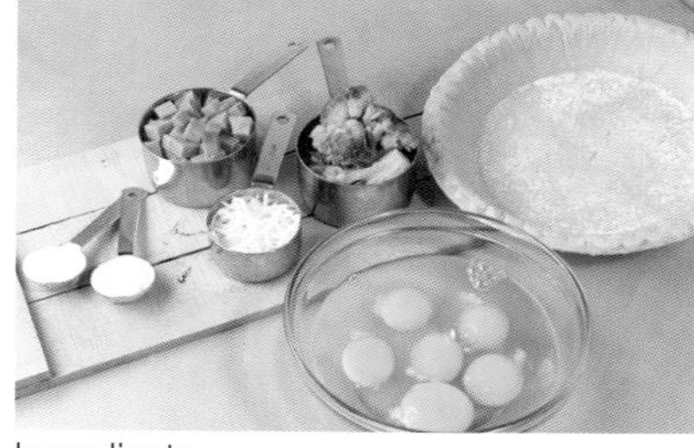
Ingredients

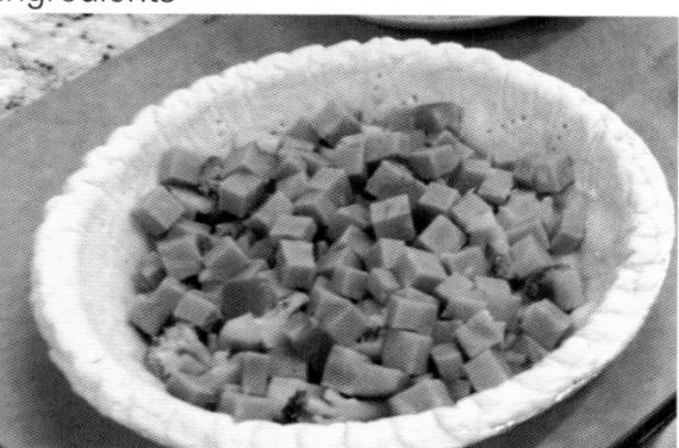
Step 3

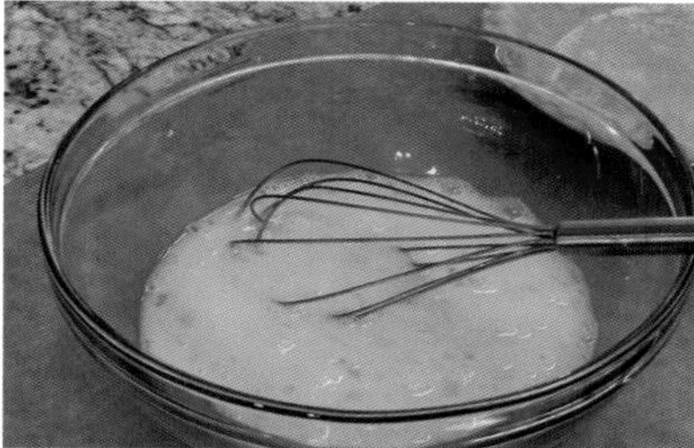
Step 4

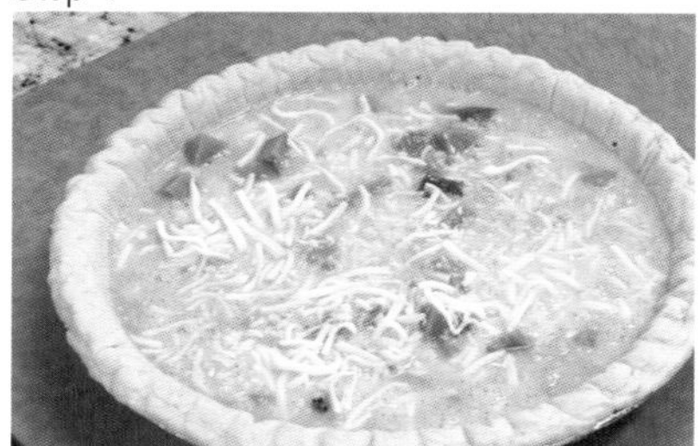
Step 4

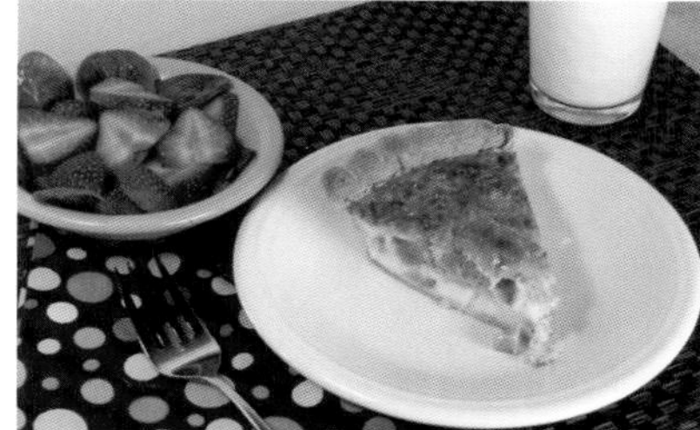
Creditable lunch/supper

Quiche
provides G/B, M/MA and VEG at lunch/supper

	Toddler	Pre-School	School Age
Quiche	1/2 slice	1/2 slice	1 slice
Spinach	1/8 cup	1/4 cup	1/2 cup
Strawberry	1/8 cup	1/4 cup	1/4 cup
Milk	1/2 cup	3/4 cup	1 cup

Quiche Cups

Prep time - 20 minutes
Cook time - 15 minutes
Total time - 35 minutes

Bake in oven

Yield - 12 quiche cups

Ingredients

6 eggs
2 tablespoons whole wheat flour
¾ cup (3 ounces) shredded mozzarella cheese
2 cups broccoli, finely chopped
1 cup turkey ham, diced small

Directions

1. Preheat oven to 375 degrees. Lightly grease a 12-cup muffin pan or coat with cooking spray.
2. In a bowl, thoroughly whisk together the eggs and flour.
3. Place portioned broccoli and ham into the muffin cups. Top each with 1 tablespoon mozzarella cheese.
4. Fill each muffin cup to about ⅔ full with eggs.
5. Bake until brown and firm, about 15-18 minutes. Quiche cups are done when a toothpick inserted into the center comes out clean.
6. Allow quiche cups to cool for 10 minutes in pan.
7. Using a dinner knife, gently run the blade around perimeter of each quiche cup to loosen and remove.

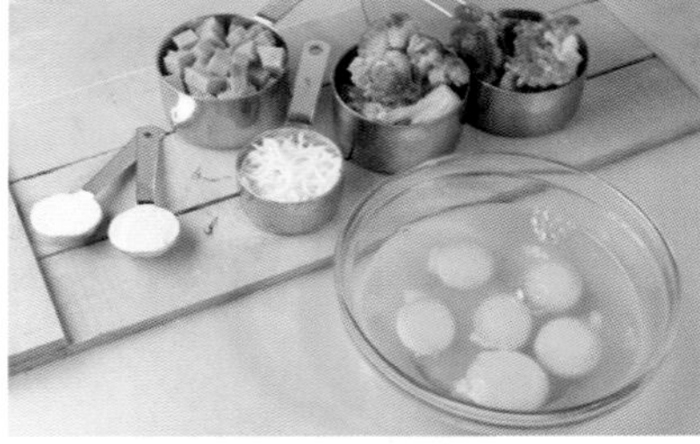
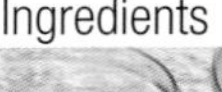

Ingredients

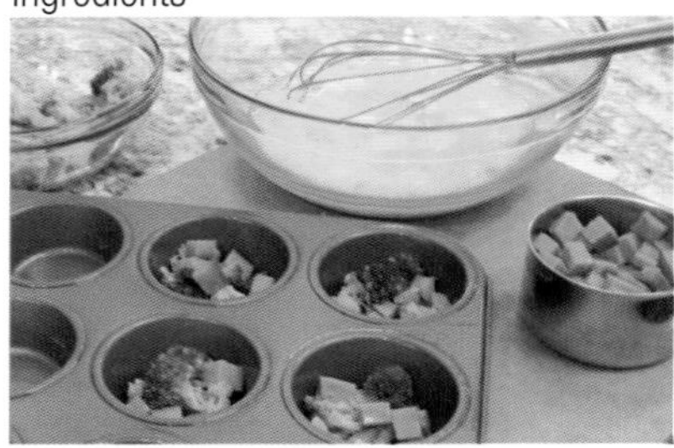

Step 2

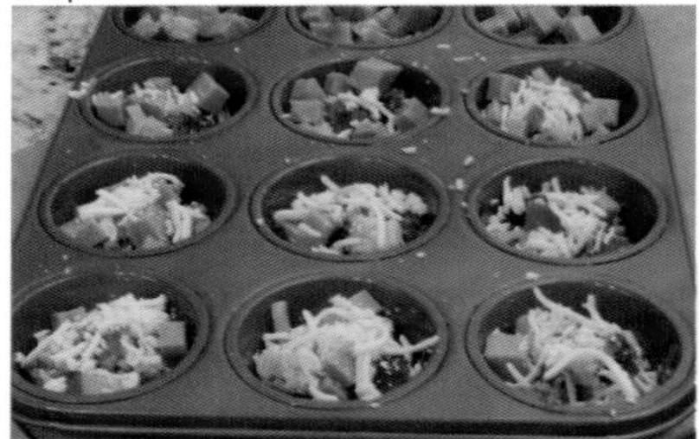

Step 3

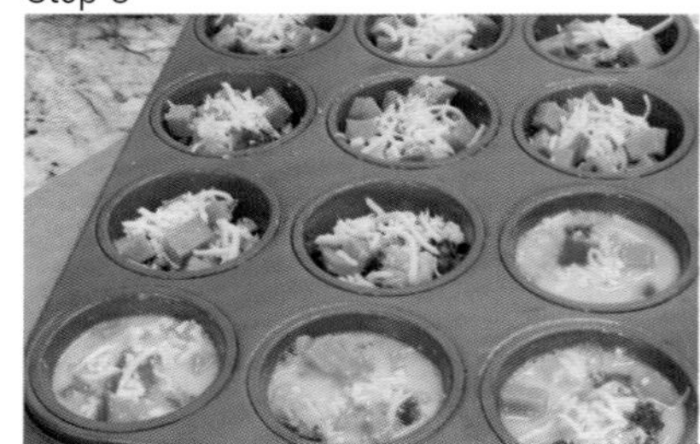

Step 4

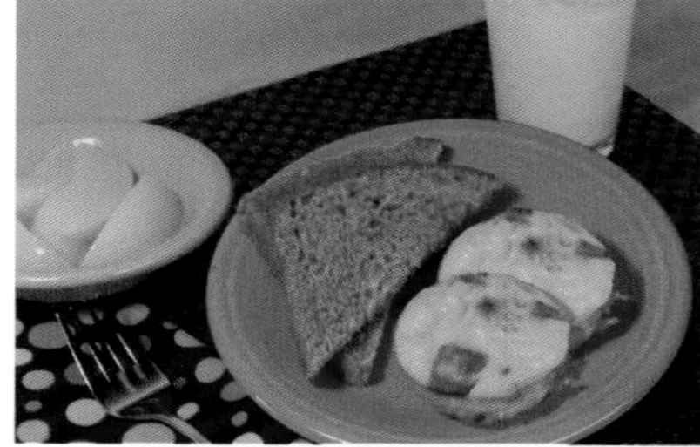

Creditable lunch/supper

Quiche Cups provide M/MA at lunch/supper			
	Toddler	Pre-School	School Age
Quiche Cups	1 quiche cup	1 quiche cup	2 quiche cups
Whole Wheat Bread	1/2 oz. or 1/2 slice	1/2 oz. or 1/2 slice	1 oz. or 1 slice
Broccoli	1/8 cup	1/4 cup	1/2 cup
Peaches	1/8 cup	1/4 cup	1/4 cup
Milk	1/2 cup	3/4 cup	1 cup

Roast Turkey Breast with Cranberry Sauce

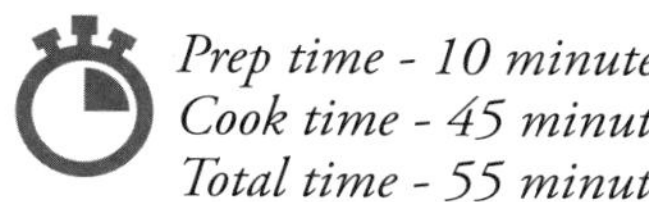

Prep time - 10 minutes
Cook time - 45 minutes
Total time - 55 minutes

Bake in oven

Yield - 9 ounces

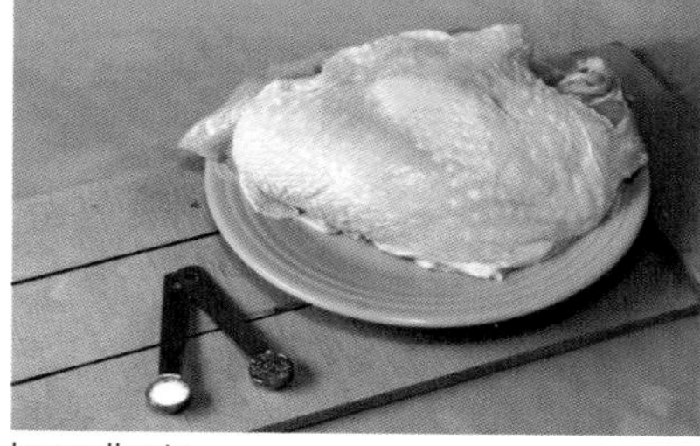

Ingredients

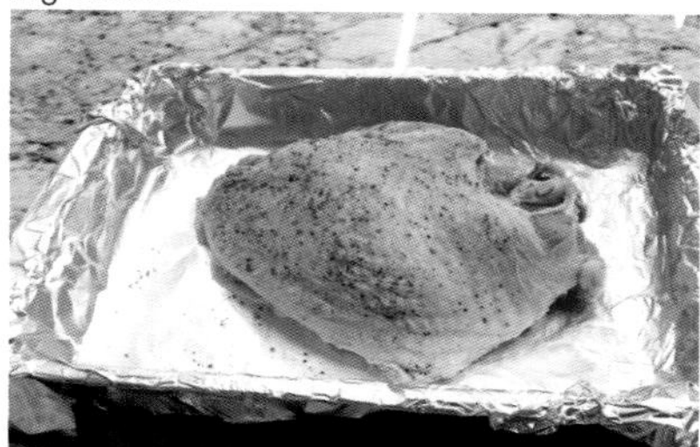

Step 1

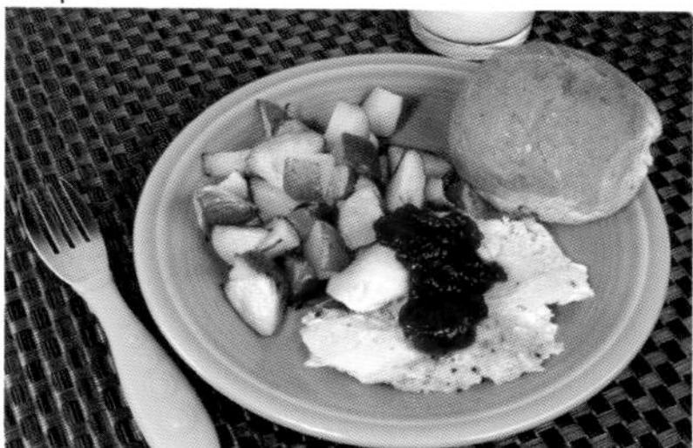

Creditable lunch/supper

Ingredients

1 pound turkey breast
¼ teaspoon kosher salt
¼ teaspoon black pepper

Ingredients for cranberry sauce

1 cup whole cranberry sauce

Directions

1. Preheat oven to 350 degrees. Line a baking pan with foil or coat with cooking spray.
2. Rub the turkey breast with the salt and pepper and place in baking pan.
3. Roast until lightly golden and firm to the touch, with an internal temperature of 165 degrees, about 45-50 minutes.
4. Just before serving, warm the cranberry sauce in a small saucepan; thin with water if desired.

Roast Turkey Breast provides M/MA at lunch/supper			
	Toddler	Pre-School	School Age
Turkey Breast	1 ounce	1-1/2 ounces	2 ounces
Cranberry Sauce	2 tablespoons	2 tablespoons	2 tablespoons
Whole Wheat Roll	1/2 ounce	1/2 ounce	1 ounce
Potatoes	1/8 cup	1/4 cup	1/2 cup
Pears	1/8 cup	1/4 cup	1/4 cup
Milk	1/2 cup	3/4 cup	1 cup

Stuffed Zucchini Boats

Prep time - 25 minutes
Cook time - 55 minutes
Total time - 80 minutes

Bake in oven

Yield - 6 zucchini boats

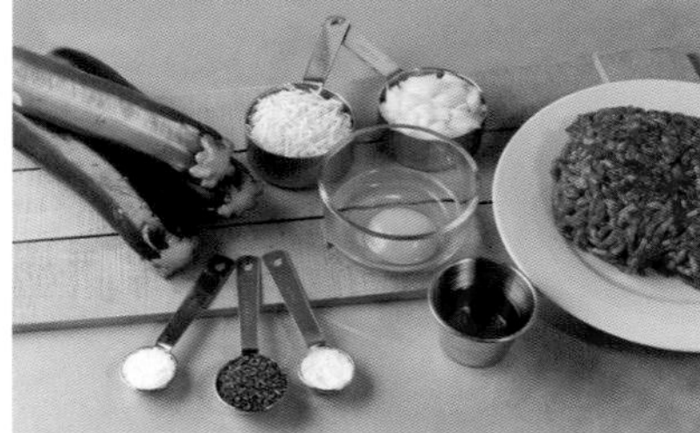
Ingredients

Ingredients

3 medium zucchini (about 1 pound)
2 tablespoons vegetable oil
1¼ pounds ground beef, at least 80% lean
½ cup onions, chopped
1 tablespoon dried basil or parsley
½ cup grated Parmesan cheese
1 egg, beaten
2 teaspoons salt

Directions

1. Preheat oven to 375 degrees. Line a baking sheet with foil or parchment paper, or coat with cooking spray.
2. Slice zucchini in half lengthwise. Scoop out the pulp of each zucchini with a small spoon (or ice cream scoop); avoid breaking the skin. Chop and reserve the pulp.
3. Heat oil in a large sauté pan over medium heat. Sauté ground beef and onions until cooked through, stirring frequently, about 10 minutes. Drain fat. Reduce heat to medium-low. Add the chopped zucchini pulp with the basil or parsley and cook an additional 5 minutes. Remove from heat and cool slightly.
4. Thoroughly combine zucchini mixture with the cheese, egg, salt and pepper. Stuff the zucchini boats with the filling and place in the baking sheet.
5. After placing pan in oven, pour water into the pan to a depth of about ¼ inch. Bake until golden brown, about 40 minutes.

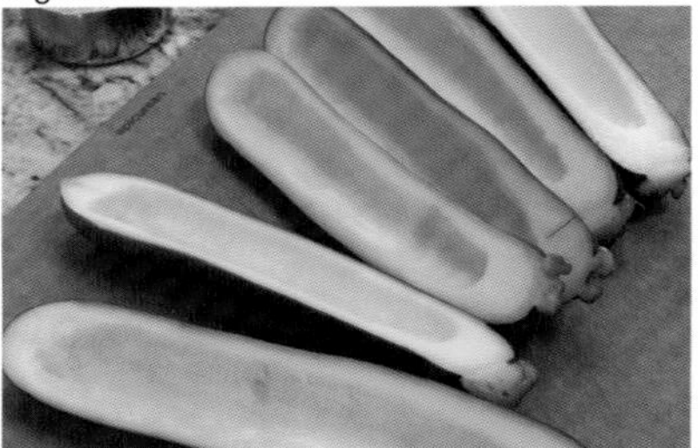
Step 2

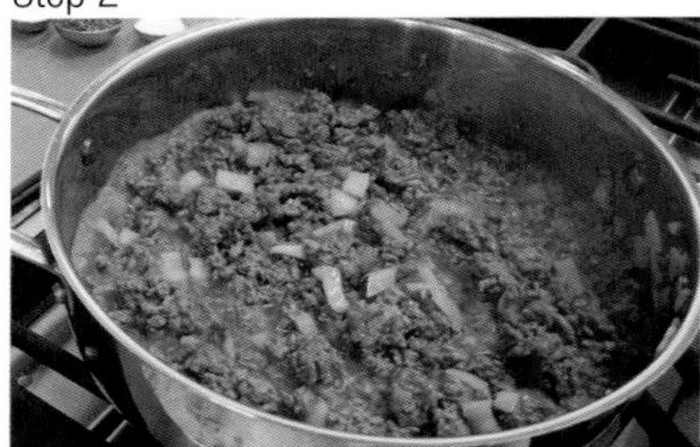
Step 3

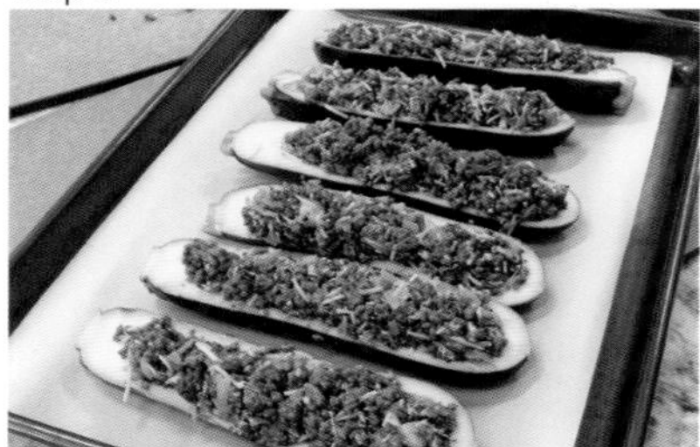
Step 4

Stuffed Zucchini Boats provide M/MA and VEG at lunch/supper			
	Toddler	Pre-School	School Age
Stuffed Zucchini	1 boat	1 boat	1-1/2 boats
Whole Grain Roll	1/2 ounce	1/2 ounce	1 ounce
Oranges	1/8 cup	1/4 cup	1/4 cup
Milk	1/2 cup	3/4 cup	1 cup

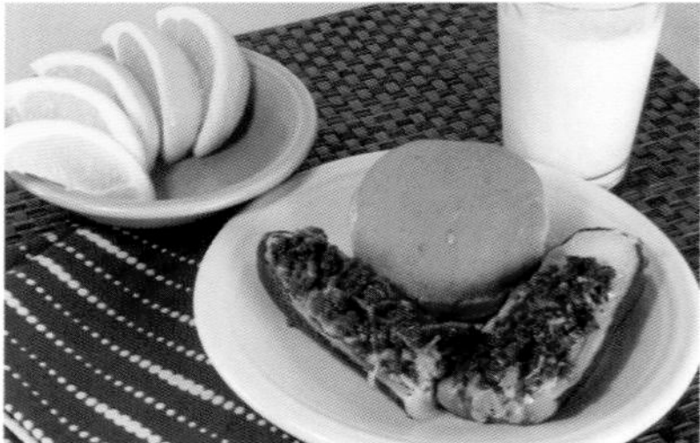
Creditable lunch/supper

Sweet and Spicy Glazed Ham

Prep time - 15 minutes
Cook time - 45 minutes
Total time - 60 minutes

Bake in oven

Yield - 11 ounces

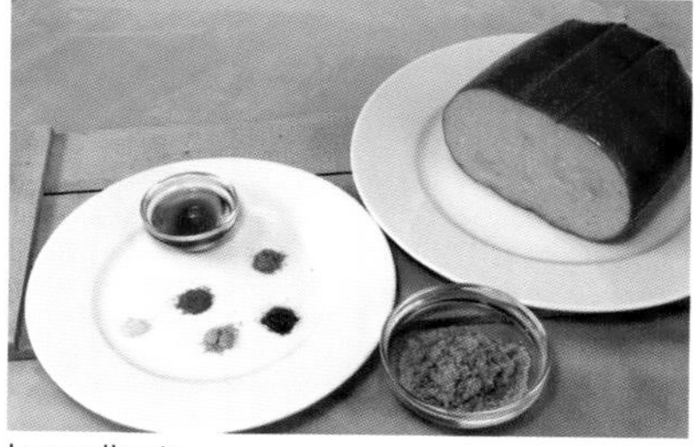
Ingredients

Ingredients

1 pound turkey ham
3 tablespoons brown sugar
2 tablespoons oil
⅛ teaspoon ground mustard
⅛ teaspoon ground cinnamon
⅛ teaspoon ground ginger
⅛ teaspoon ground cloves
⅛ teaspoon ground nutmeg

Directions

1. Heat oven to 325 degrees. Line a baking pan with foil or parchment paper, or coat with cooking spray.
2. Place turkey ham in pan, cut side down. Bake, uncovered, until ham is heated through, with an internal temperature of 140 degrees, about 45 minutes.
3. To make basting sauce, mix the oil, sugar and spices in a small bowl. Brush sauce over ham twice during the last 20 minutes of baking.
4. Remove from oven and slice for serving.

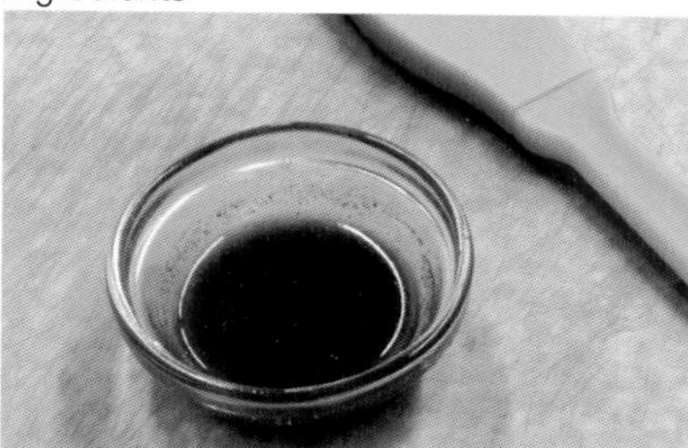
Step 4

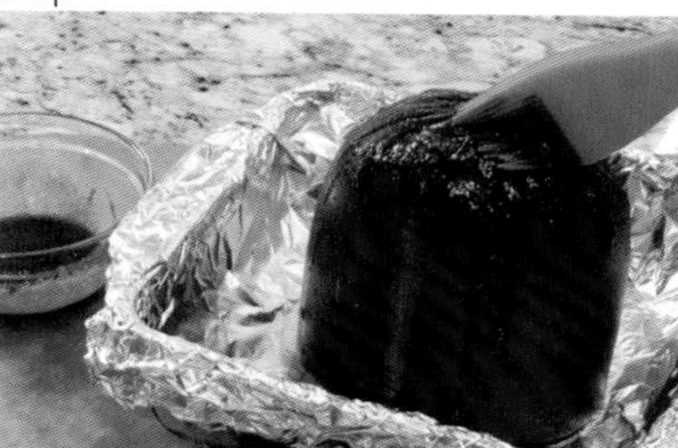
Step 4

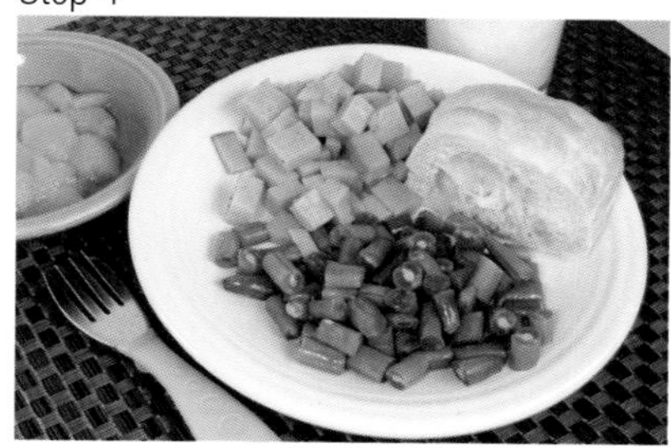
Creditable lunch/supper

Sweet and Spicy Glazed Ham
provides M/MA at lunch/supper

	Toddler	Pre-School	School Age
Glazed Ham	1 ounce	1-1/2 ounces	2 ounces
Whole Grain Roll	1/2 ounce	1/2 ounce	1 ounce
Green Beans	1/8 cup	1/4 cup	1/2 cup
Apricots	1/8 cup	1/4 cup	1/4 cup
Milk	1/2 cup	3/4 cup	1 cup

Tuna Casserole

Prep time - 20 minutes
Cook time - 35 minutes
Total time - 55 minutes

Cook on stovetop and in oven

Yield - 6 cups

Ingredients

3 ounces (2¼ cups) dry whole grain egg noodles
Water for boiling pasta
1 10¾-ounce can condensed cream of mushroom soup
10 ounces water-packed tuna, drained
1½ cups frozen green peas
½ cup onions, chopped
1 cup (4 ounces) shredded cheddar cheese, divided

Directions

1. Preheat oven to 350 degrees. Grease an 11x7-inch baking dish or coat with cooking spray.
2. Cook noodles according to package directions, about 10 minutes; drain.
3. In a large bowl, mix together the cooked noodles, mushroom soup, tuna, peas, onions, and ½ cup of the cheese. Mix well and pour into baking dish.
4. Sprinkle remaining cheese on top of casserole
5. Bake, uncovered, until lightly golden and heated through, about 25 minutes.

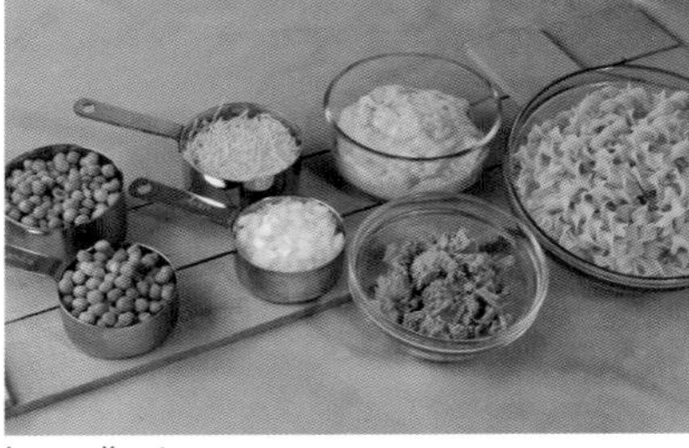

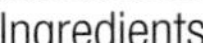

Ingredients

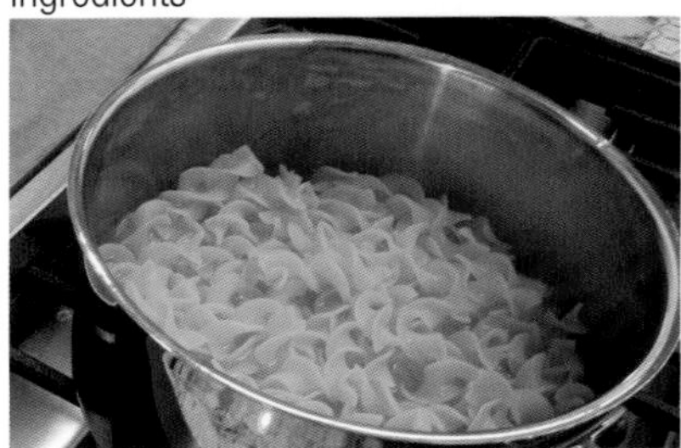

Step 2

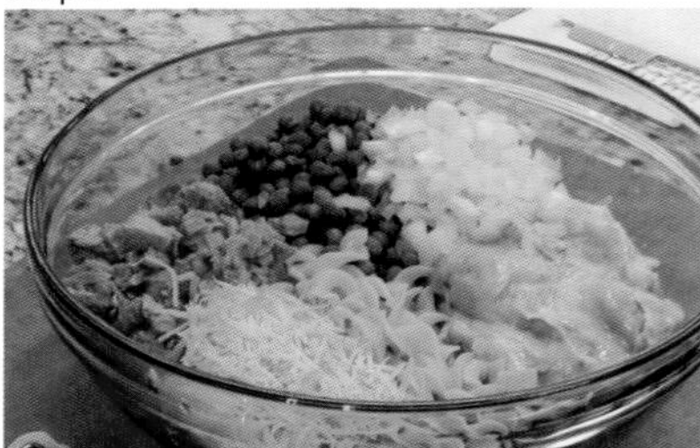

Step 3

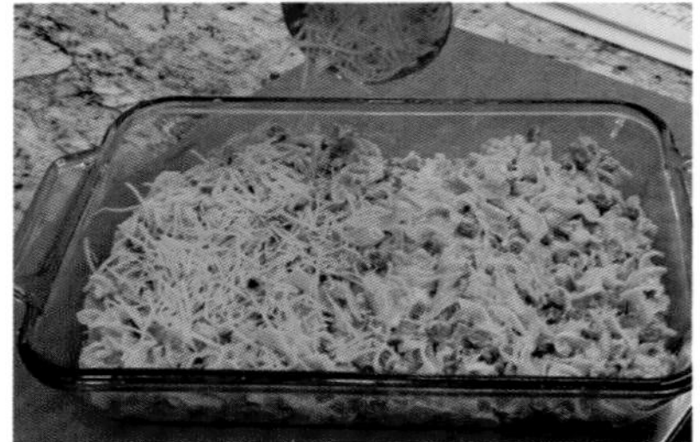

Step 4

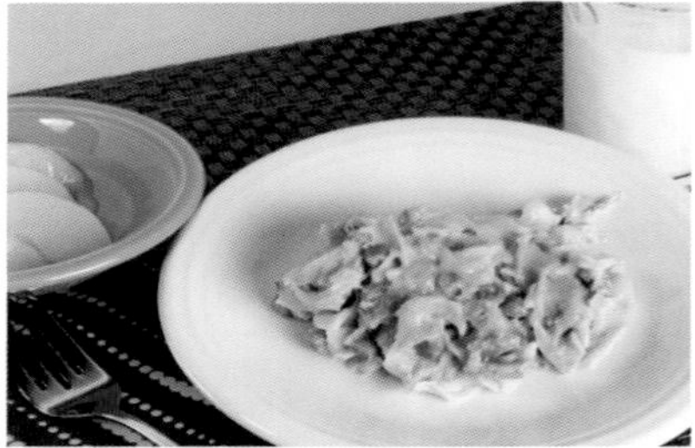

Creditable lunch/supper

Tuna Casserole provides G/B, M/MA and VEG at lunch/supper			
	Toddler	Pre-School	School Age
Tuna Casserole	2/3 cup	1 cup	1-1/3 cups
Peaches	1/8 cup	1/4 cup	1/4 cup
Milk	1/2 cup	3/4 cup	1 cup

Veggie Lasagna

Prep time - 25 minutes
Cook time - 40 minutes
Total time - 65 minutes

Cook on stovetop and in oven

Yield - 12 cups

Ingredients

7 ounces (9 noodles) whole grain lasagna noodles
Water for boiling
3 cups frozen mixed vegetables
3 cups marinara sauce
2 cups ricotta cheese
½ cup grated Parmesan cheese
1 egg
1 teaspoon black pepper
½ teaspoon salt
2 cups (8 ounces) shredded mozzarella cheese

Directions

1. Preheat oven to 350 degrees. Grease a 9x13-inch pan.
2. To cook noodles, bring a large pot of water to a rolling boil. Cook until almost tender, about 12 minutes, then drain.
3. Meanwhile, in a large skillet over medium-high heat, cook the frozen vegetables until warmed through. Add the marinara sauce and simmer over low heat, about 8 minutes.
4. In a bowl, stir together the ricotta, Parmesan, egg, black pepper and salt; set aside.
5. To assemble, lay three cooked noodles in the pan and spread evenly with one-third of the cheese mixture, marinara sauce and mozzarella. Make 2 more layers with remaining ingredients.
6. Bake for 30 minutes. Then increase oven temperature to 375 degrees and bake another 10 minutes.
7. When done, remove from oven and cool for 10 minutes before cutting and serving. Cut into 12 portions.

Veggie Lasagna
provides G/B, M/MA and VEG at lunch/supper

	Toddler	Pre-School	School Age
Veggie Lasagna	2/3 cup	1 cup	1-1/3 cups
Mixed Fruit	1/8 cup	1/4 cup	1/4 cup
Milk	1/2 cup	3/4 cup	1 cup

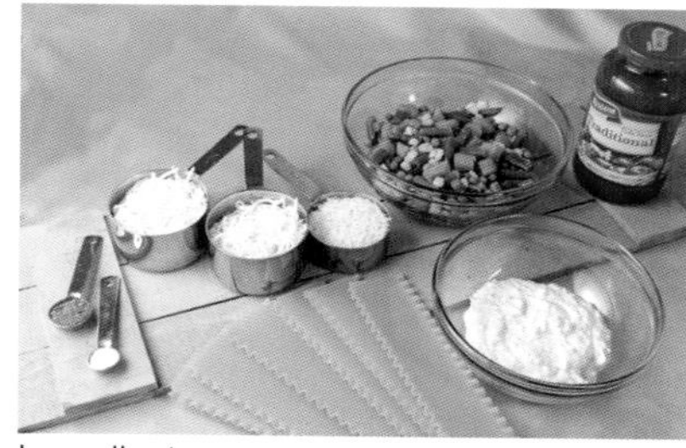

Ingredients

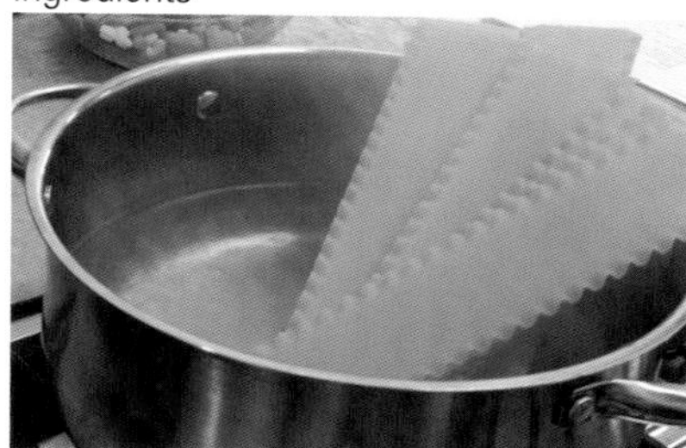

Step 2

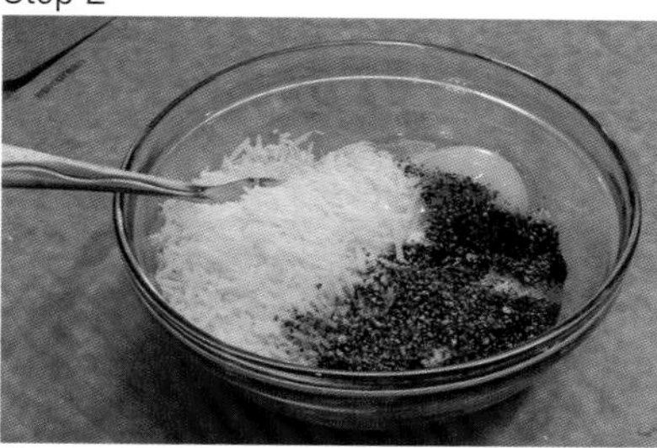

Step 4

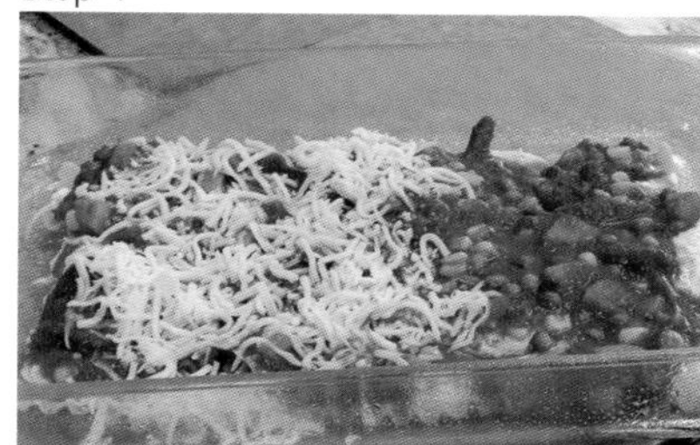

Step 5

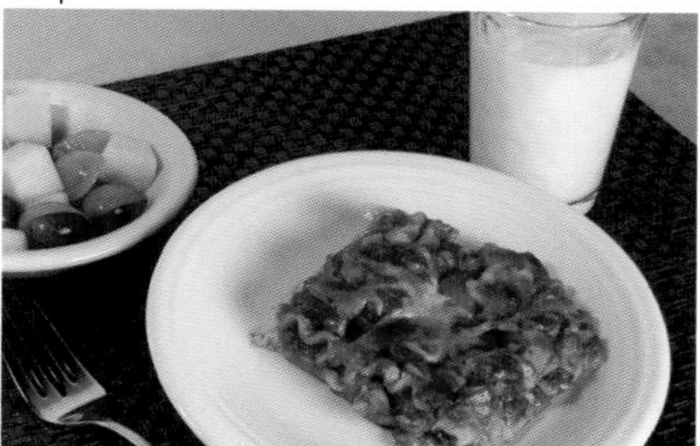

Creditable lunch/supper

Asian Beef Stir-Fry

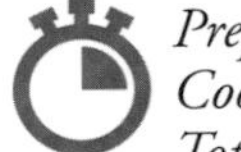

Prep time - 15 minutes
Cook time - 20 minutes
Total time - 35 minutes

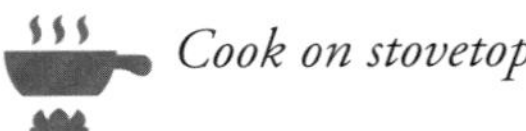

Cook on stovetop

Yield - 4 cups

Ingredients

1½ cups cooked Savory Brown Rice
¼ cup soy sauce
1 tablespoon cornstarch
2 tablespoons vegetable oil
1 pound ground beef, at least 80% lean
½ teaspoon garlic powder
2 cups green pepper, diced
1½ cups onions, diced

Directions

1. Prepare Savory Brown Rice; recipe is on next page.
2. In a bowl, combine soy sauce and cornstarch; set aside.
3. Heat large skillet over medium heat; add oil and beef. Cook until browned, stirring frequently, about 10 minutes.
4. Add garlic powder and mix well. Add onions and peppers and cook until peppers are tender-crisp, stirring occasionally, about 5 minutes.
5. Add soy sauce mixture to pan; bring to a boil, then reduce heat and simmer until sauce thickens, about 5 minutes.
6. Serve over Savory Brown Rice.

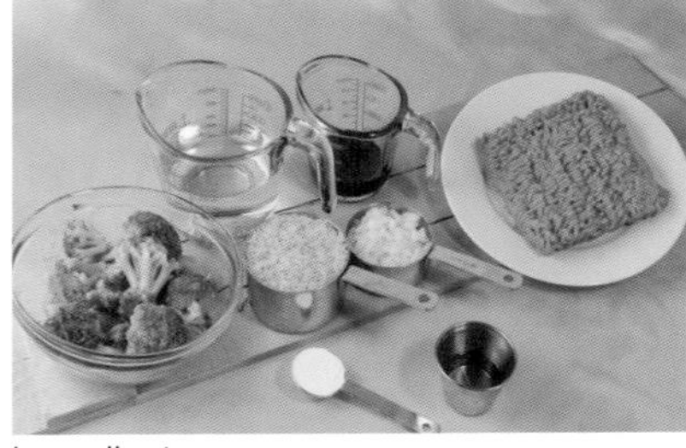

Ingredients

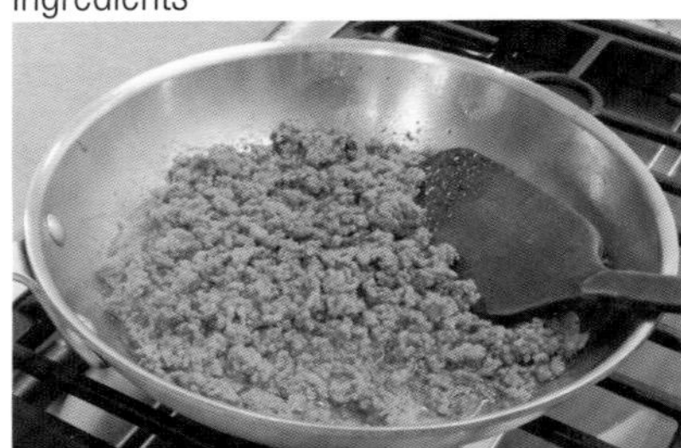

Step 3

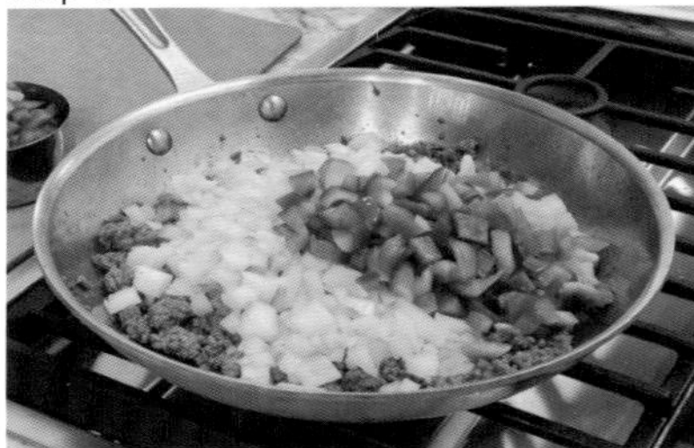

Step 4

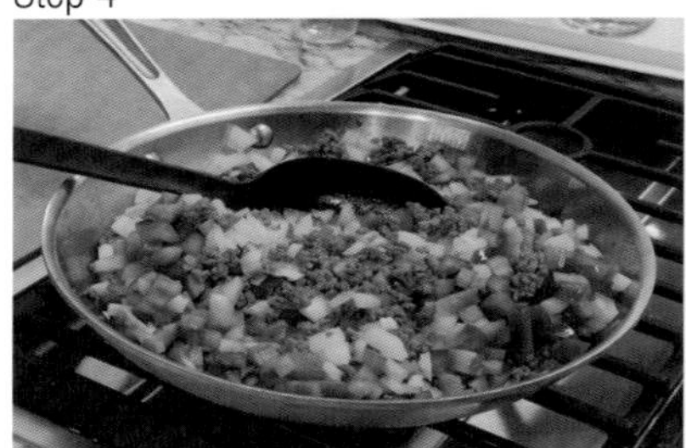

Step 5

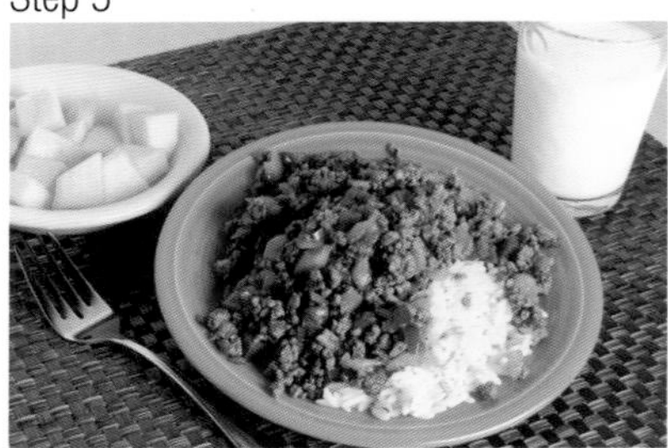

Creditable lunch/supper

Asian Beef Stir-Fry provides G/B, M/MA and VEG at lunch/supper			
	Toddler	Pre-School	School Age
Beef Stir-Fry	1/2 cup	2/3 cup	1-1/4 cups
Savory Brown Rice	1/4 cup	1/4 cup	1/2 cup
Melon	1/8 cup	1/4 cup	1/4 cup
Milk	1/2 cup	3/4 cup	1 cup

Savory Brown Rice

Prep time - 5 minutes
Cook time - 35 minutes
Resting time - 5 minutes
Total time - 45 minutes

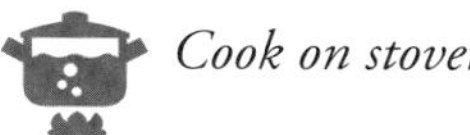
Cook on stovetop

Yield - 1¾ cups

Ingredients

1 cup long-grain brown rice
2 cups water or vegetable/chicken broth
½ teaspoon salt, optional

Directions

1. Rinse rice in water and drain.
2. In medium sauce pan over high heat, add brown rice, salt and water/broth and bring to a boil. Cover and reduce heat to low.
3. Simmer until all the water has been absorbed, rice is tender, and there are "eyes" –small holes covering the surface–about 35-40 minutes.
4. Remove from heat, cover and let stand 5 minutes before serving.

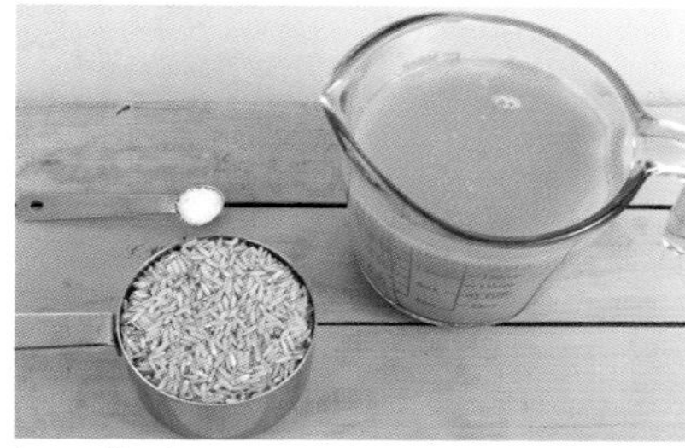
Ingredients

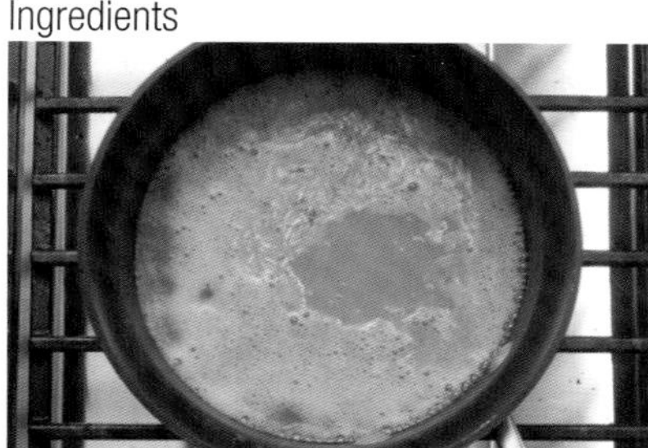
Step 2

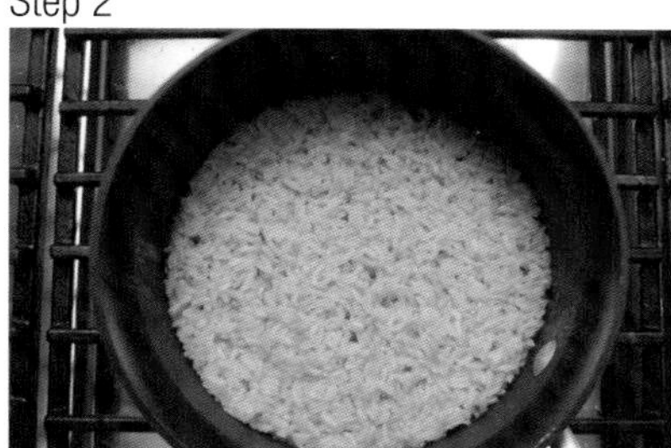
Step 3

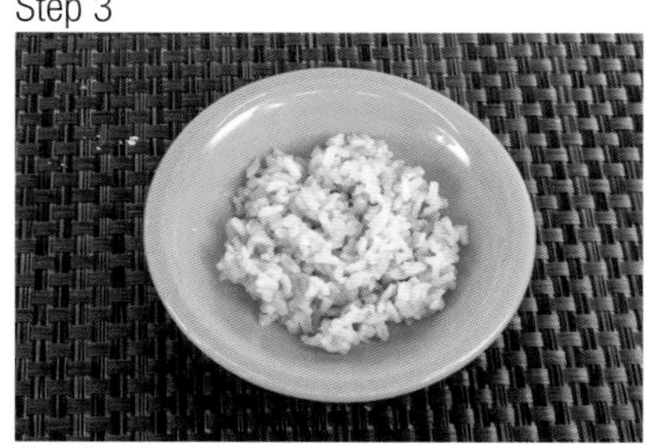
Creditable side

Savory Brown Rice provides G/B at lunch/supper			
	Toddler	Pre-School	School Age
Savory Brown Rice	1/4 cup	1/4 cup	1/2 cup

Beef Burritos

Prep time - 20 minutes
Cook time - 10 minutes
Total time - 30 minutes

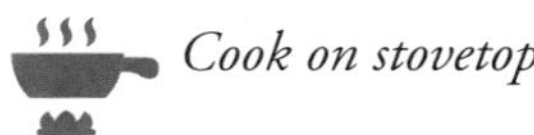

Cook on stovetop

Yield - 3 burritos

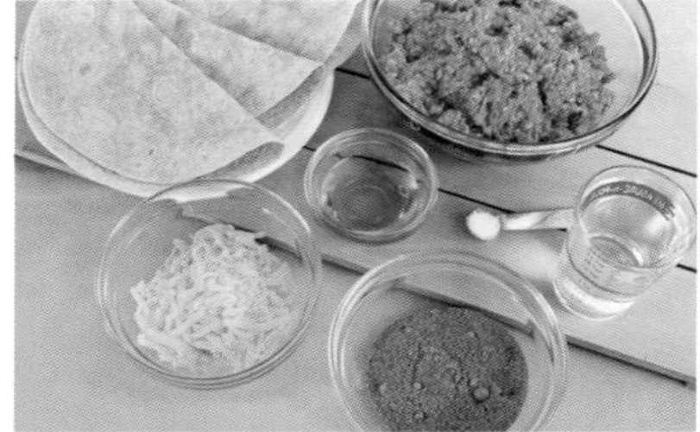
Ingredients

Ingredients

2 tablespoons vegetable oil
1 pound ground beef, at least 80% lean
2 tablespoons taco seasoning (1 packet)
½ cup water
½ cup (2 ounces) shredded cheddar cheese
3 8-inch whole wheat tortillas

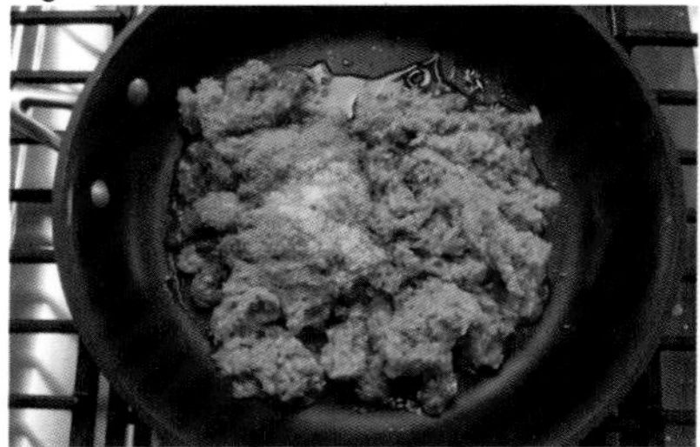
Step 1

Directions

1. Heat a large skillet over medium heat, then add oil, beef, taco seasoning, salt and water. Mix well.
2. Stirring frequently, cook until beef is cooked, with an internal temperature of 160 degrees, about 10 minutes.
3. Lay tortillas on work surface. Place one third of the seasoned beef down the center of each tortilla and top with 2 tablespoons of cheese. Roll up and cut in half to serve.

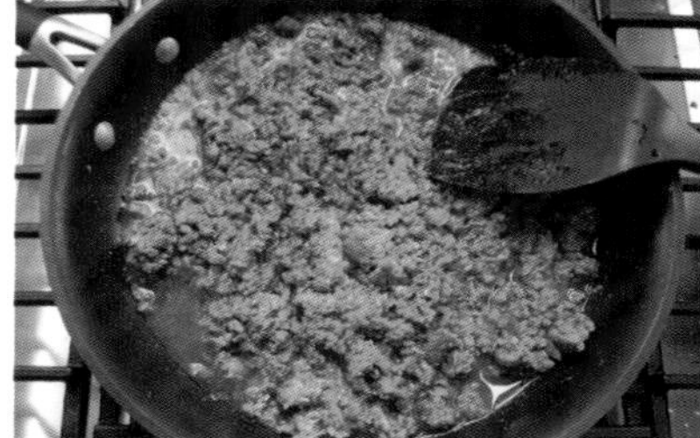
Step 2

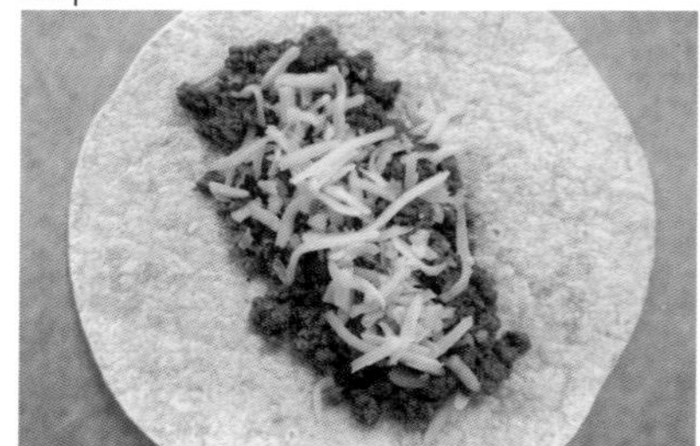
Step 3

Beef Burritos provide G/B and M/MA at lunch/supper			
	Toddler	Pre-School	School Age
Beef Burritos	1/2 burrito	1/2 burrito	1 burrito
Lettuce	1/8 cup	1/4 cup	1/2 cup
Grapes	1/8 cup	1/4 cup	1/4 cup
Milk	1/2 cup	3/4 cup	1 cup

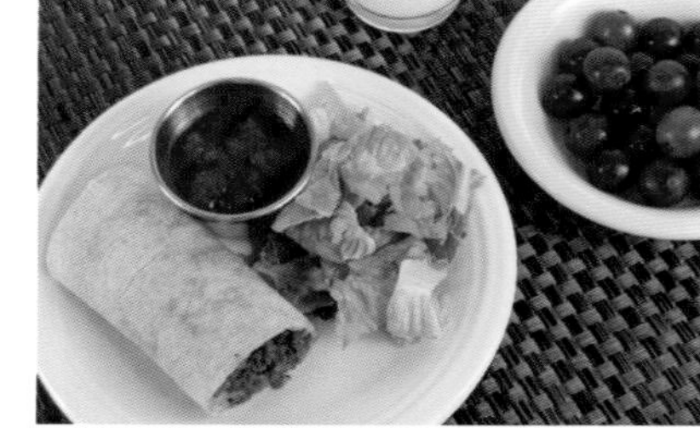
Creditable lunch/supper

Black Bean Burritos

Prep time - 20 minutes
Cook time - 40 minutes
Total time - 60 minutes

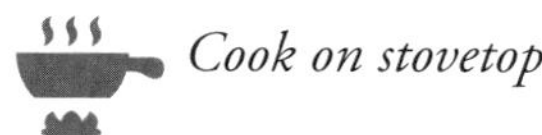

Cook on stovetop

Yield - 3 burritos

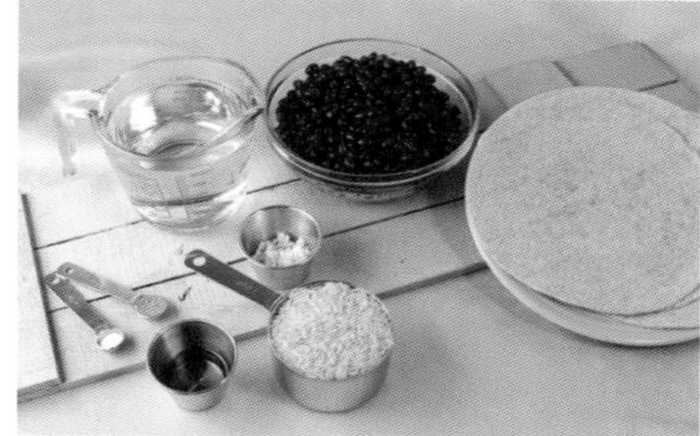

Ingredients

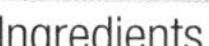

Ingredients

1 cup long-grain brown rice
2 cups water for cooking rice
2 tablespoons vegetable oil
2 teaspoons garlic, minced
½ teaspoon ground cumin
⅛ teaspoon salt
2¼ cups black beans, rinsed and drained
⅓ cup water
3 8-inch whole wheat tortillas

Directions

1. Cook rice according to package directions, about 35 minutes.
2. While rice is cooking, in large skillet over medium heat, combine oil, cumin, salt, garlic and beans.
3. Add ⅓ cup of water and simmer for 20 minutes; remove from heat.
4. Add cooked rice to skillet and mix well. Return to stovetop and cook until warmed through, stirring occasionally, about 5 minutes.
5. Lay tortillas on a work surface. Place 1¼ cups of beans and rice down the center of each burrito and roll up.

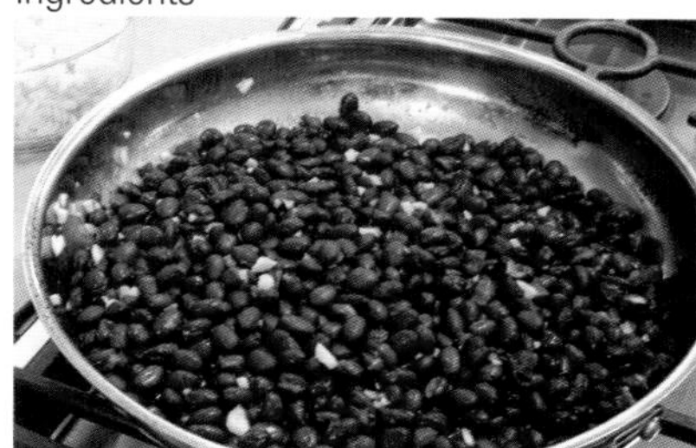

Step 2

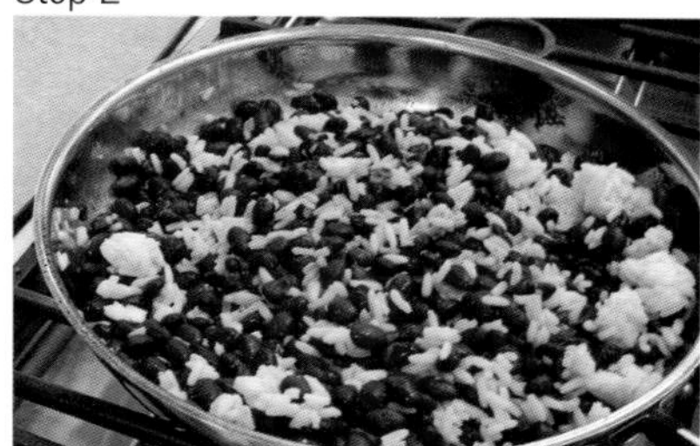

Step 5

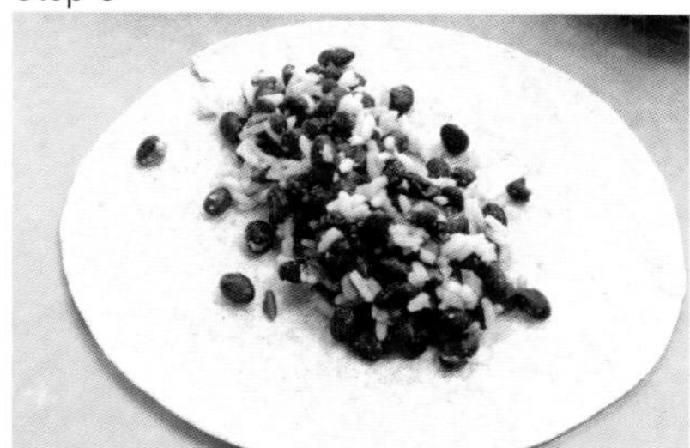

Step 6

Black Bean Burritos provide G/B and M/MA at lunch/supper			
	Toddler	Pre-School	School Age
Black Bean Burrito	1/2 burrito	1/2 burrito	1 burrito
Green Peppers	1/8 cup	1/4 cup	1/2 cup
Melon	1/8 cup	1/4 cup	1/4 cup
Milk	1/2 cup	3/4 cup	1 cup

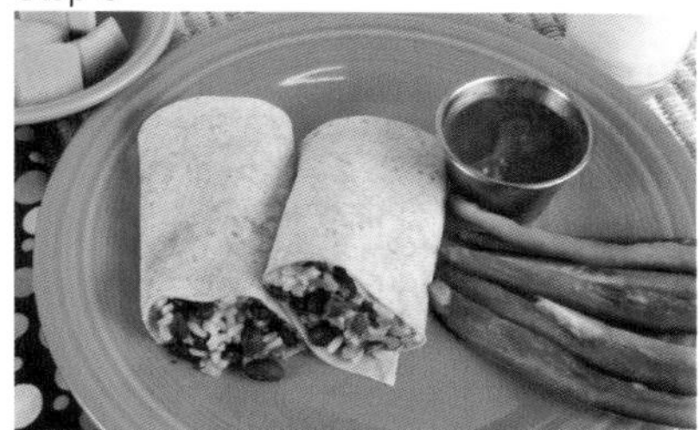

Creditable lunch/supper

Cheese Enchiladas

Prep time - 20 minutes
Cook time - 35 minutes
Total time - 55 minutes

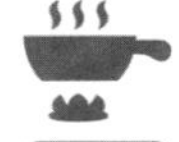

Cook on stovetop and in oven

Yield - 6 enchiladas

Ingredients

2 tablespoons vegetable oil
½ cup onions, diced
½ teaspoon garlic powder
2 teaspoons taco seasoning
1 15-ounce can tomato sauce
2½ cups (10 ounces) grated cheddar cheese, reserve ¼ cup
6 6-inch whole grain corn tortillas

Directions

1. Preheat oven to 350 degrees. Grease an 8x8-inch baking dish, or coat with cooking spray.
2. Heat oil in sauce pan over medium heat. Add onions, garlic powder and taco seasoning. Stirring frequently, cook until onions are tender, about 5 minutes.
3. Add tomato sauce. Cover and simmer 5 minutes.
4. Warm tortillas in oven or microwave to make pliable.
5. Lay tortillas on work surface and place ⅜ cup cheese down the middle of each. Roll up tightly and place in the baking dish.
6. Cover the enchiladas with the sauce, then sprinkle with the reserved ¼ cup cheese.
7. Bake until cheese is melted and bubbly, about 25-30 minutes.

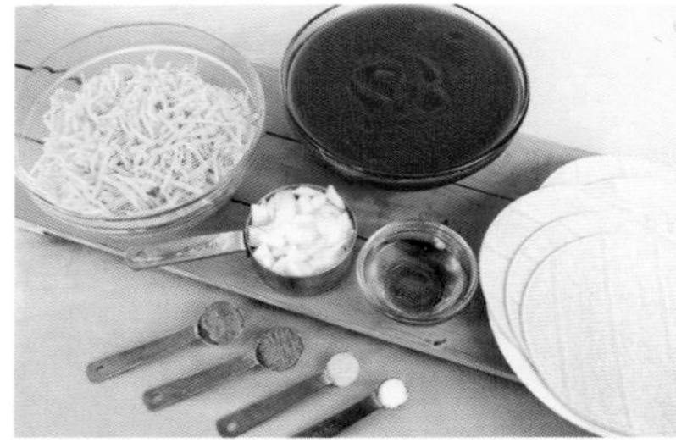

Ingredients

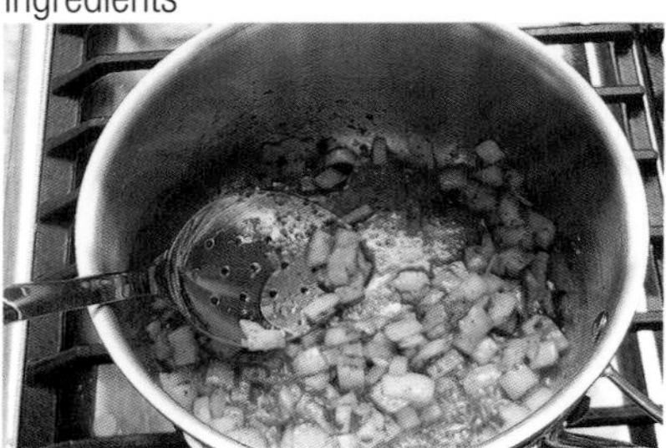

Step 2

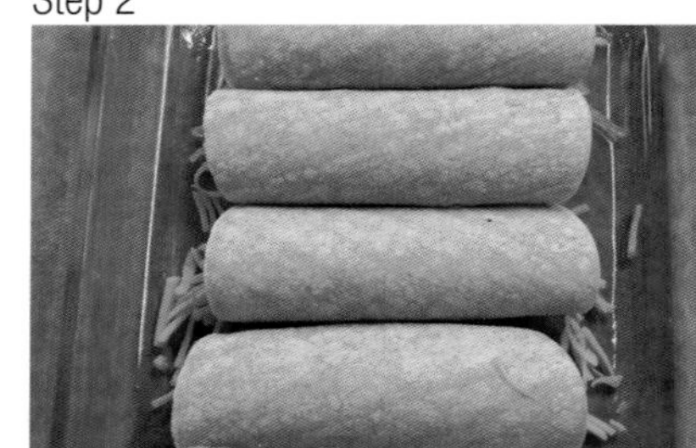

Step 5

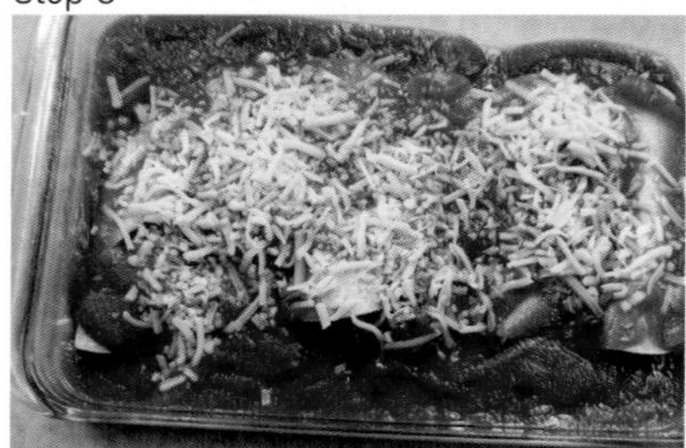

Step 6

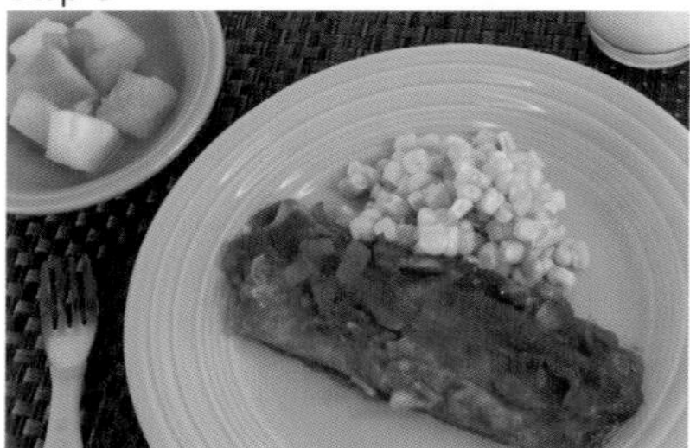

Creditable lunch/supper

Cheese Enchiladas provide G/B and M/MA at lunch/supper			
	Toddler	Pre-School	School Age
Cheese Enchiladas	1 enchilada	1 enchilada	1-1/2 enchilada
Corn	1/8 cup	1/4 cup	1/2 cup
Tropical Fruit	1/8 cup	1/4 cup	1/4 cup
Milk	1/2 cup	3/4 cup	1 cup

Chicken Chow Mein

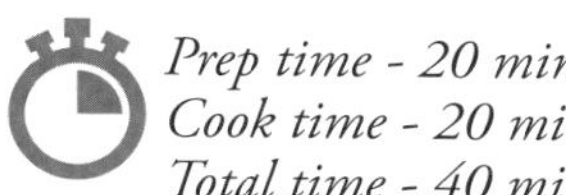

Prep time - 20 minutes
Cook time - 20 minutes
Total time - 40 minutes

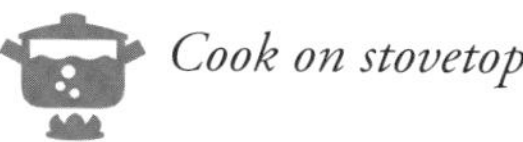

Cook on stovetop

Yield - 6 cups

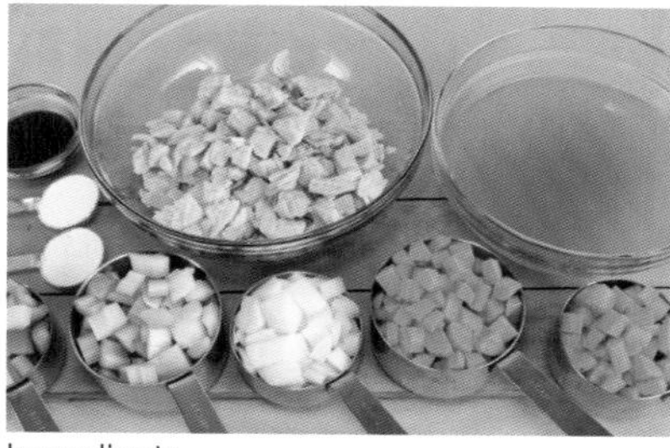

Ingredients

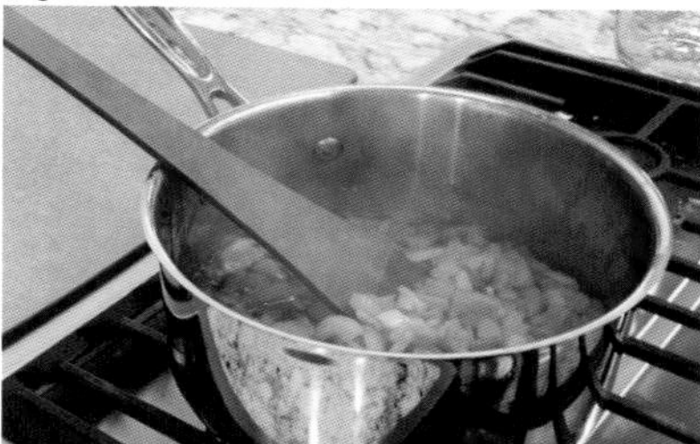

Step 1

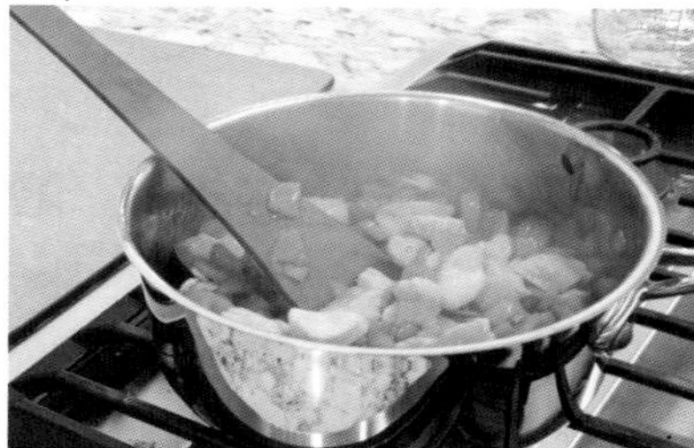

Step 3

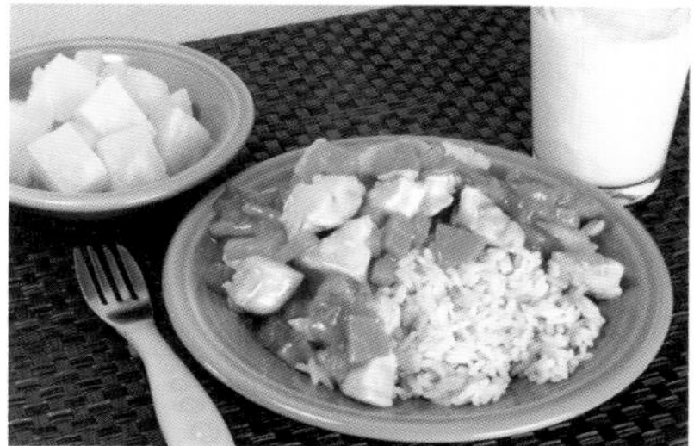

Creditable lunch/supper

Ingredients

2 cups cooked brown rice
4 teaspoons soy sauce
2 cups chicken broth, 3 tablespoons reserved
1½ cups celery, diced
1½ cups carrots, diced
½ cup onions, chopped, optional
2 tablespoons cornstarch
12 ounces cooked chicken, cubed

Directions

1. In a large saucepan over medium-high heat, combine the soy sauce and broth, except for the reserved broth.
2. Add celery, carrots and onions and cook until tender, about 10 minutes.
3. In a small bowl, combine cornstarch and reserved chicken broth; add to the vegetable mixture and cook, stirring constantly, until the liquid thickens, about 5 minutes.
4. Add chicken and mix well; cook until the chicken is heated through, about 5 minutes.
5. Serve over rice.

Chicken Chow Mein provides M/MA and VEG at lunch/supper			
	Toddler	Pre-School	School Age
Chicken Chow Mein	1/2 cup	3/4 cup	1 cup
Rice	1/4 cup	1/4 cup	1/2 cup
Pineapple	1/8 cup	1/4 cup	1/4 cup
Milk	1/2 cup	3/4 cup	1 cup

Chicken Fajitas

Prep time - 20 minutes
Marinate time - 30 minutes
Cook time - 20 minutes
Total time - 70 minutes

Cook on stovetop

Yield - 3 fajitas

Ingredients

2 tablespoons lime juice
3 tablespoons vegetable oil
¼ teaspoon garlic powder
½ teaspoon cumin
½ teaspoon chili powder
¼ teaspoon salt
1 pound boneless, skinless chicken breast, sliced in thin strips
1 cup onions, thinly sliced
2 cups green peppers, thinly sliced
3 8-inch whole wheat tortillas

Directions

1. Make the marinade by whisking together the lime juice, oil, garlic powder, cumin, chili powder and salt.
2. Place sliced chicken into a sturdy, resealable bag or a baking dish. Pour marinade over the chicken, seal the bag (or cover the dish) and marinate for 30-60 minutes in the refrigerator.
3. In a large skillet over medium heat, boil the chicken and marinade for 1 minute, then lower heat and cook until chicken reaches an internal temperature of 165 degrees, about 10 minutes. Remove from pan and set aside.
4. Add onions and peppers to the same skillet and cook until tender, about 5 minutes. Return chicken to pan, combine well with onions and peppers and heat through, about 5 minutes.
5. Lay tortillas on a work surface. Place one-third of the fajita filling down the center of each tortilla, then roll up.

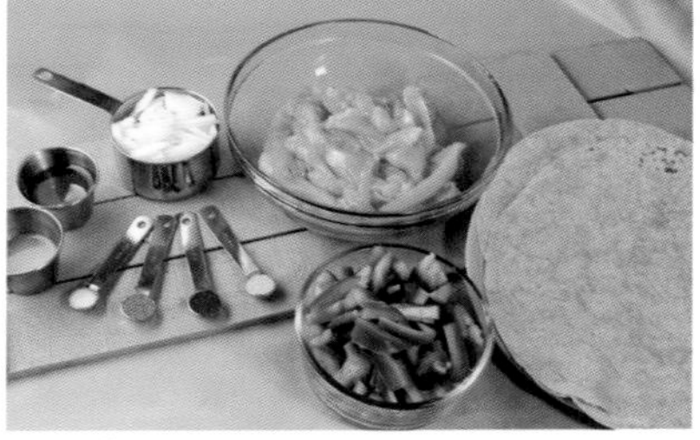

Ingredients

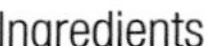

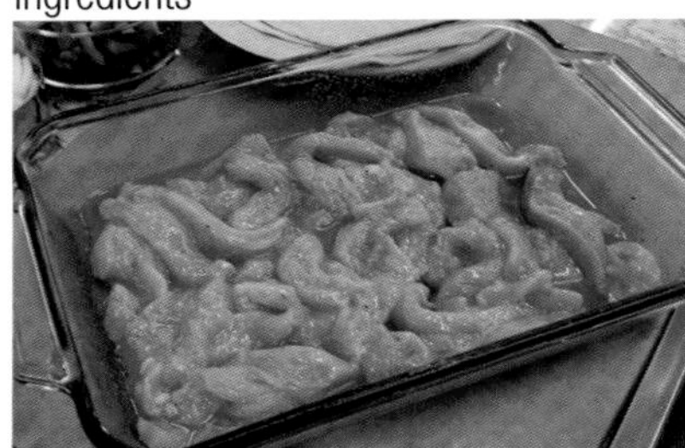

Step 2

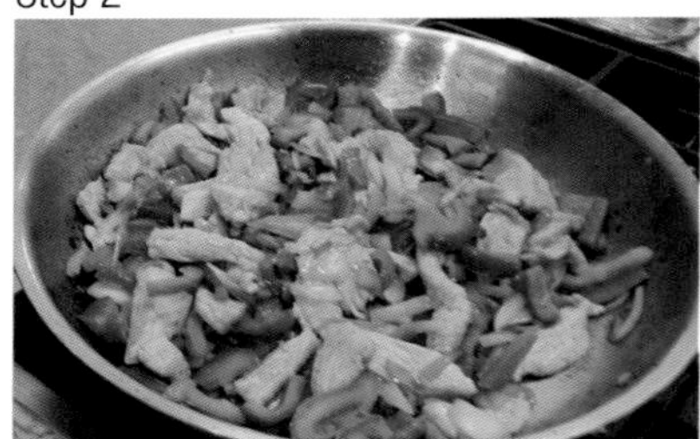

Step 4

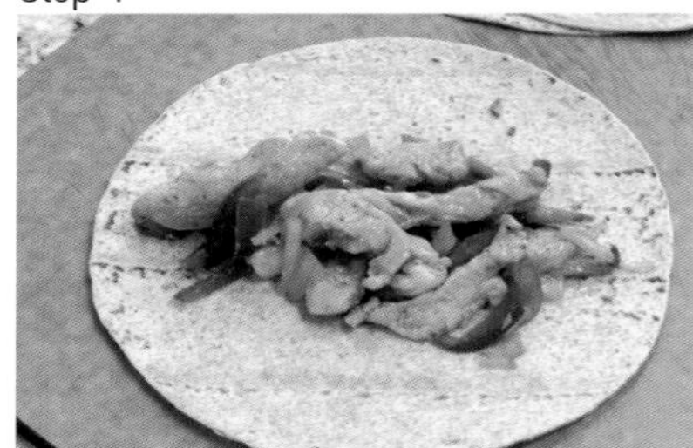

Step 5

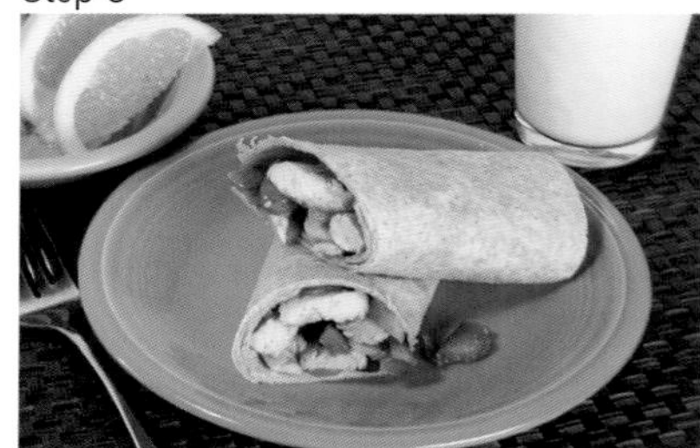

Creditable lunch/supper

Chicken Fajitas provides G/B, M/MA and VEG at lunch/supper			
	Toddler	Pre-School	School Age
Chicken Fajitas	1/2 fajita	1/2 fajita	1 fajita
Oranges	1/8 cup	1/4 cup	1/4 cup
Milk	1/2 cup	3/4 cup	1 cup

Chicken-Broccoli Quesadillas

Prep time - 20 minutes
Cook time -15 minutes
Total time - 35 minutes

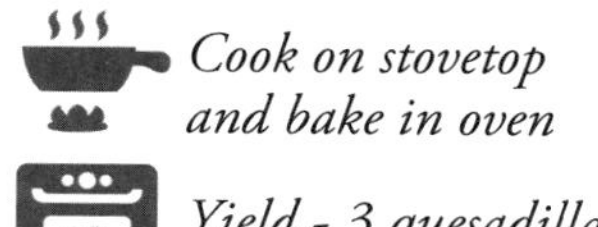

Cook on stovetop and bake in oven

Yield - 3 quesadillas

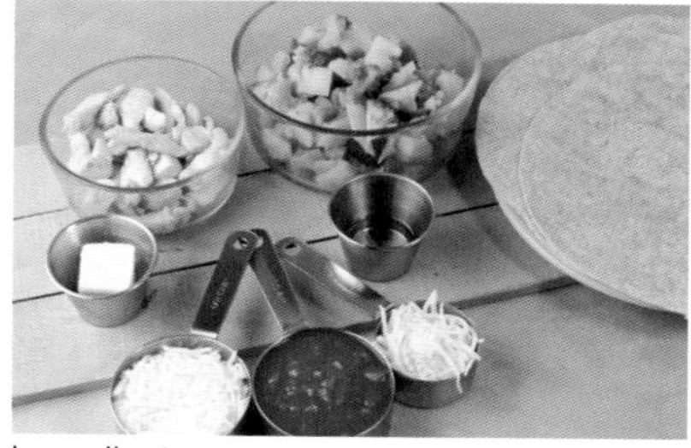

Ingredients

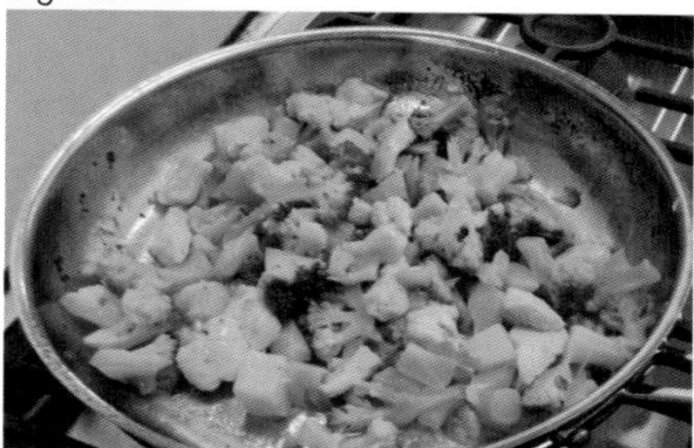

Step 1

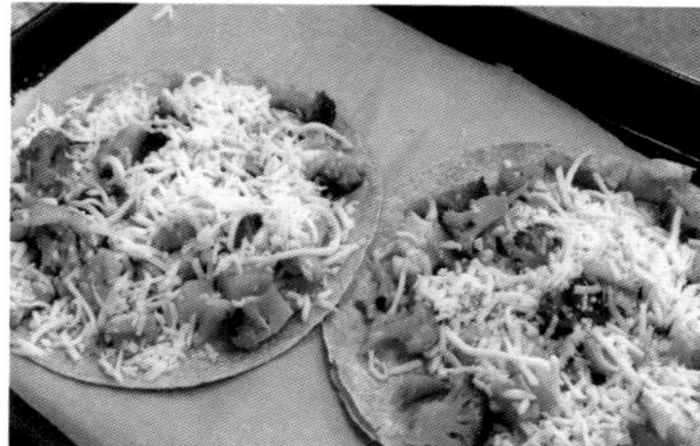

Step 4

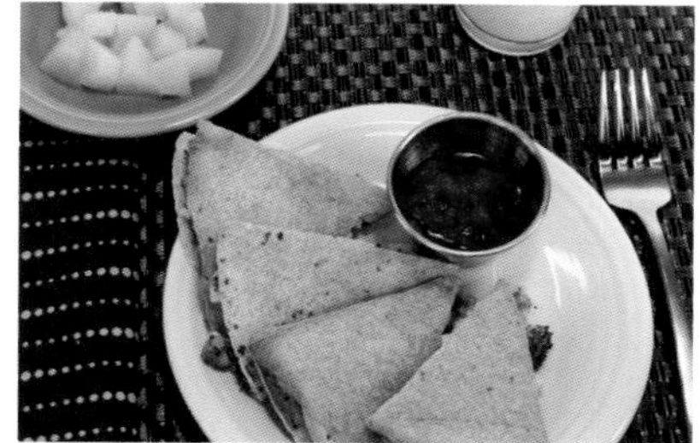

Creditable lunch/supper

Ingredients

2 tablespoons butter
3 cups broccoli, finely chopped
9 ounces cooked chicken, chopped
6 6-inch whole grain tortillas
¾ cup (3 ounces) shredded mozzarella cheese
¾ cup salsa

Directions

1. Preheat oven to 400 degrees. Line a baking sheet with parchment paper or foil.
2. Melt butter in a large skillet over medium heat. Add broccoli and chicken and cook until broccoli is tender, about 8 minutes.
3. Brush one side of each tortilla with the oil and place 3 tortillas on baking sheet, oiled side down.
4. Spread the broccoli and chicken evenly over the 3 tortillas, followed by ¼ cup of the cheese. Top each with a second tortilla, oiled side up, and place on baking sheet.
5. Bake until the cheese is melted, about 6-8 minutes. Rotate pan halfway through baking.
6. Serve with 2 tablespoons of salsa.

Chicken-Broccoli Quesadillas
provide G/B, M/MA and VEG at lunch/supper

	Toddler	Pre-School	School Age
Quesadillas	1/3 quesadilla	1/2 quesadilla	1 quesadilla
Pears	1/8 cup	1/4 cup	1/4 cup
Milk	1/2 cup	3/4 cup	1 cup

Chinese Beef & Broccoli

Prep time - 15 minutes
Cook time - 25 minutes
Total time - 40 minutes

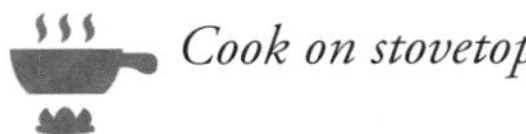

Cook on stovetop

Yield - 4 cups

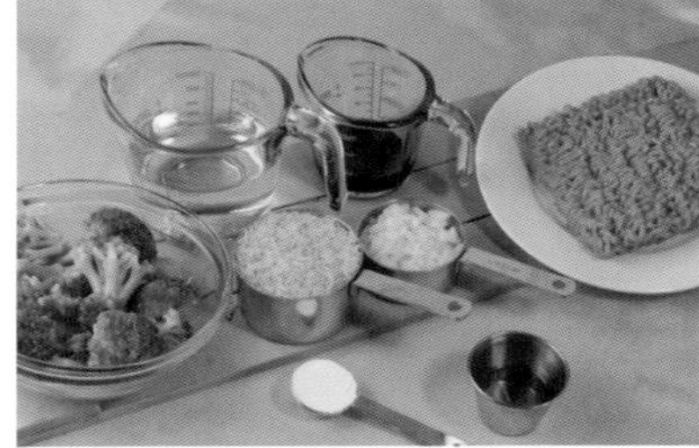

Ingredients

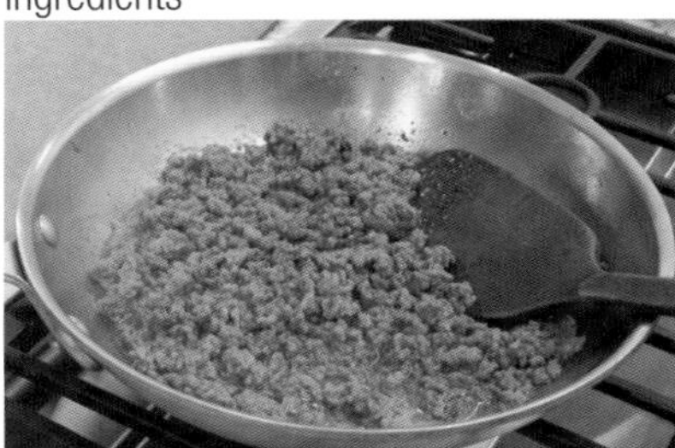

Step 1

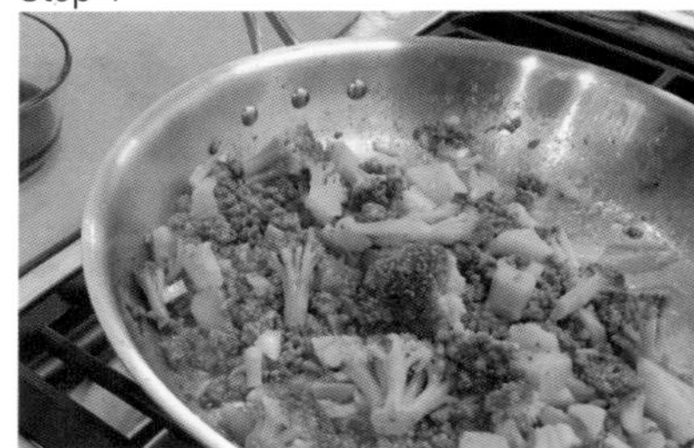

Step 2

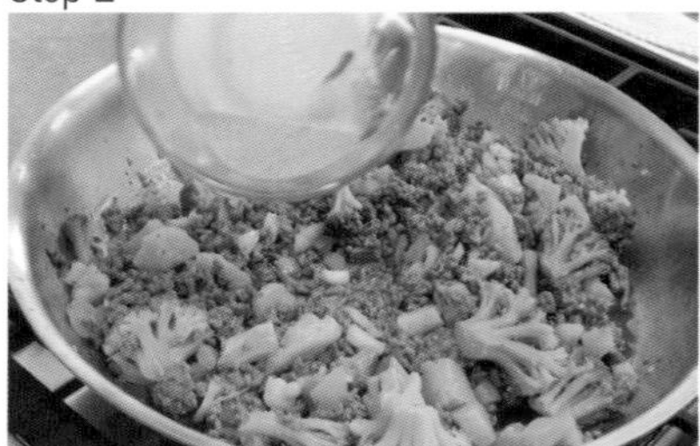

Step 3

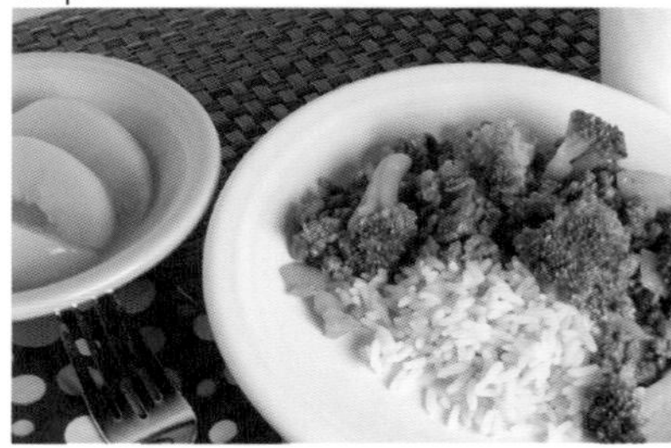

Creditable lunch/supper

Ingredients

2 cups cooked brown rice
¼ cup soy sauce
1 tablespoon cornstarch
2 tablespoons vegetable oil
1¼ pounds lean ground beef, at least 80% lean
½ cup onions, chopped
3 cups frozen broccoli florets
¼ cup water

Directions

1. In a small mixing bowl, combine soy sauce and cornstarch.
2. Heat a large skillet over medium heat; add oil and beef and cook, stirring frequently, until beef is done, with an internal temperature of 160, about 10 minutes.
3. Add onions and broccoli to beef and cook, stirring occasionally, until broccoli is crisp-tender, about 10 minutes. To speed up cooking, add ¼ cup water to pan and cover.
4. Add soy sauce mixture to pan and bring to a boil. Turn the heat down and simmer until thick, about 5 minutes.
5. Serve over rice.

Chinese Beef & Broccoli
provides G/B, M/MA and VEG at lunch/supper

	Toddler	Pre-School	School Age
Beef & Broccoli	1/3 cup	1/2 cup	3/4 cup
Rice	1/4 cup	1/4 cup	1/2 cup
Peaches	1/8 cup	1/4 cup	1/4 cup
Milk	1/2 cup	3/4 cup	1 cup

Fiesta Chicken

Prep time - 15 minutes
Marinate time - 15 minutes
Cook time - 35 minutes
Total time - 65 minutes

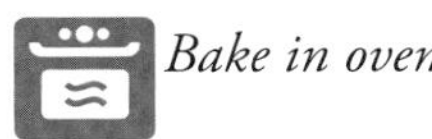

Bake in oven

Yield - 12 ounces

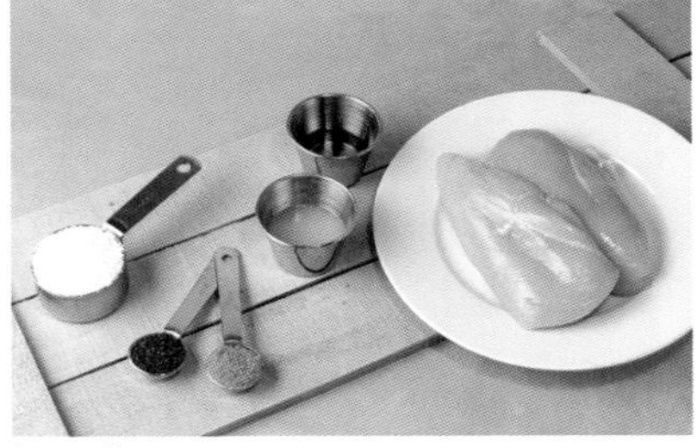
Ingredients

Ingredients

1 teaspoon chili powder
1 teaspoon ground cumin
¼ cup grated Parmesan cheese
2 tablespoons lemon or lime juice
2 tablespoons vegetable oil
1 pound boneless, skinless chicken breasts (about 3 breasts)

Directions

1. In a large mixing bowl, whisk together chili powder, cumin, cheese, lemon or lime juice and oil.
2. Add chicken and toss to coat. Cover bowl and marinate in the refrigerator for 15 minutes.
3. Preheat oven to 350 degrees. Line a baking pan with foil or parchment paper.
4. Lay marinated chicken breasts in a single layer in baking pan and bake until golden brown and firm to the touch, with an internal temperature of 165 degrees, about 35-45 minutes.
5. Remove from oven and slice.

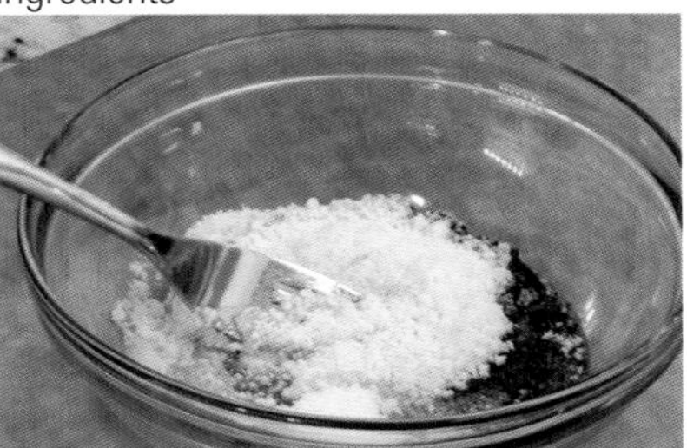
Step 1

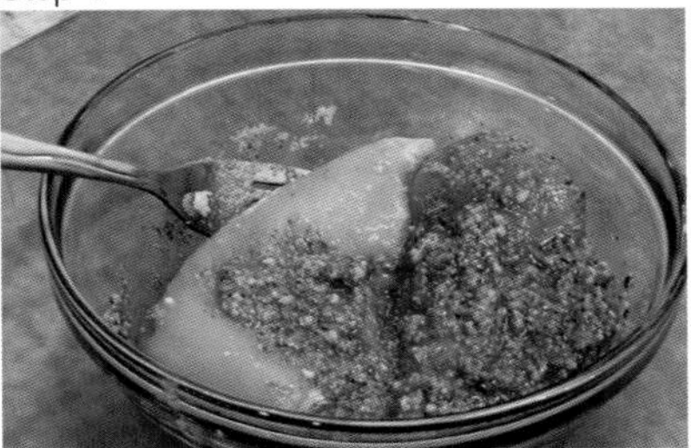
Step 2

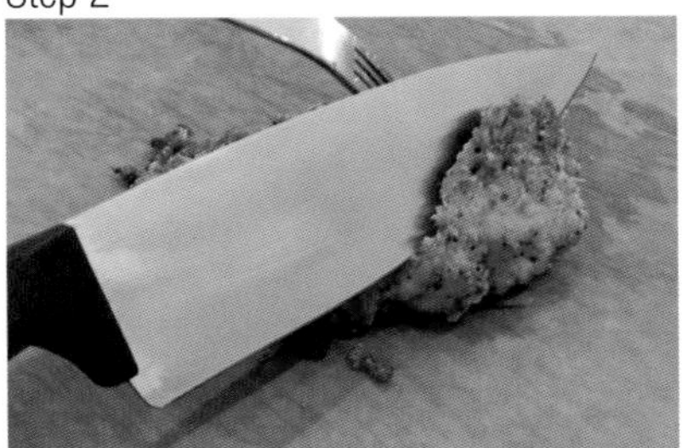
Step 6

Fiesta Chicken provides M/MA at lunch/supper			
	Toddler	Pre-School	School Age
Fiesta Chicken	1 ounce	1-1/2 ounces	2 ounces
Pasta or Rice	1/4 cup	1/4 cup	1/2 cup
Corn	1/8 cup	1/4 cup	1/2 cup
Oranges	1/8 cup	1/4 cup	1/4 cup
Milk	1/2 cup	3/4 cup	1 cup

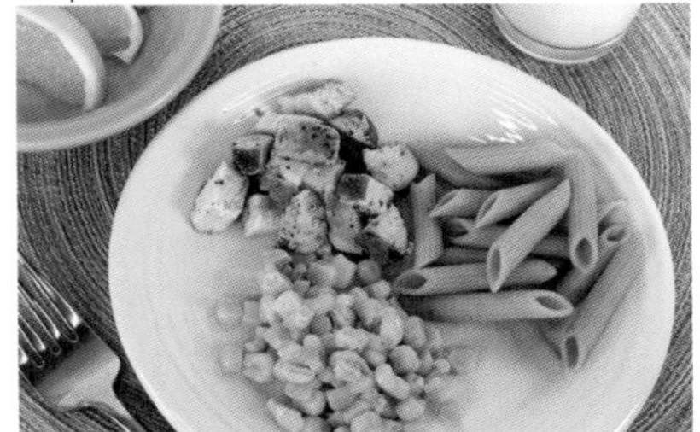
Creditable lunch/supper

Fish Tacos

Prep time - 15 minutes
Cook time - 20 minutes
Total time - 35 minutes

Bake in oven

Yield - 6 fish tacos

Ingredients

5 4-ounce fish portions, frozen, breaded*
¼ cup mayonnaise or salad dressing
1 tablespoon taco seasoning mix (½ packet)
1½ cups coleslaw mix
6 taco shells
Taco sauce

Directions

1. Bake fish portions as directed on package, about 20-25 minutes. When internal temperature reaches 145 degrees, remove from oven and cut each portion into bite-size pieces.
2. Heat taco shells in oven as directed on box.
3. In medium bowl, stir together the mayonnaise and taco seasoning. Add coleslaw mix and combine thoroughly. Let stand 5 minutes.
4. Fill taco shells with 3 ounces of fish and top with ¼ cup coleslaw mixture. Sprinkle with taco sauce, if desired.

**65% fish, not minced fish or pre-cooked fish.*
Or use a CN-labeled breaded fish product.

Fish Tacos provide G/B, M/MA and VEG at lunch/supper			
	Toddler	Pre-School	School Age
Fish Tacos	1 taco	1 taco	2 tacos
Tropical Fruit	1/8 cup	1/4 cup	1/4 cup
Milk	1/2 cup	3/4 cup	1 cup

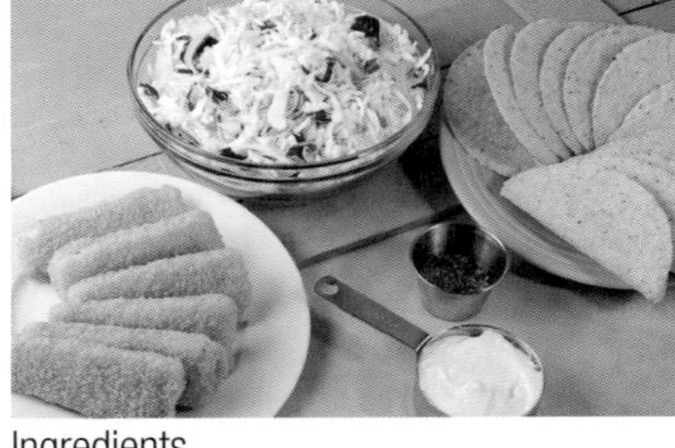
Ingredients

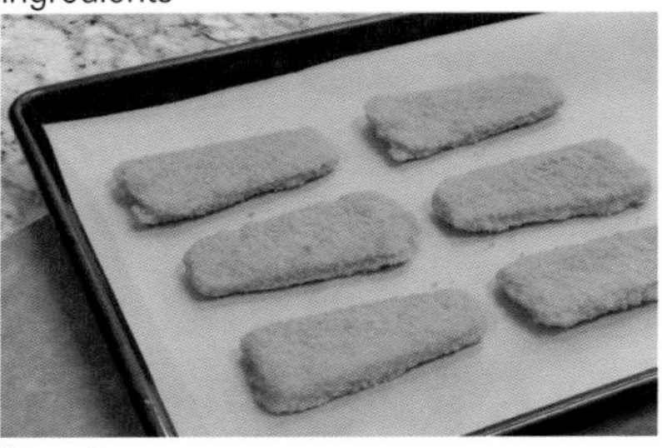
Step 1

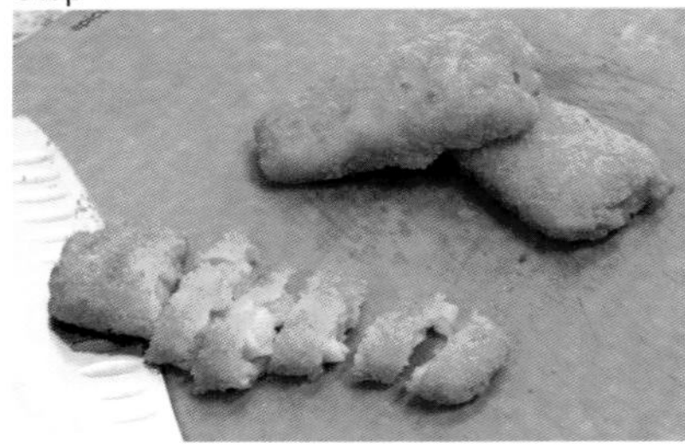
Step 2

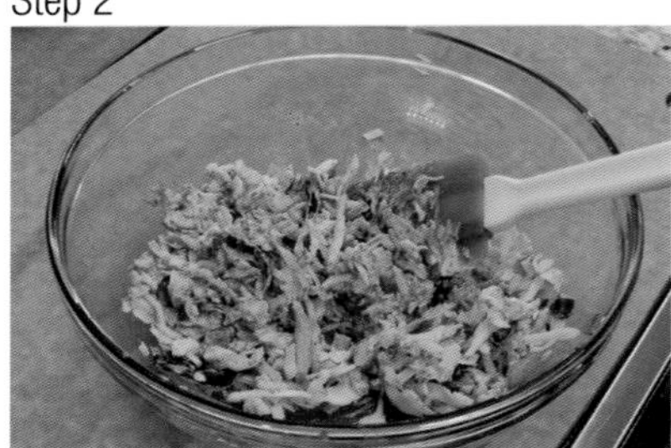
Step 3

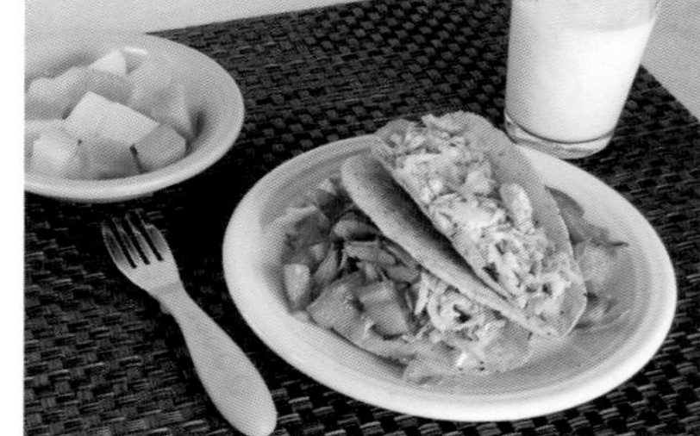
Creditable lunch/supper

Jambalaya

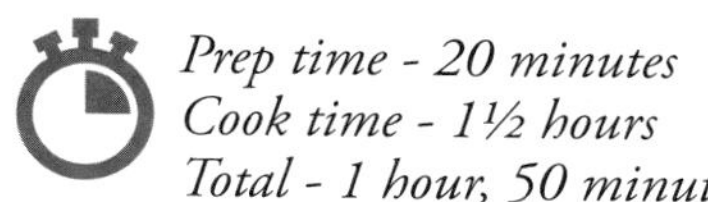

Prep time - 20 minutes
Cook time - 1½ hours
Total - 1 hour, 50 minutes

Bake in oven

Yield - 8 cups

Ingredients

1 pound boneless, skinless chicken breasts, diced —about 2 breasts
8 ounces fresh pork sausage, diced
½ cup green peppers, diced
½ cup celery, diced
2 cups canned petite diced tomatoes, with juice
1½ teaspoons creole or cajun spice blend
1 cup long-grain brown rice
2 cups chicken broth
1 cup water

Directions

1. Preheat oven to 350 degrees. Grease 11x7-inch baking pan or coat with cooking spray.
2. Add all ingredients to the baking pan and stir to combine.
3. Bake until the jambalaya reaches an internal temperature of 165 degrees, about 1½ hours.

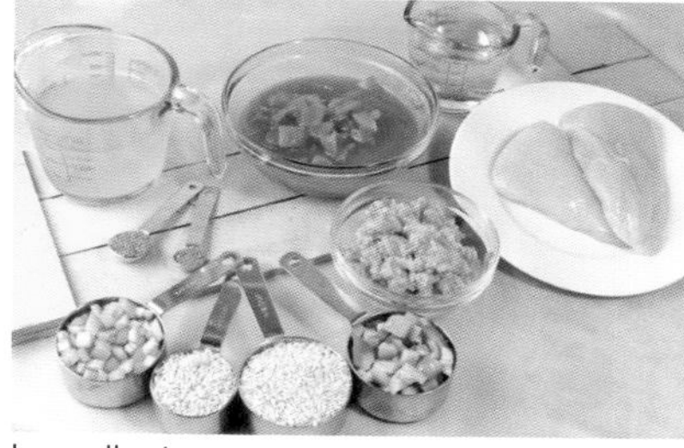

Ingredients

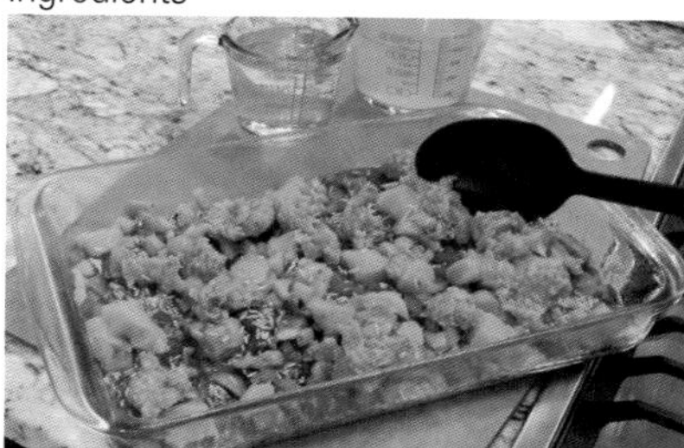

Step 1

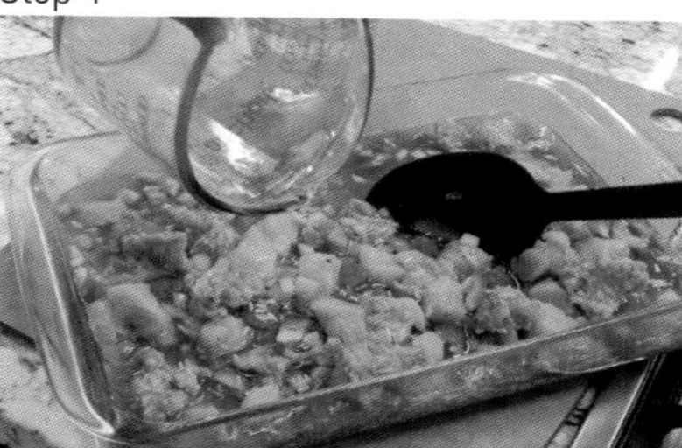

Step 2

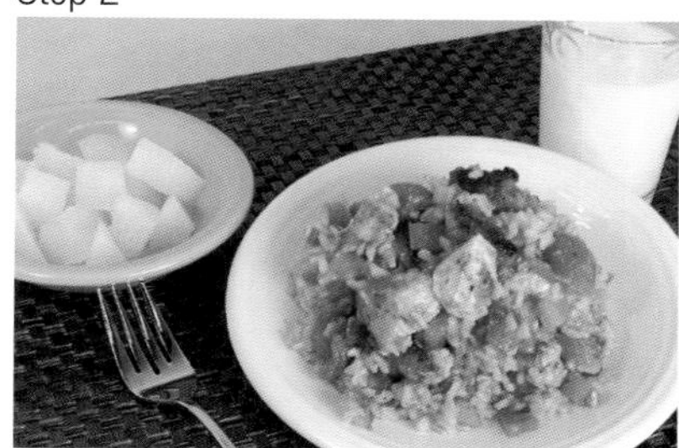

Creditable lunch/supper

***Batch Cooking Tip** - Make ahead, freeze and reheat.*
This recipe makes 10 1-cup servings of M/MA.

Jambalaya provides G/B, M/MA and VEG at lunch/supper			
	Toddler	Pre-School	School Age
Jambalaya	2/3 cup	1 cup	1-1/3 cups
Pears	1/8 cup	1/4 cup	1/4 cup
Milk	1/2 cup	3/4 cup	1 cup

Lentil Curry

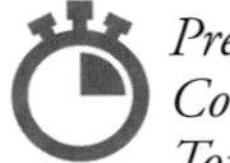
Prep time - 15 minutes
Cook time - 65 minutes
Total time -
1 hour, 20 minutes

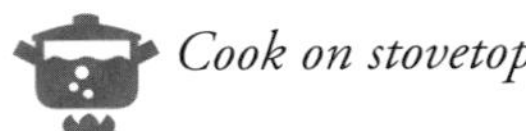
Cook on stovetop

Yield - 6½ cups

Ingredients

1½ cups cooked brown rice
1 tablespoon vegetable oil
1 cup onions, diced
½ teaspoon ground cumin
½ teaspoon curry powder
¼ teaspoon paprika
2 cups raw lentils, rinsed
1½ teaspoons garlic, minced
6 cups vegetable or chicken stock/broth
¾ teaspoon salt, or to taste

Directions

1. Heat oil in stock pot over medium-high heat.
2. Add oil, then onions, cumin, curry powder and paprika. Cook until onions are softened, about 5 minutes.
3. Stir in lentils, garlic and broth.
4. Bring to a boil, then lower heat and simmer until lentils are tender, about 1 hour.
5. Add salt. Thin with water or stock as desired.
6. Serve over rice.

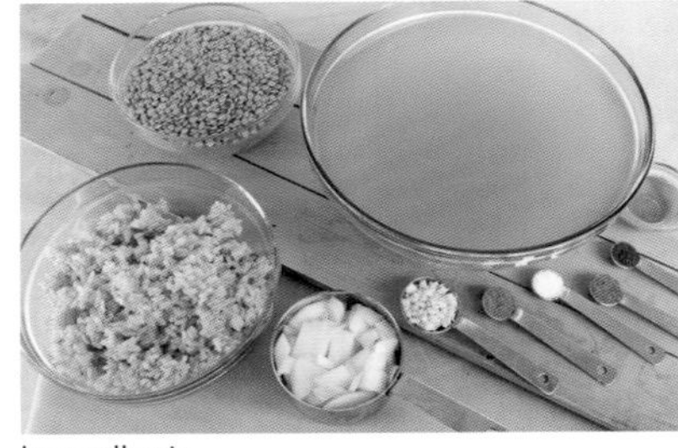
Ingredients

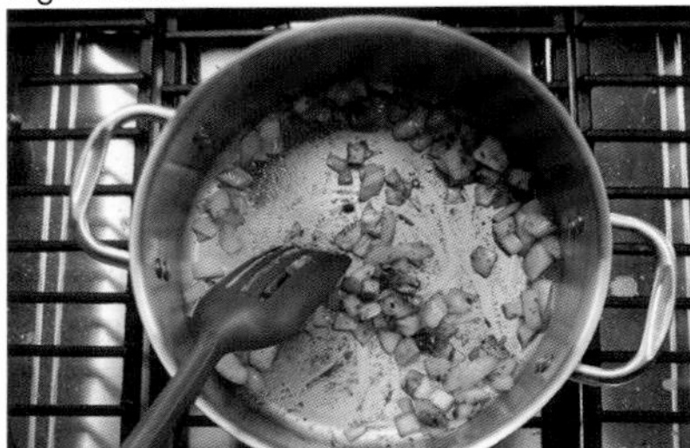
Step 2

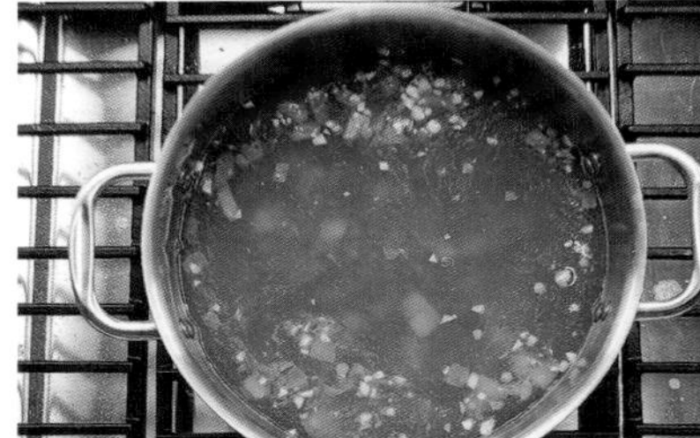
Step 3

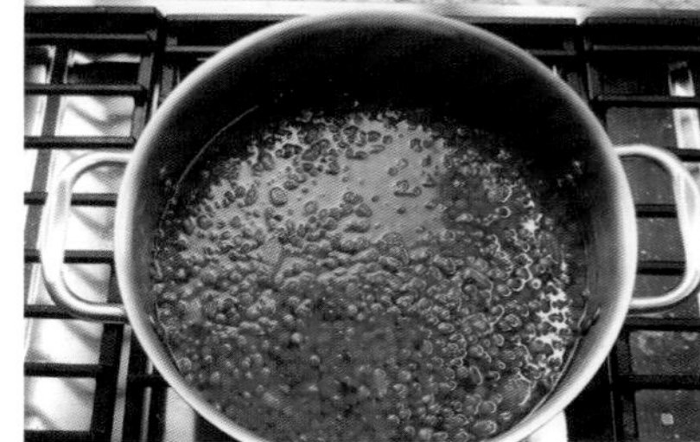
Step 4

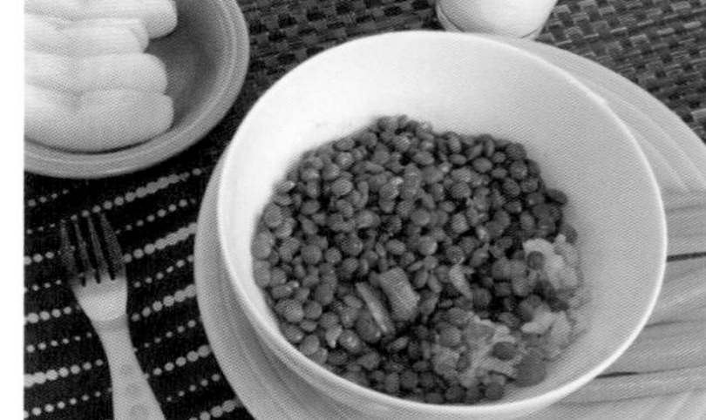
Creditable lunch/supper

Lentil Curry provides M/MA at lunch/supper			
	Toddler	Pre-School	School Age
Lentil Curry	1/2 cup	3/4 cup	1 cup
Rice	1/4 cup	1/4 cup	1/2 cup
Carrots	1/4 cup	1/2 cup	1/2 cup
Apples	1/8 cup	1/4 cup	1/4 cup
Milk	1/2 cup	3/4 cup	1 cup

Mexican Beans & Rice

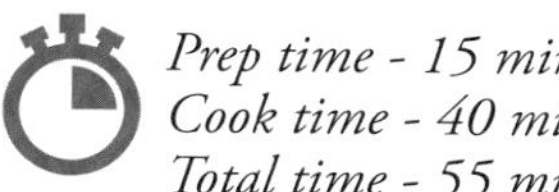
Prep time - 15 minutes
Cook time - 40 minutes
Total time - 55 minutes

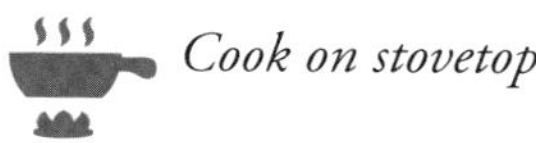
Cook on stovetop

Yield - 4 cups

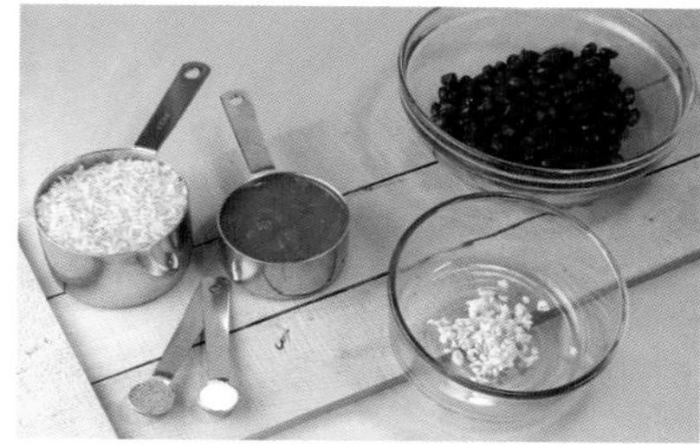
Ingredients

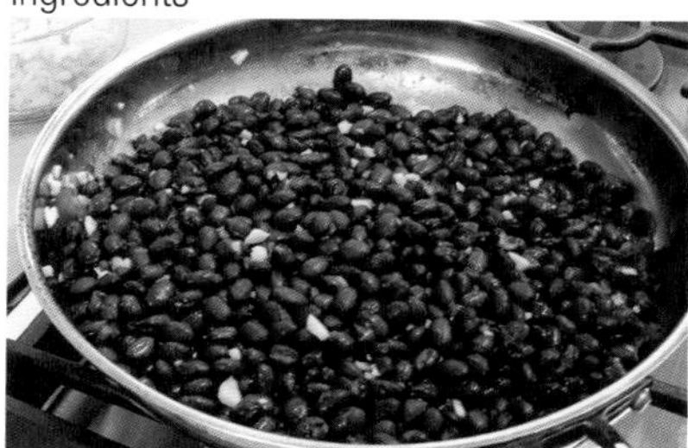
Step 2

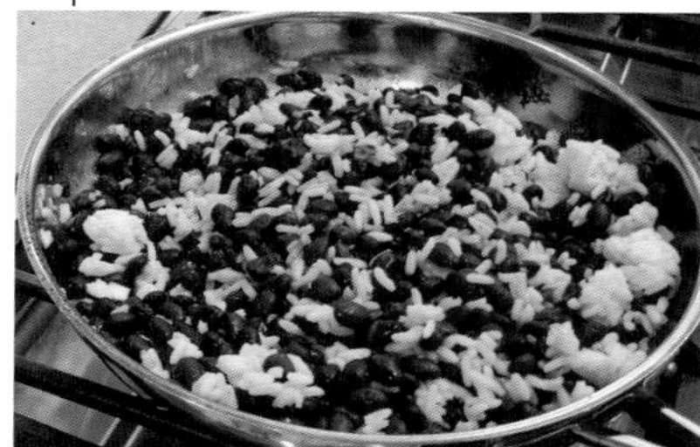
Step 3

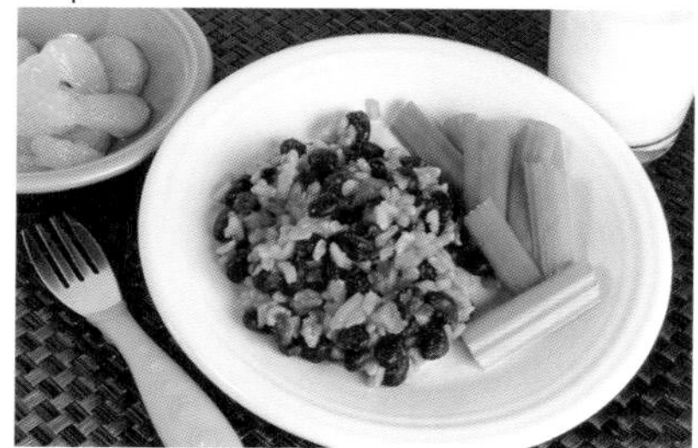
Creditable lunch/supper

Ingredients

1 cup long-grain brown rice
2 cups water for cooking rice
2 tablespoons vegetable oil
2 teaspoons garlic, minced
½ teaspoon ground cumin
½ teaspoon salt
2¼ cups black beans, rinsed and drained
½ cup salsa

Directions

1. Cook rice according to package directions; set aside.
2. To a large skillet over medium heat, add oil, garlic, cumin and salt. Stir briefly to mix, then add beans. Cook about 1 minute, then stir in salsa. Simmer over low heat for 15-20 minutes, stirring occasionally.
3. Add cooked rice to beans and mix well. Cook until heated through, about 5 minutes.

Mexican Beans & Rice provides G/B and M/MA at lunch/supper			
	Toddler	Pre-School	School Age
Beans & Rice	1/2 cup	2/3 cup	1 cup
Celery	1/4 cup	1/2 cup	1/2 cup
Mandarin Oranges	1/8 cup	1/4 cup	1/4 cup
Milk	1/2 cup	3/4 cup	1 cup

Mexican Dip

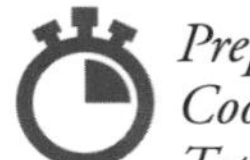
Prep time - 10 minutes
Cook time - 5 minutes
Total time - 15 minutes

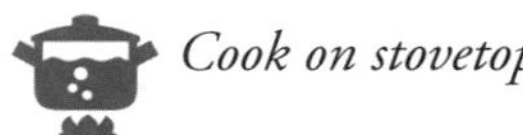
Cook on stovetop

Yield - 4½ cups

Ingredients

1½ cups refried beans
1 teaspoon ground cumin
½ cup salsa
1½ cups plain yogurt
1½ cups shredded lettuce

Directions

1. Heat refried beans in small saucepan over medium heat, about 5 minutes. Add cumin and mix well.
2. Transfer beans to an 8x8-inch casserole dish and spread evenly.
3. Top beans with yogurt, salsa and shredded lettuce.

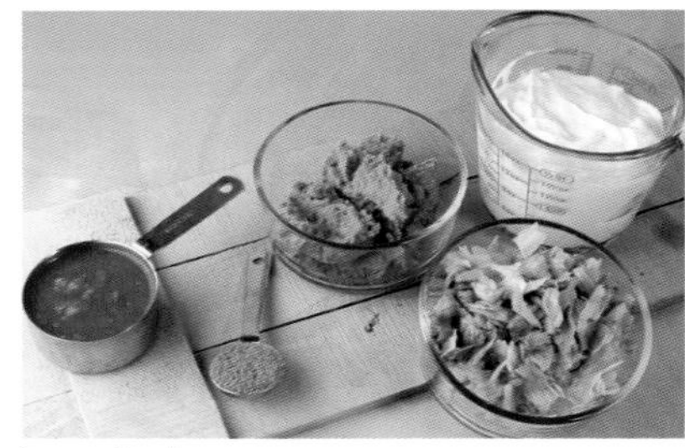
Ingredients

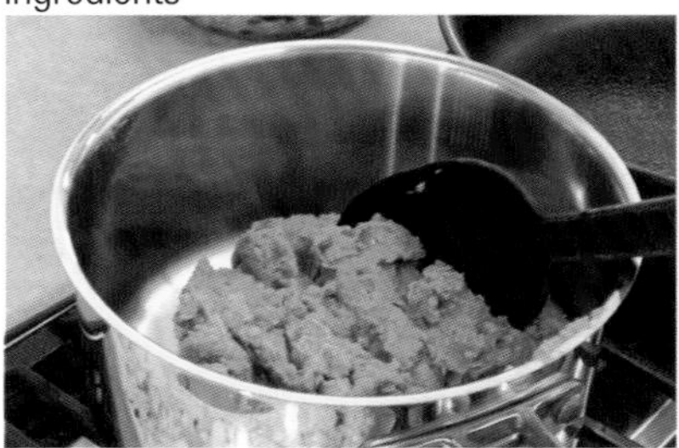
Step 1

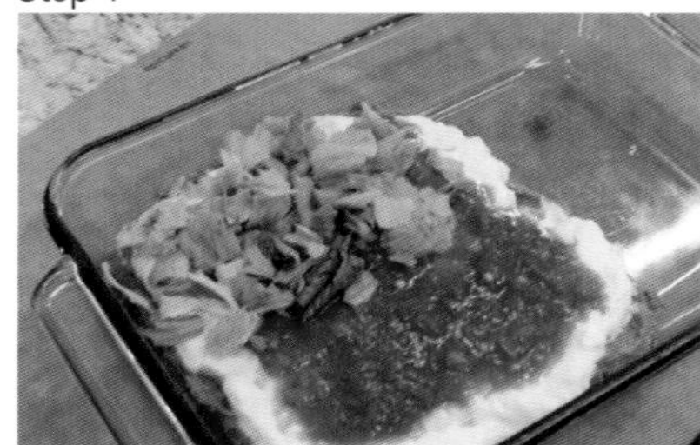
Step 4

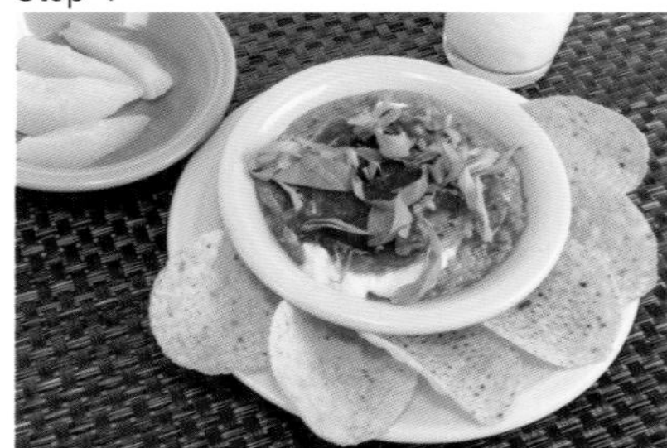
Creditable lunch/supper

Mexican Dip provides M/MA and VEG at lunch/supper			
	Toddler	Pre-School	School Age
Mexican Dip	1/2 cup	3/4 cup	1 cup
Tortilla Chips	1/2 ounce	1/2 ounce	1 ounce
Pears	1/8 cup	1/4 cup	1/4 cup
Milk	1/2 cup	3/4 cup	1 cup

Orange Chicken

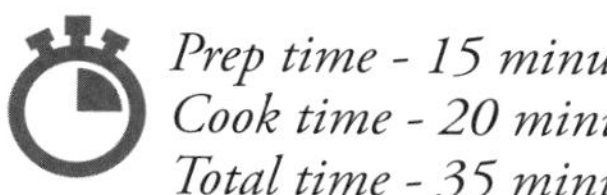
Prep time - 15 minutes
Cook time - 20 minutes
Total time - 35 minutes

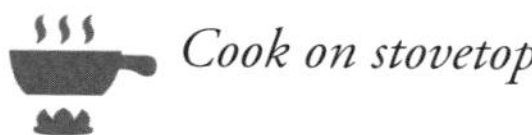
Cook on stovetop

Yield - 12 ounces

Ingredients

1½ cups cooked brown rice
1 pound boneless, skinless chicken breasts, diced
1 cup orange juice
2 tablespoons cornstarch
3 tablespoons soy sauce
⅛ teaspoon cayenne pepper, optional

Directions

1. To a large skillet over medium heat, add chicken and cook until it is no longer pink in the center, with an internal temperature of 165 degrees, about 10 minutes. When done, transfer to a plate and cover to keep warm.
2. To make the sauce, whisk together the orange juice, cornstarch, soy sauce and cayenne in a small bowl.
3. Pour sauce into the skillet and cook over medium-low heat for 5-10 minutes, stirring constantly, or until the sauce has thickened and is reduced by about a third.
4. Reduce heat to low, add the chicken, and stir until it is coated in sauce. Cook until chicken is heated through, about 5-10 minutes.
5. Serve over rice.

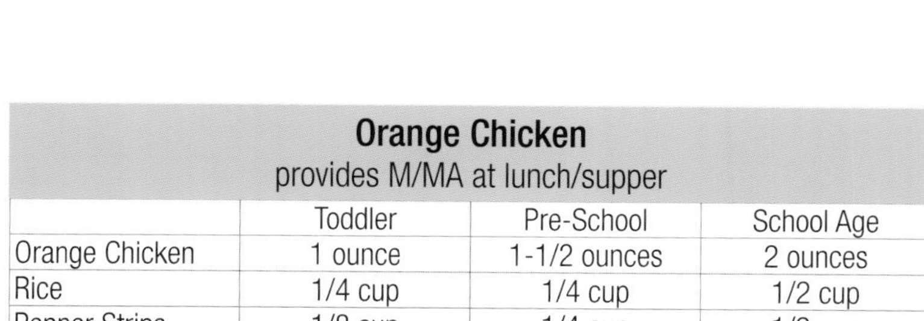

Orange Chicken provides M/MA at lunch/supper			
	Toddler	Pre-School	School Age
Orange Chicken	1 ounce	1-1/2 ounces	2 ounces
Rice	1/4 cup	1/4 cup	1/2 cup
Pepper Strips	1/8 cup	1/4 cup	1/2 cup
Bananas	1/8 cup	1/4 cup	1/4 cup
Milk	1/2 cup	3/4 cup	1 cup

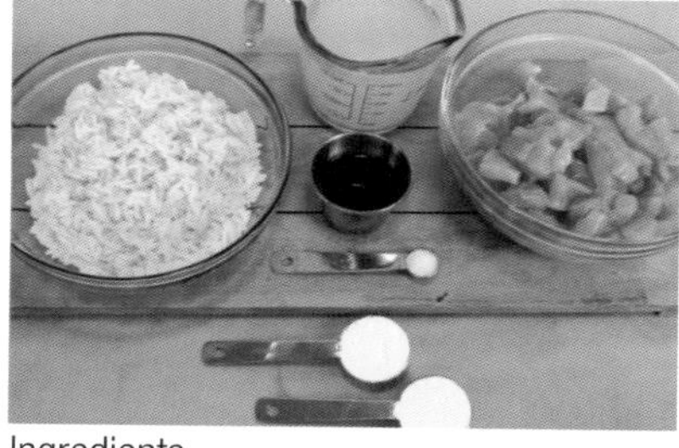
Ingredients

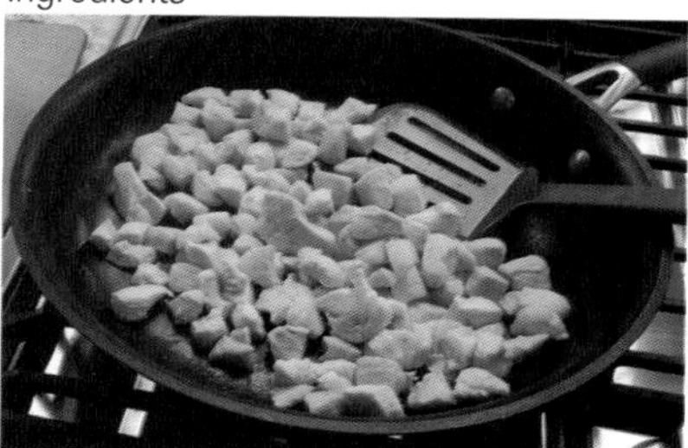
Step 1

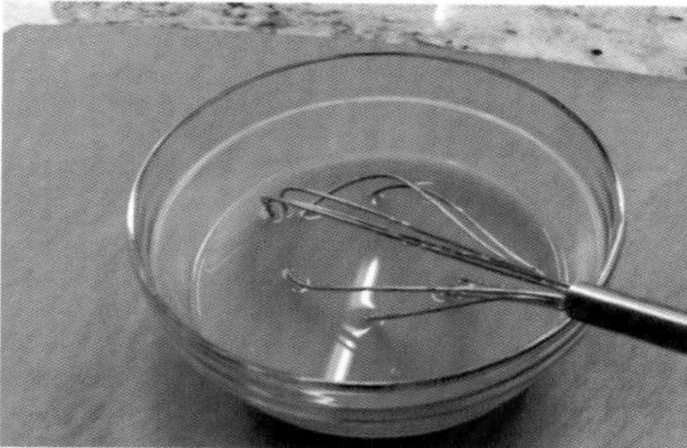
Step 2

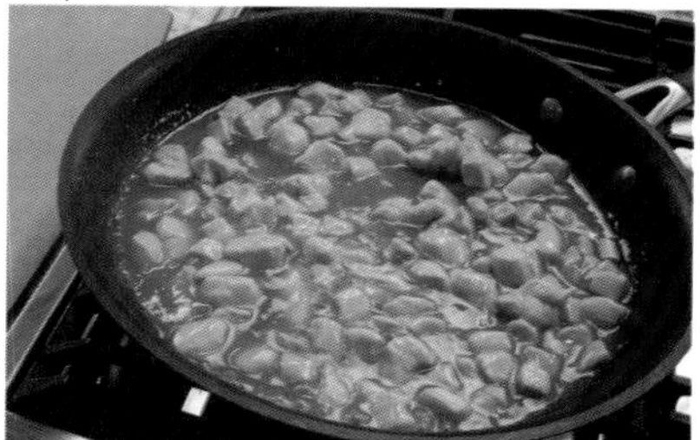
Step 3

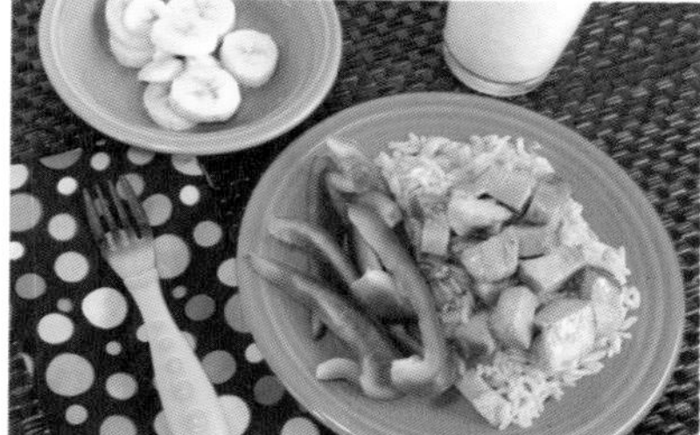
Creditable lunch/supper

Pork Fried Rice

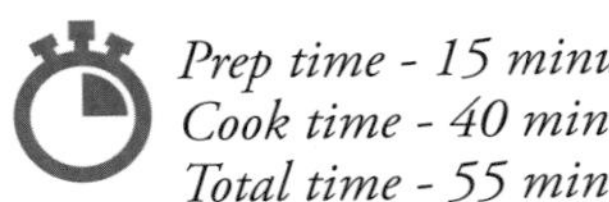

Prep time - 15 minutes
Cook time - 40 minutes
Total time - 55 minutes

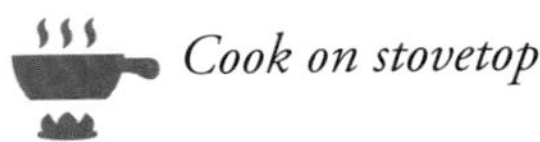

Cook on stovetop

Yield - 5 cups

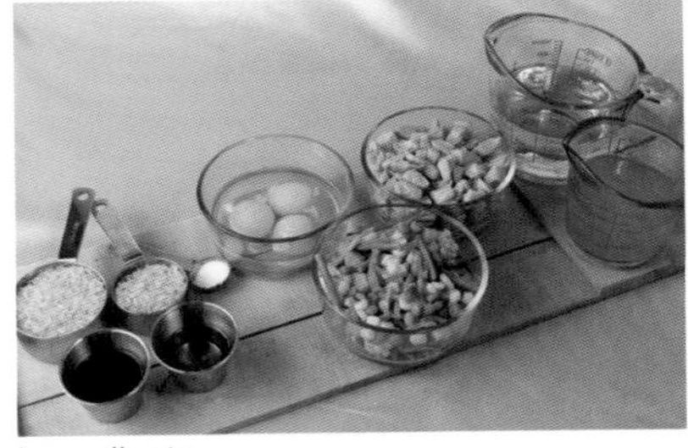

Ingredients

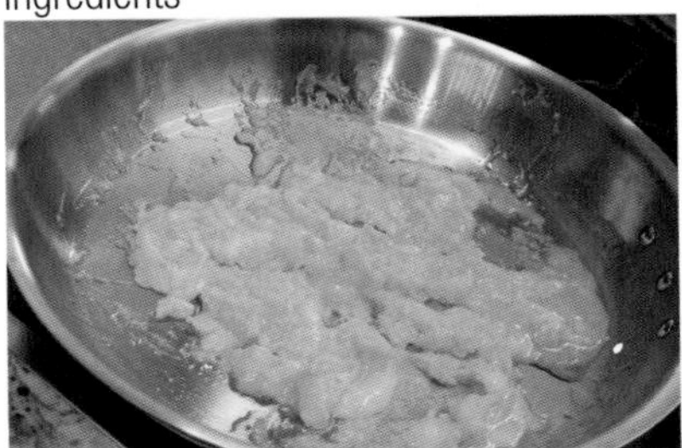

Step 2

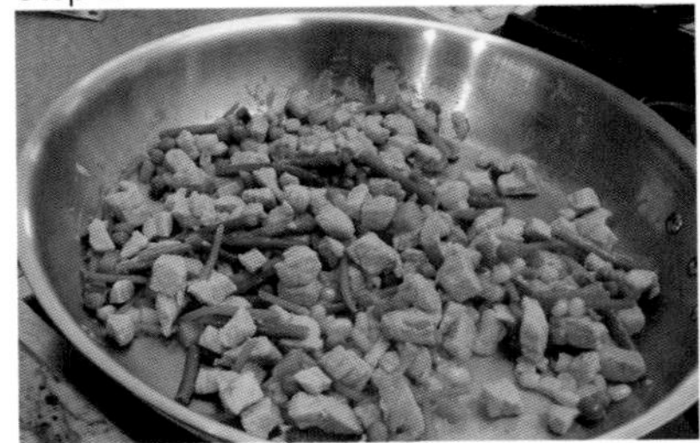

Step 3

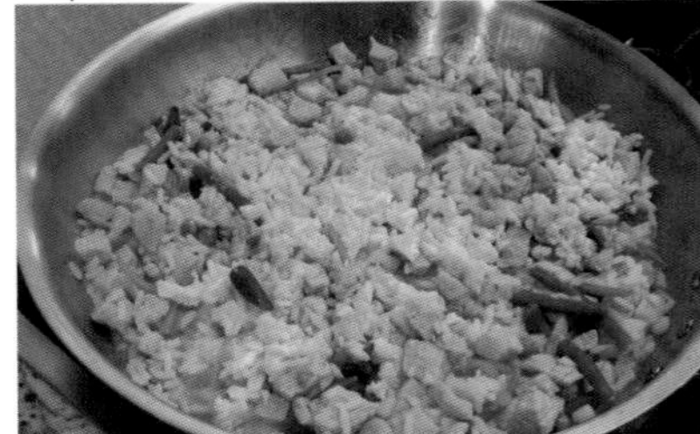

Step 4-5

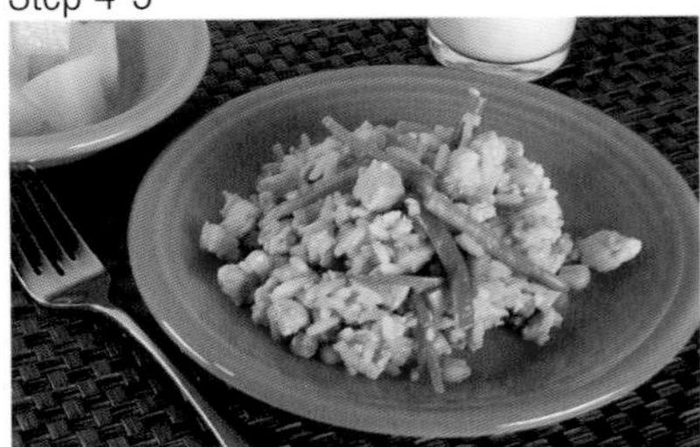

Creditable lunch/supper

Ingredients

1¼ cups long-grain brown rice
2½ cups water for cooking rice
3 tablespoons vegetable oil
3 eggs, lightly beaten
6 ounces cooked pork, diced
2¼ cups frozen mixed vegetables,
—carrot, corn and green bean blend
¾ cup chicken broth
3 tablespoons soy sauce
¾ teaspoon sugar

Directions

1. Cook rice according to package directions, about 35 minutes.
2. Heat oil in a large skillet over medium-high heat, then add eggs. Cook until firm to the touch, about 5 minutes. Transfer to a plate.
3. Add pork and mixed vegetables to the skillet. Heat for 5 minutes.
4. Add cooked rice and broth. Cover and cook until heated through, about 5 minutes.
5. Chop the cooked egg into small pieces and add to the skillet.
6. In a small bowl, stir the soy sauce and sugar together. Pour into skillet and stir to mix.

Pork Fried Rice provides G/B, M/MA and VEG at lunch/supper			
	Toddler	Pre-School	School Age
Pork Fried Rice	1/2 cup	2/3 cup	1 cup
Pineapple	1/8 cup	1/4 cup	1/4 cup
Milk	1/2 cup	3/4 cup	1 cup

Summer Veggie Rice Bowl

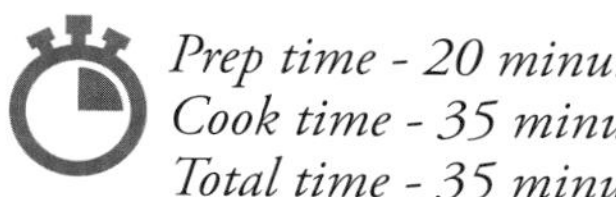

Prep time - 20 minutes
Cook time - 35 minutes
Total time - 35 minutes

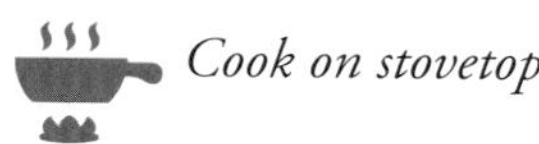

Cook on stovetop

Yield - 3 cups

Ingredients

1¼ cups brown rice
2½ cups water for cooking rice
¼ cup teriyaki sauce
1 tablespoon cornstarch
2 tablespoons vegetable oil
1 cup onions, diced
1½ cups carrots, diced
1½ cups zucchini, diced
½ teaspoon garlic powder
¼ teaspoon ground ginger

Directions

1. Cook rice according to package directions, about 35 minutes.
2. In a small bowl, whisk teriyaki sauce and cornstarch together; set aside.
3. Heat oil in large skillet over medium-high heat. Add onions and carrots and cook, stirring frequently, until carrots are tender-crisp, about 5 minutes.
4. Add zucchini, garlic powder and ginger powder and cook until zucchini is tender, about 5 minutes.
5. Add teriyaki sauce to pan. Bring to a boil, then reduce heat and simmer until thickened, about 5 minutes.
6. Serve over rice.

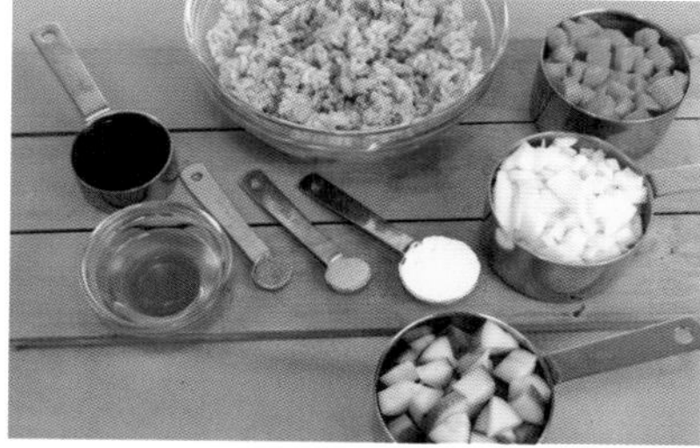

Ingredients

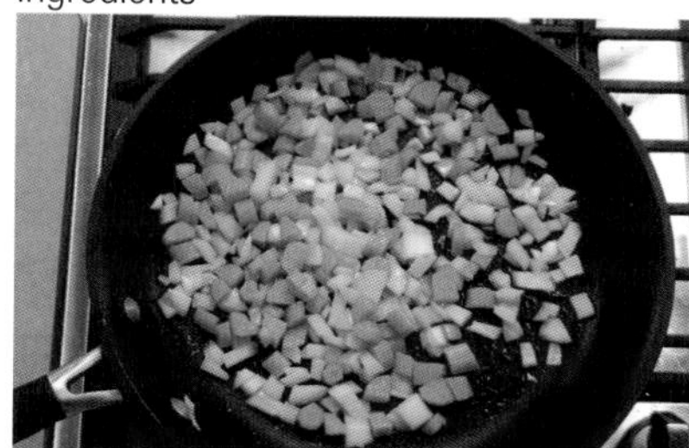

Step 3

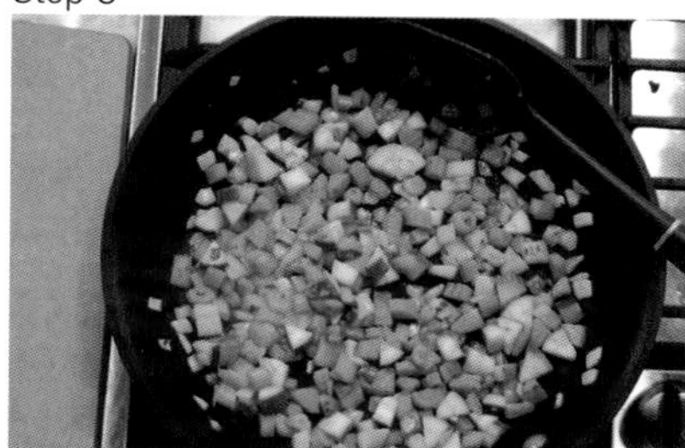

Step 4

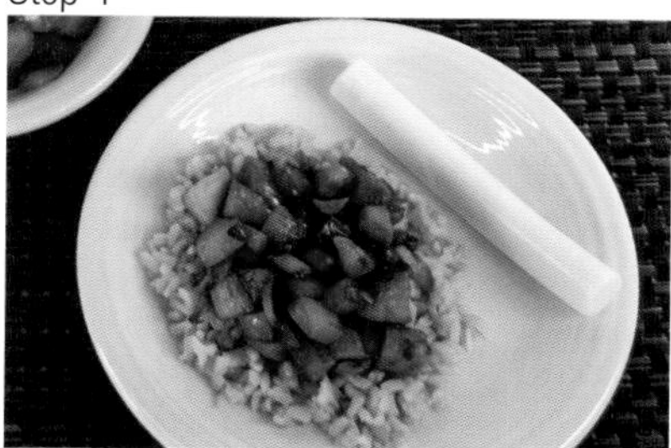

Creditable lunch/supper

Summer Veggie Rice Bowl
provides G/B and VEG at lunch/supper

	Toddler	Pre-School	School Age
Veggie Bowl	1/4 cup	1/2 cup	1 cup
Rice	1/4 cup	1/4 cup	1/2 cup
String Cheese	1 ounce	1-1/2 ounces	2 ounces
Strawberries	1/8 cup	1/4 cup	1/4 cup
Milk	1/2 cup	3/4 cup	1 cup

Sweet & Sour Chicken

Prep time - 15 minutes
Cook time - 40 minutes
Total time - 55 minutes

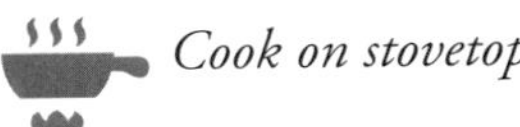

Cook on stovetop

Yield - 6 cups

Ingredients

1 cup long-grain brown rice
2 cups water for cooking rice
1½ tablespoons oil
1 pound boneless, skinless chicken breast, sliced into strips
2 cups frozen stir-fry vegetables
1 cup pineapple chunks, with juice
¼ cup sweet and sour sauce
1½ cups water

Directions

1. Cook rice according to package directions, about 35 minutes. Cover and set aside.
2. Heat a large skillet over medium-high heat. Add oil and chicken and cook, stirring frequently, until chicken reaches an internal temperature of 165 degrees, about 10 minutes.
3. Add the vegetables, pineapple with juice and the sweet and sour sauce. Mix well. Stir in the water and bring to boil.
4. Stir in the cooked rice. Cover and reduce heat to medium-low. Simmer 5 minutes until rice is heated through.

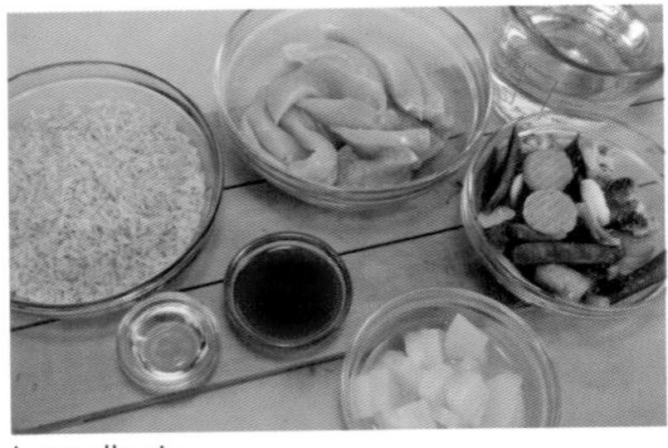
Ingredients

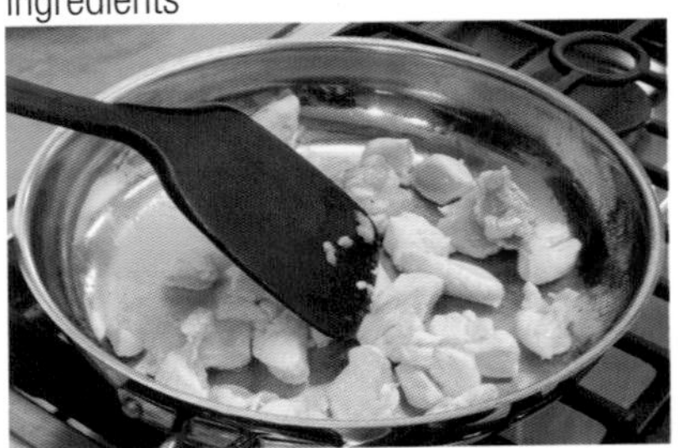
Step 1

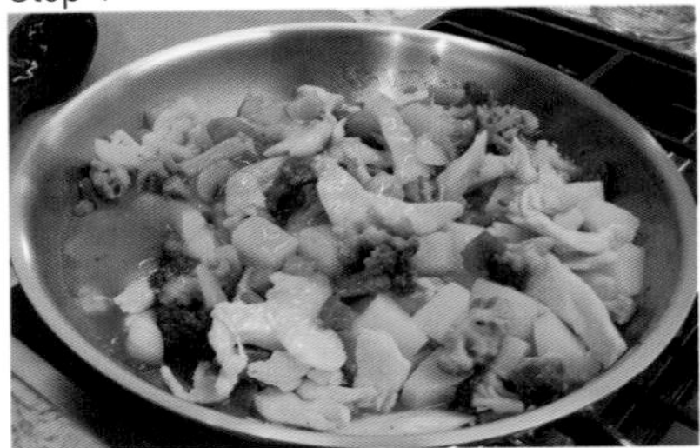
Step 2

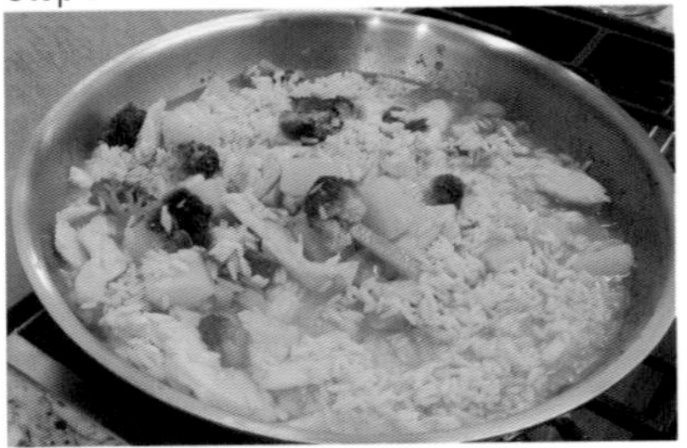
Step 3

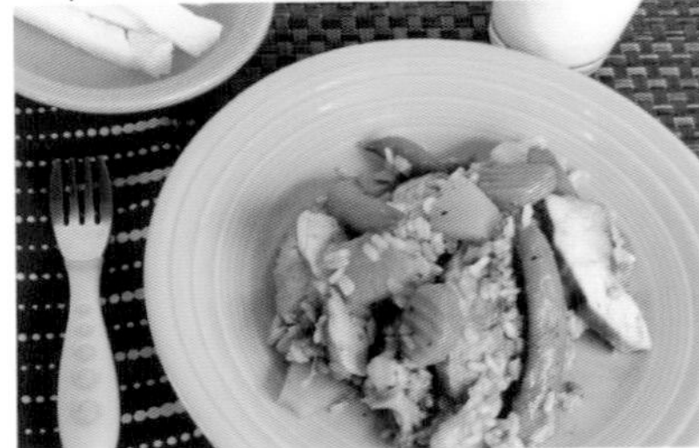
Creditable lunch/supper

Sweet & Sour Chicken
provides G/B, M/MA and VEG at lunch/supper

	Toddler	Pre-School	School Age
Chicken	2/3 cup	1 cup	1-1/3 cups
Jicama	1/8 cup	1/4 cup	1/2 cup
Milk	1/2 cup	3/4 cup	1 cup

Vegetarian Taco Pizza

Prep time - 10 minutes
Cook time - 5 minutes
Total time - 15 minutes

Bake in oven

Yield - 12 pizza wedges

Ingredients

1½ cups refried beans
2 tablespoons taco seasoning (1 packet)
2 whole wheat pita bread rounds, at least 1½ ounces each
½ cup whole kernel corn, cooked
½ cup cherry tomatoes, sliced
¾ cup (3 ounces) finely shredded cheddar cheese
½ cup lettuce, finely shredded
Taco sauce

Directions

1. Preheat oven to 400 degrees. Line a baking sheet with foil or parchment paper, or coat with cooking spray.
2. In a bowl, mix beans and taco seasoning.
3. Lay pita rounds on baking sheet. Spread bean mixture evenly over both.
4. Top with ¼ cup of corn and tomatoes and ⅜ cup cheese.
5. Bake until heated through and cheese is melted, 5-7 minutes.
6. Remove from oven and sprinkle each round with ¼ cup of lettuce.
7. Cut each round into 6 wedges and serve with taco sauce.

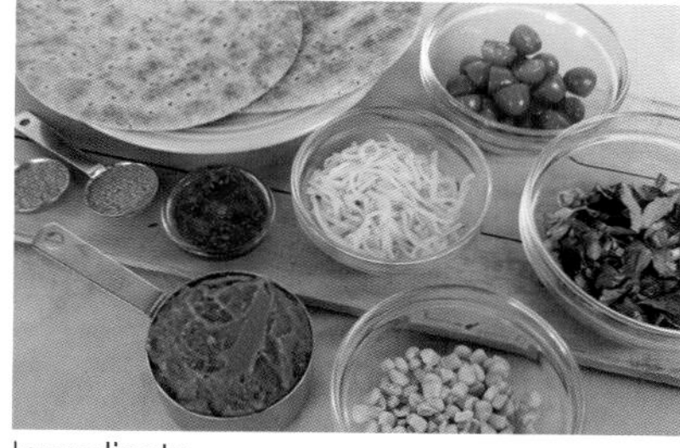

Ingredients

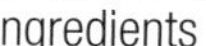

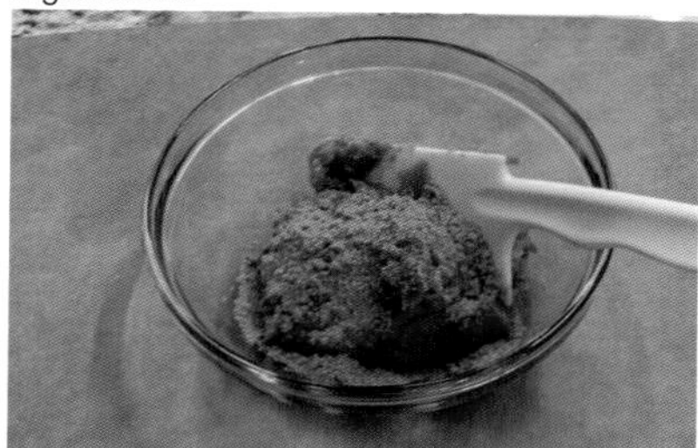

Step 2

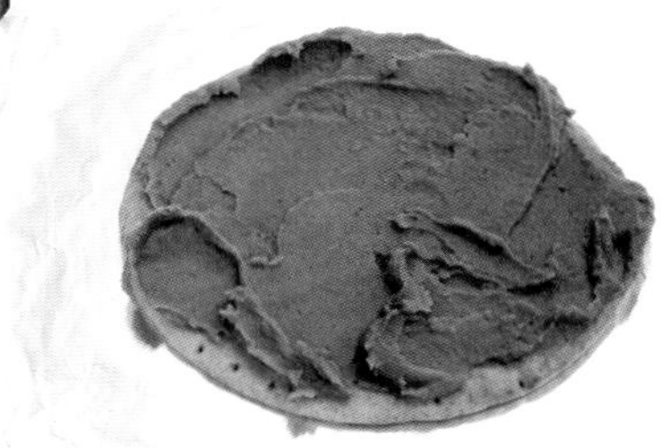

Step 3

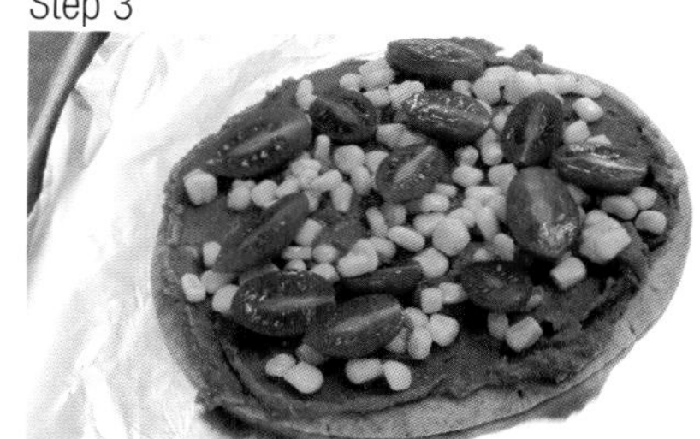

Step 4

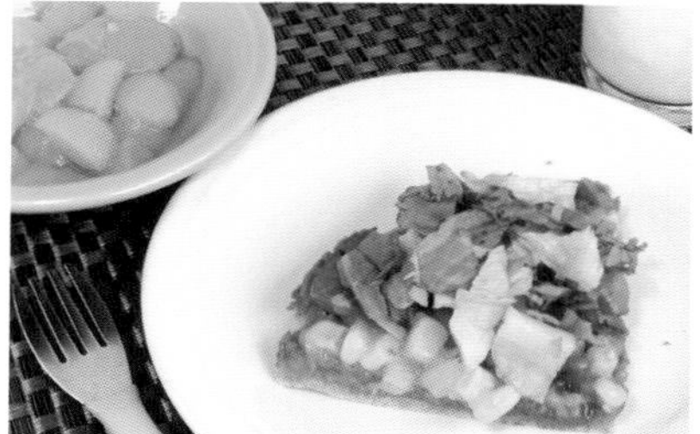

Creditable lunch/supper

Vegetarian Taco Pizza
provides G/B, M/MA and VEG at lunch/supper

	Toddler	Pre-School	School Age
Taco Pizza	2 wedges	2 wedges	4 wedges
Apricots	1/8 cup	1/4 cup	1/4 cup
Milk	1/2 cup	3/4 cup	1 cup

Snacks

Apple Pie Bites

Prep time - 20 minutes
Cook time - 20 minutes
Total time - 40 minutes

Bake in oven

Yield - 6 slices

Ingredients

½ cup whole wheat flour
½ teaspoon baking powder
½ teaspoon sugar
⅛ teaspoon salt
1 tablespoon butter, cut into small pieces
2½ tablespoons milk
4 cups apples, diced
3 tablespoons brown sugar
½ teaspoon of ground cinnamon or apple pie spice

Directions

1. Preheat oven to 375 degrees. Grease pie plate or coat with cooking spray.
2. Mix flour, baking powder, sugar and salt in a bowl. Cut in butter or mix with clean hands until texture is crumbly.
3. Add milk slowly, just until all ingredients are wet. Do not add all the milk at once.
4. Once the dough is formed, press into the bottom of the pie plate. Top dough with diced apples and sprinkle with brown sugar and cinnamon or apple pie spice.
5. Bake for 20 minutes. When cooled slightly, cut into 6 slices.

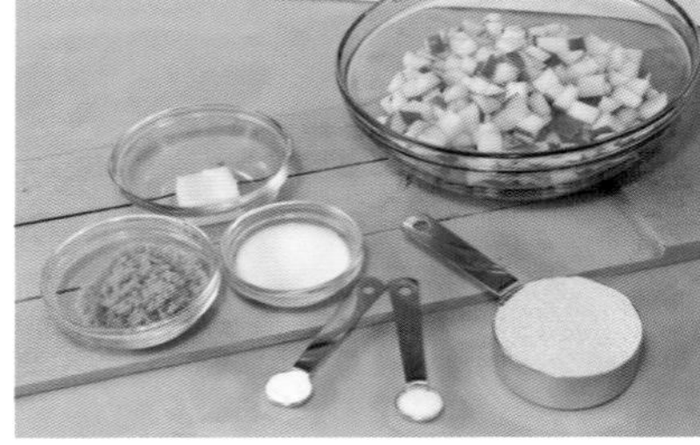

Ingredients

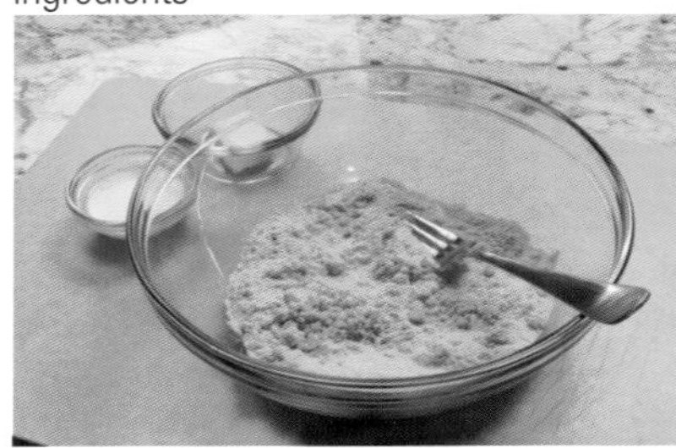

Step 2

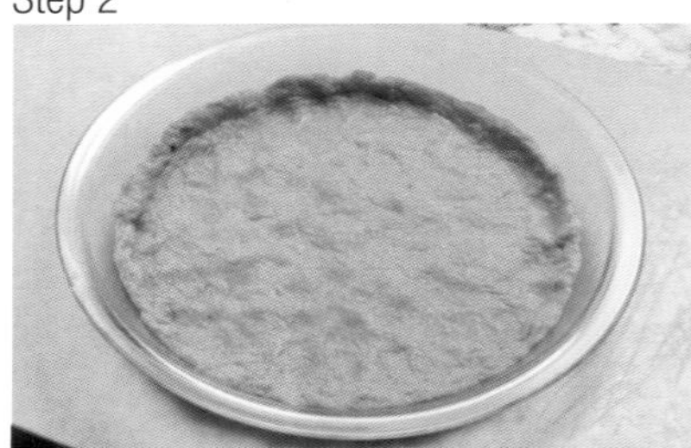

Step 3

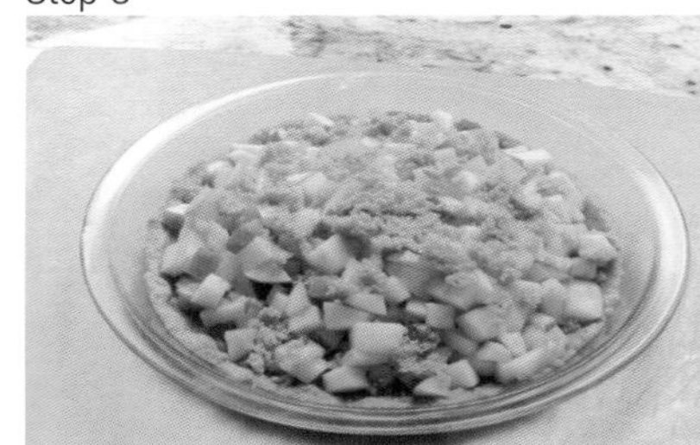

Step 4

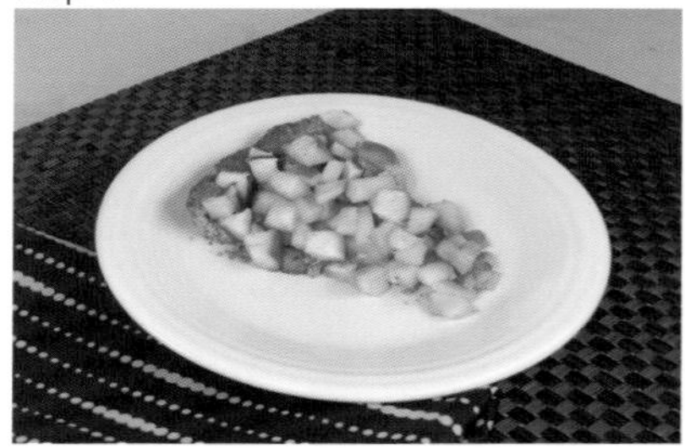

Creditable snack

Apple Pie Bites provide G/B AND FR at snack			
	Toddler	Pre-School	School Age
Apple Pie Bites	1 slice	1 slice	2 slices

Applesauce-Bran Muffins

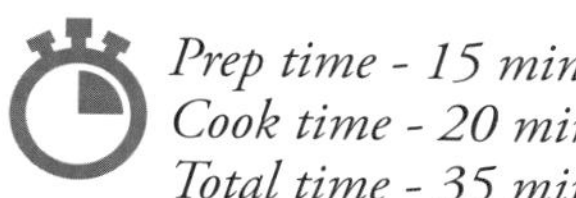

Prep time - 15 minutes
Cook time - 20 minutes
Total time - 35 minutes

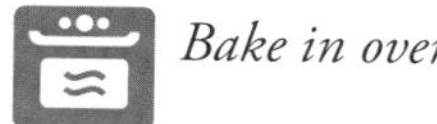

Bake in oven

Yield - 12 muffins

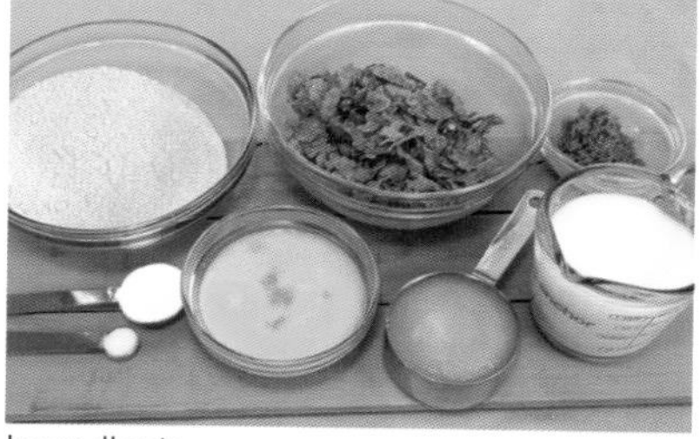
Ingredients

Ingredients

1⅓ cups whole wheat flour
1 tablespoon baking powder
¼ teaspoon salt
2 cups bran and raisin cereal
1 cup milk
2 eggs, beaten
½ cup applesauce
⅜ cup brown sugar

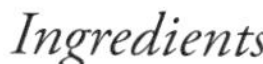

Directions

1. Preheat oven to 400 degrees. Grease muffin pans or coat with cooking spray.
2. Mix flour, baking powder and salt in large bowl.
3. Mix cereal and milk in medium bowl; let stand 3 minutes, stirring once.
4. Add the egg, applesauce and sugar to the cereal.
5. Add cereal mixture to flour and stir just until moistened. Batter will be lumpy.
6. Spoon batter into muffin pans, filling each cup two-thirds full.
7. Bake until golden brown, about 20 minutes. Serve warm.

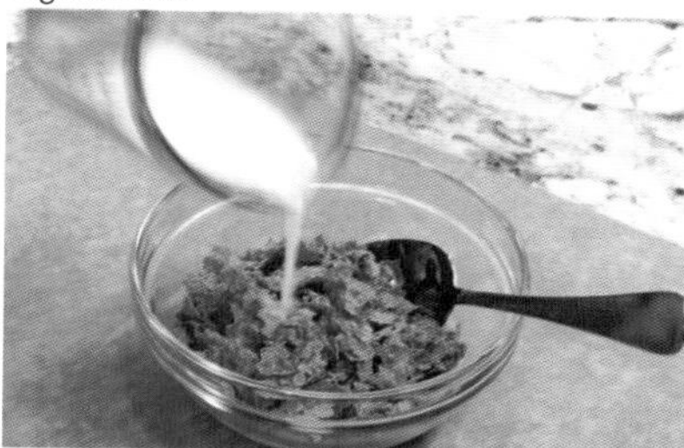
Step 3

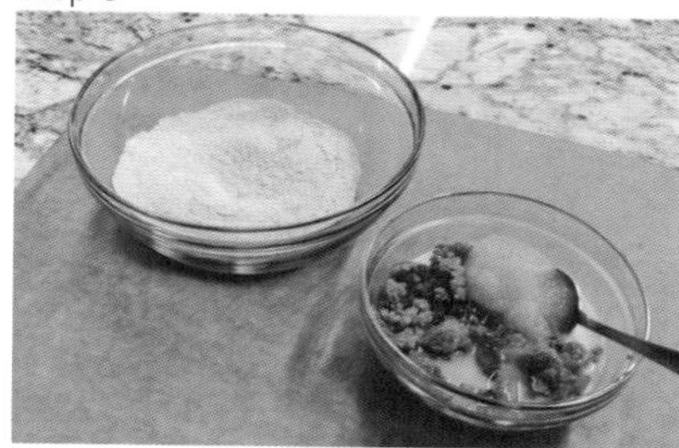
Step 4

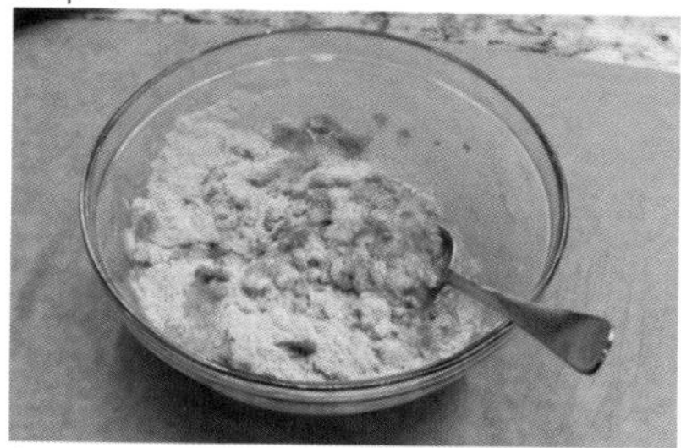
Step 5

Applesauce-Bran Muffins
provide G/B at snack

	Toddler	Pre-School	School Age
Applesauce Muffins	1/2 oz. or 1/2 muffin	1/2 oz. or 1/2 muffin	2 oz. or 2 muffins
Milk	1/2 cup	1/2 cup	1 cup

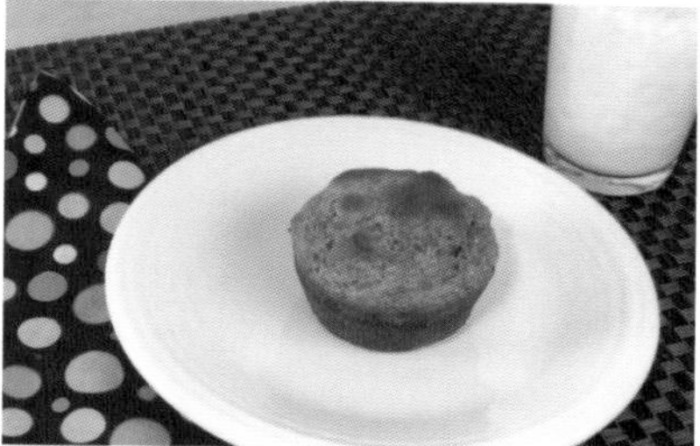
Creditable snack

Autumn Apple Squares

Prep time - 20 minutes
Cook time - 30 minutes
Total time - 50 minutes

Bake in oven

Yield - 16 squares

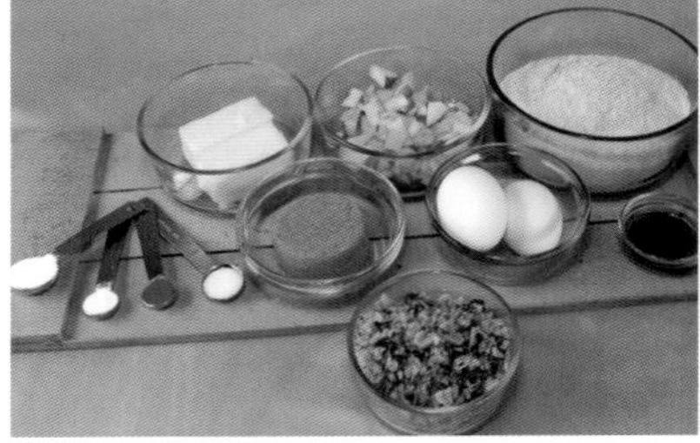
Ingredients

Ingredients

½ cup butter, softened
⅓ cup packed brown sugar
2 eggs
2 teaspoons vanilla extract
2 cups whole wheat flour
1½ teaspoons baking powder
½ teaspoon salt
½ teaspoon ground cinnamon
1 cup apples, chopped
3 ounces walnuts, finely chopped

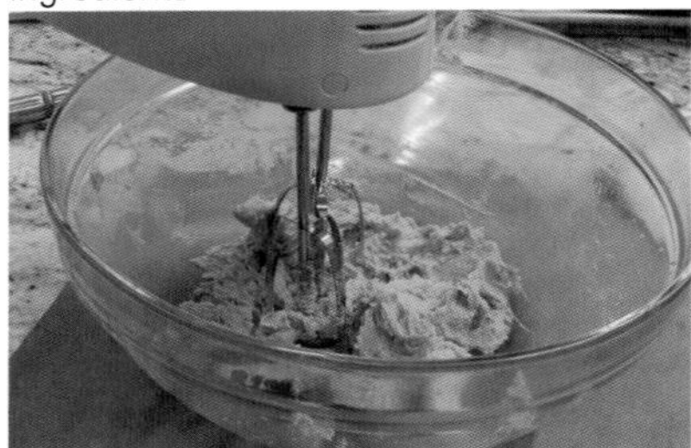
Step 2

Directions

1. Preheat oven to 350 degrees. Grease and flour a 9x13-inch pan or coat with cooking spray and flour.
2. In a large bowl, cream the butter and brown sugar with a mixer until smooth and fluffy, about 3 minutes.
3. Beat in the eggs and vanilla.
4. Combine flour, baking powder, salt and cinnamon in a bowl. Add to the creamed butter and mix until just combined.
5. Fold in the apples and walnuts.
6. Pour batter into the pan and spread evenly.
7. Bake until golden brown, about 30-35 minutes. Bars should spring back when lightly touched.
8. Cool in the pan, then cut into 16 squares.

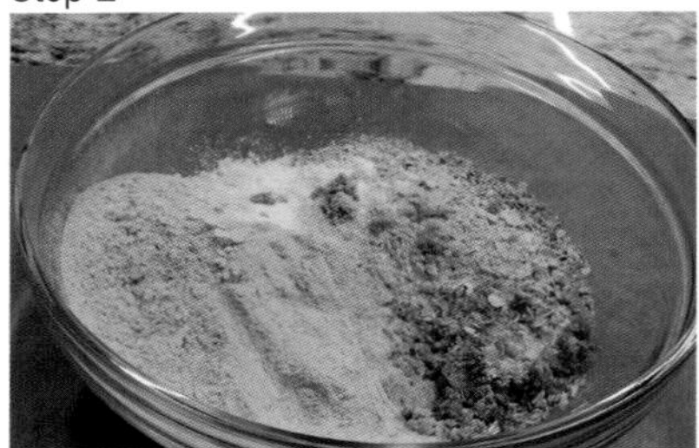
Step 4

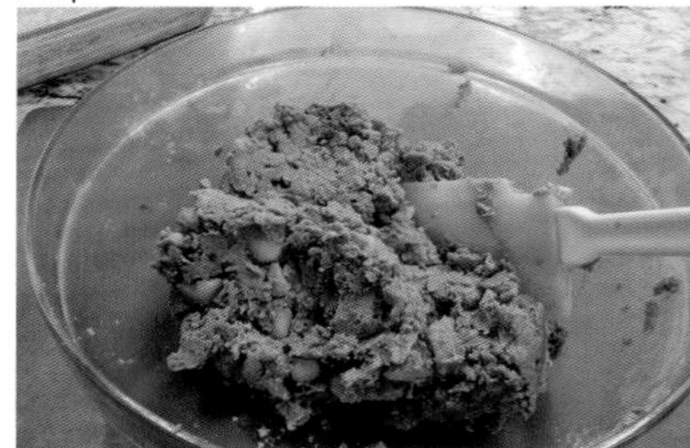
Step 5

Autumn Apple Squares provide G/B at snack			
	Toddler	Pre-School	School Age
Apple Squares	1/2 square	1/2 square	1 square
Milk	1/2 cup	1/2 cup	1 cup

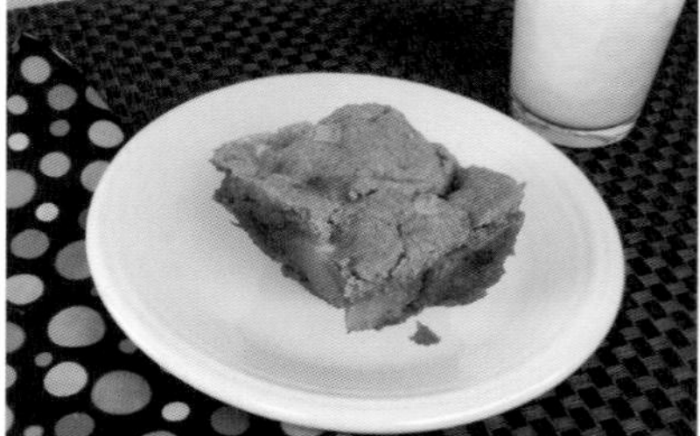
Creditable snack

Breadsticks

Prep time - 25 minutes
Resting time - 35 minutes
Cook time - 10 minutes
Total time - 70 minutes

Bake in oven

Yield - 12 breadsticks

Ingredients

¼ teaspoon sugar
¾ cup warm water
1¼ teaspoons active dry yeast (½ packet)
1¾ cups whole wheat flour
Flour for kneading
⅛ teaspoon garlic powder
1 teaspoon salt
1 tablespoon butter, melted
Marinara sauce for dipping

Directions

1. Preheat oven to 400 degrees. Line a baking sheet with foil or parchment paper, or coat with cooking spray.
2. Combine sugar, water and yeast; let sit until mixture rises and becomes foamy, about 7 minutes.
3. In a large mixing bowl, thoroughly combine flour, garlic powder and salt.
4. Stir yeast mixture into flour with a spoon. As the dough starts to stick together, mix it with your hands.
5. Once dough takes shape, move it from bowl to a lightly floured surface and knead for 3-5 minutes, adding flour as needed so it doesn't stick. Dough should be elastic, not gooey.
6. Roll dough into a foot-long log and cut into 12 equal portions. Roll each portion into a 6-inch breadstick.
7. Arrange breadsticks on baking sheet, cover with a towel and let rise until volume doubles, about 35 minutes.
8. Brush breadsticks with melted butter. Bake until firm and lightly browned, about 10-12 minutes.

Breadsticks provide G/B at snack			
	Toddler	Pre-School	School Age
Breadsticks	1/2 oz or 1/2 stick	1/2 oz. or 1/2 stick	1 oz. or 1 stick
Marinara Sauce	2 tablespoons	2 tablespoons	4 tablespoons
Grapes	1/2 cup	1/2 cup	3/4 cup

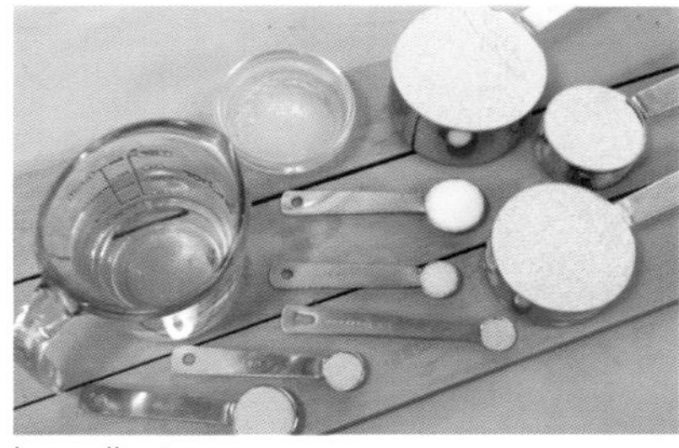

Ingredients

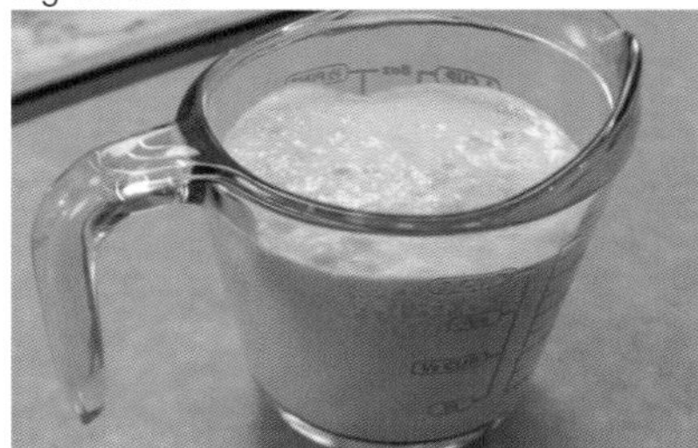

Step 2

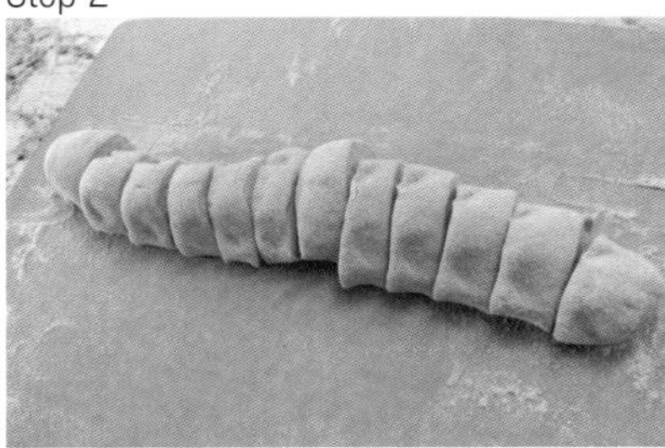

Step 4

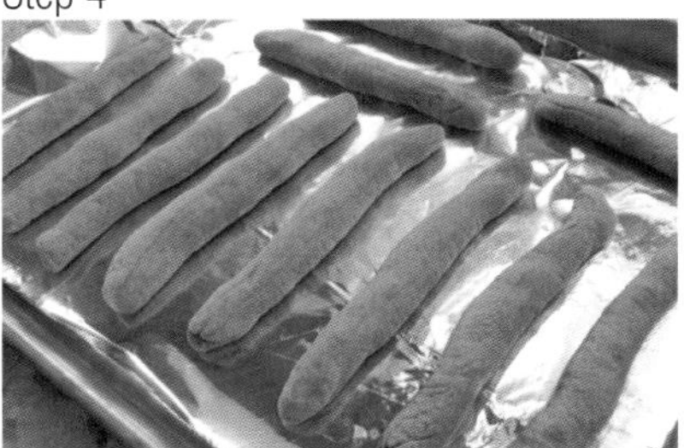

Step 5

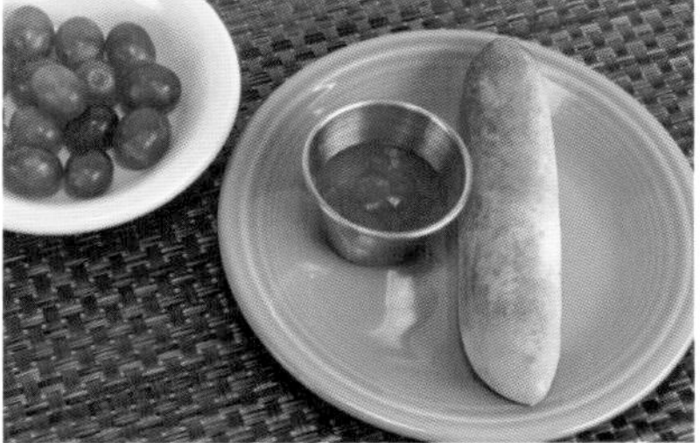

Creditable snack

Polka Dot Twisters

Prep time - 25 minutes
Cook time - 15 minutes
Total time - 40 minutes

Bake in oven

Yield - 12 twisters

Ingredients

2 cups whole wheat flour
1 tablespoon baking powder
1 teaspoon salt
¼ cup butter
1 cup milk
½ cup raisins
Flour for working dough
2 eggs, beaten
2 tablespoons sugar
2 teaspoons ground cinnamon

Directions

1. Preheat oven to 425 degrees. Line a baking sheet with foil or parchment paper, or coat with cooking spray.
2. Combine flour, baking powder and salt. Then cut in butter with a pastry cutter or pulse in a food processor until crumbly.
3. In a large mixing bowl, coat raisins with flour mixture. Add milk and stir for 1 to 2 minutes until soft dough forms. Dough will become less sticky as it is stirred.
4. Transfer dough onto a well-floured surface. With floured hands, shape into a ball, using extra flour as needed to keep from sticking. Divide dough into 12 equal pieces.
5. Roll each piece into a rope 12 inches long. Fold each rope in half and gently twist together.
6. Place on baking sheet and brush with egg. Mix together sugar and cinnamon and sprinkle ½ teaspoon over each twister.
7. Bake for until light golden brown, about 15 minutes. Cool slightly before serving.

Polka Dot Twisters
provide G/B at snack

	Toddler	Pre-School	School Age
Twister	1/2 oz or 1/2 twist	1/2 oz or 1/2 twist	1 oz. or 1 twist
Milk	1/2 cup	1/2 cup	1 cup

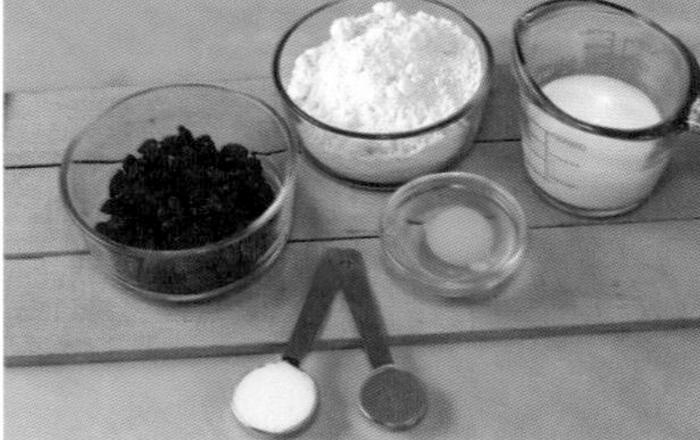

Ingredients

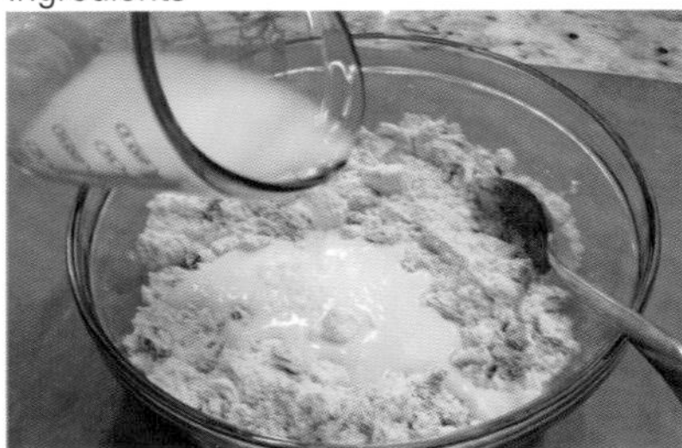

Step 3

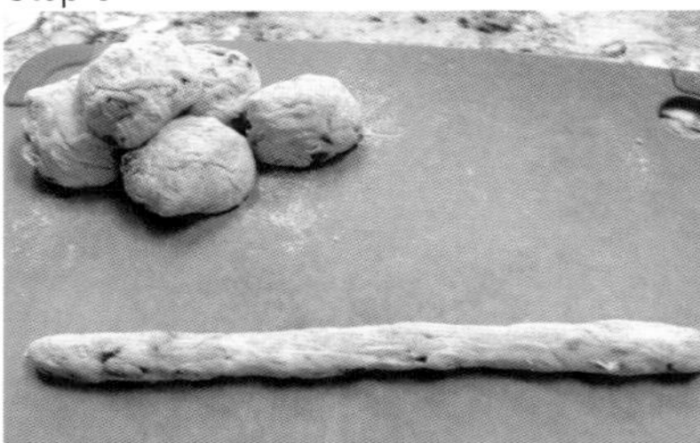

Step 5

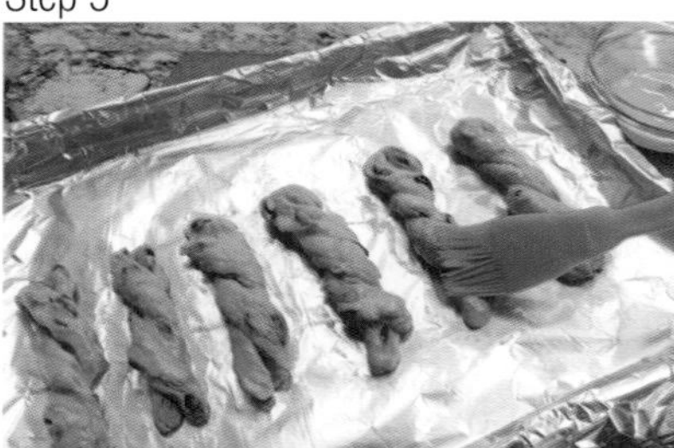

Step 6

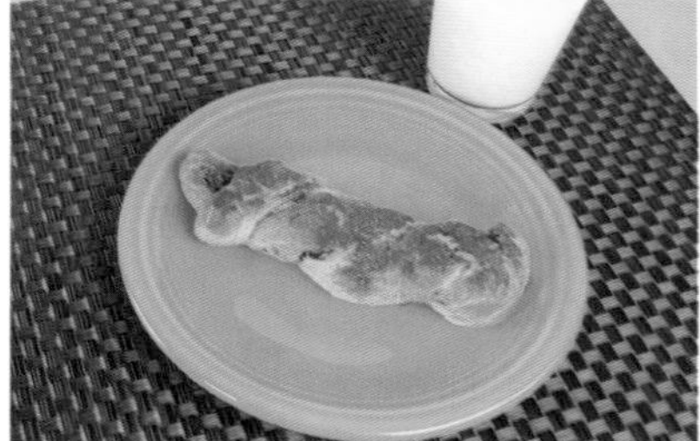

Creditable snack

Pretzel Sticks

Prep time - 15 minutes
Cook time - 10 minutes
Total time - 25 minutes

Bake in oven

Yield - 12 pretzel sticks

Ingredients

1 cup whole wheat flour
1 teaspoon sugar
1 teaspoon baking powder
⅛ teaspoon salt
¼ cup butter, cut into small pieces
¼ cup milk

Directions

1. Preheat oven to 350 degrees. Line a baking sheet with foil or parchment paper, or coat with cooking spray.
2. Mix together the flour, baking powder, sugar and salt. Cut in the butter with two knives or a pastry cutter.
3. Add milk slowly, stirring until all ingredients are wet. All of the milk may not be needed.
4. Once the dough is formed, divide into 12 small balls. Roll balls into 6-inch lengths.
5. Bake for 10-12 minutes or until golden brown.

Pretzel Sticks provide G/B at snack			
	Toddler	Pre-School	School Age
Pretzel Sticks	1 pretzel	1 pretzel	2 pretzels
Nectarines	1/2 cup	1/2 cup	3/4 cup

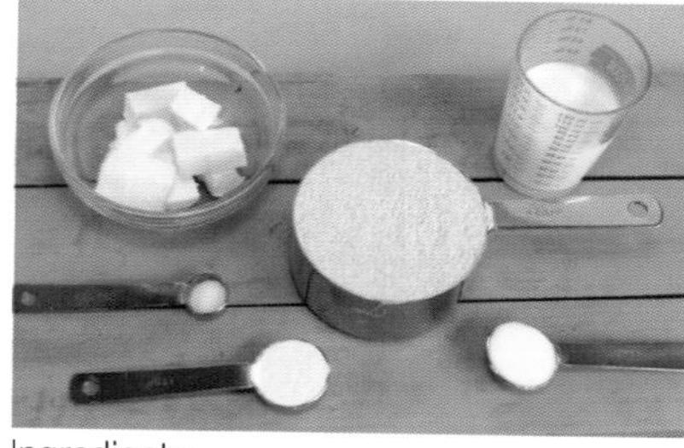

Ingredients

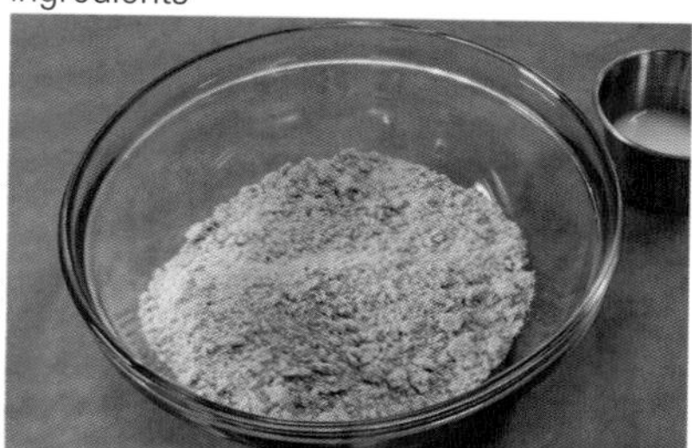

Step 3

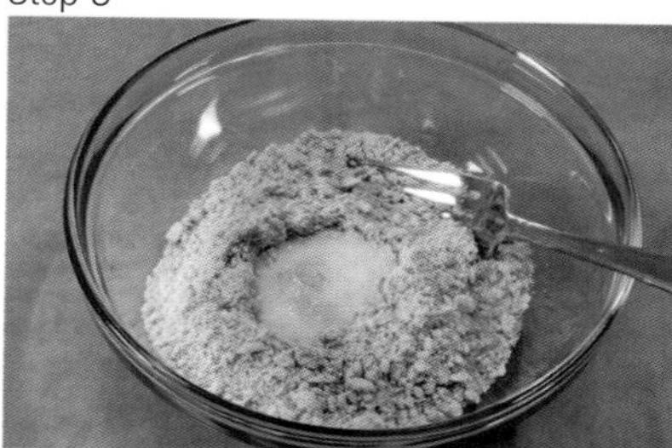

Step 5

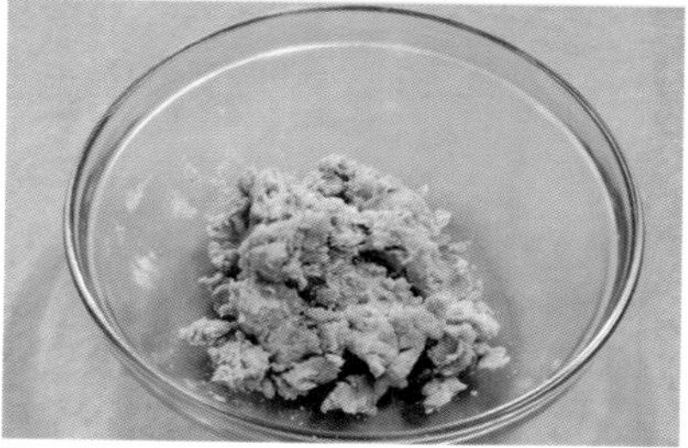

Step 6

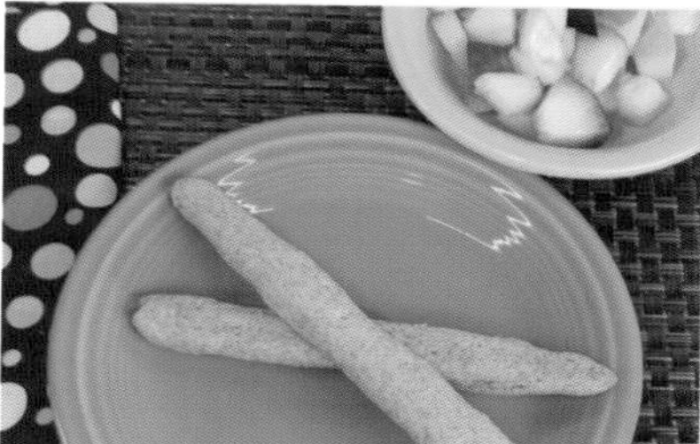

Creditable snack

Pretzel Knots

Prep time - 25 minutes
Cook time - 10 minutes
Total time - 35 minutes

Bake in oven

Yield - 12 pretzel knots

Ingredients

1¼ teaspoons sugar, divided
¾ cup water
1¼ teaspoons active dry yeast (½ packet)
1¾ cups whole wheat flour
Flour for kneading
1 teaspoon salt
1 egg, beaten
⅛ teaspoon kosher salt

Directions

1. Preheat to 425 degrees. Line a baking sheet with foil or parchment paper, or coat with cooking spray.
2. Combine ¼ teaspoon of the sugar with water and yeast; let sit until mixture rises and becomes foamy, about 7 minutes.
3. In a large mixing bowl, thoroughly combine remaining sugar, flour and salt.
4. Stir water mixture into flour mixture with a spoon. When mixture starts to stick together, mix it with your hands.
5. Once dough takes shape, move from bowl to lightly floured surface and knead for 3-5 minutes, adding flour as needed to keep it from sticking to your hands. Dough should be elastic, not gooey.
6. Roll dough into a foot-long log and cut into 12 equal portions. Roll each portion into a 1-foot rope and shape into a knot.

continued on next page

Pretzel Knots provide G/B at snack			
	Toddler	Pre-School	School Age
Pretzel Knots	1/2 pretzel	1/2 pretzel	1 pretzel
Milk	1/2 cup	1/2 cup	3/4 cup

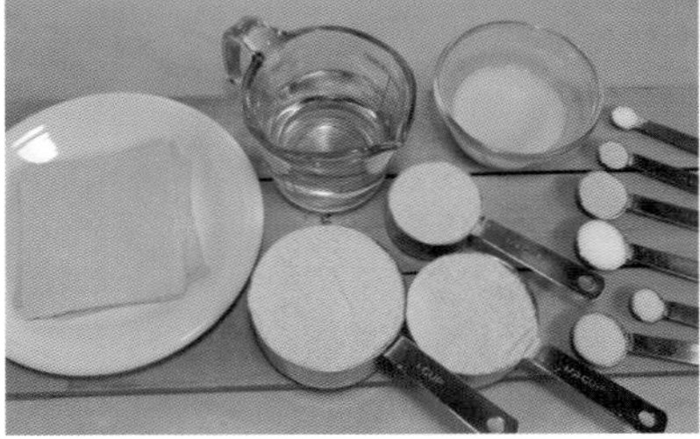

Ingredients

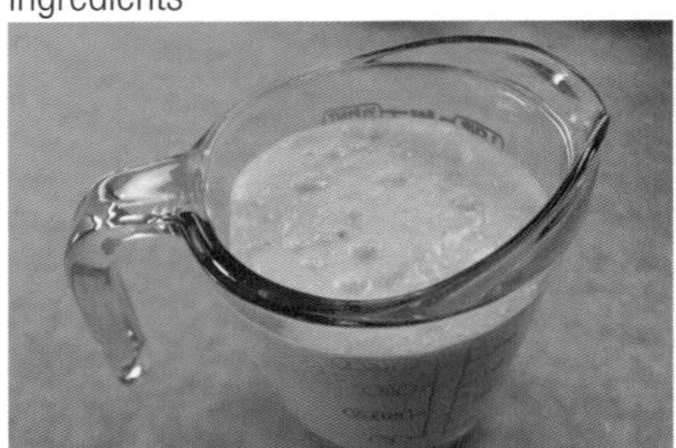

Step 2

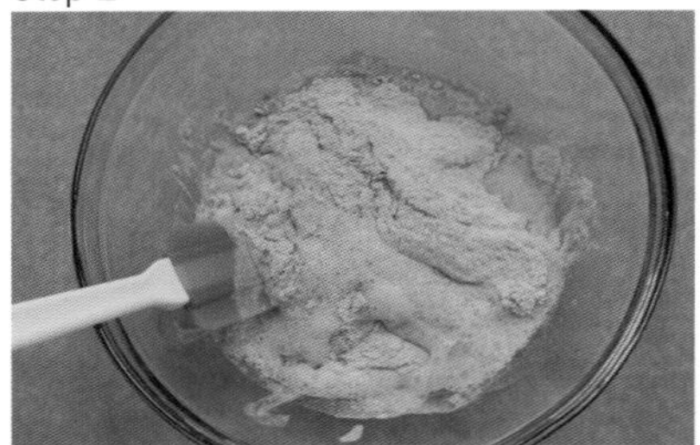

Step 3

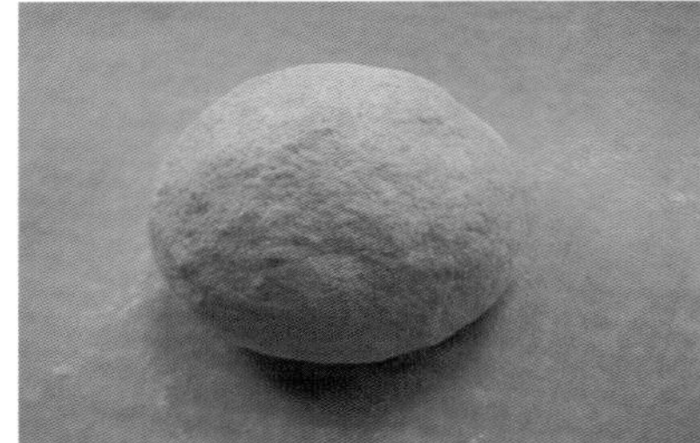

Step 5

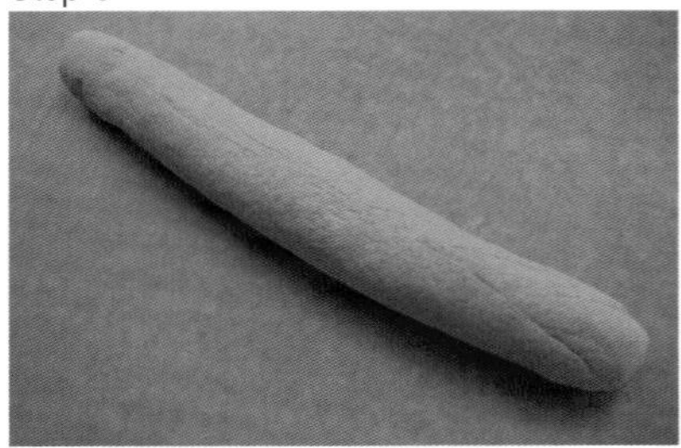

Step 6a

7. Place on baking sheet; brush with whisked egg and sprinkle with kosher salt.
8. Bake about 10 minutes, until pretzels have expanded, are firm to the touch and just beginning to brown. Remove from oven.
9. Reposition oven rack to about 6 inches below the broiler element and preheat broiler.
10. Place baking sheet under broiler for 30-60 seconds, until pretzels are browned. Remove from oven and cool.

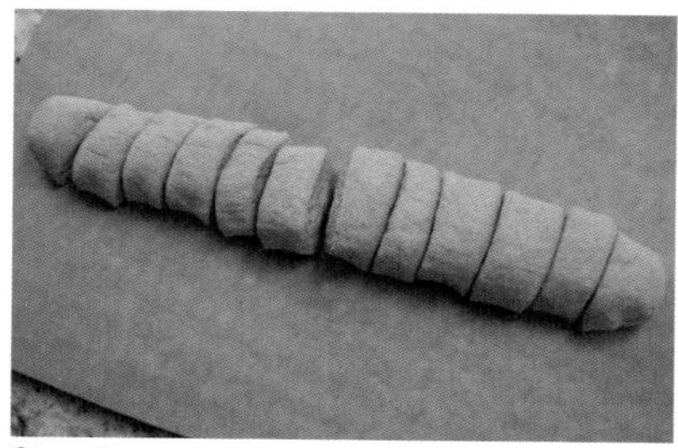
Step 6b

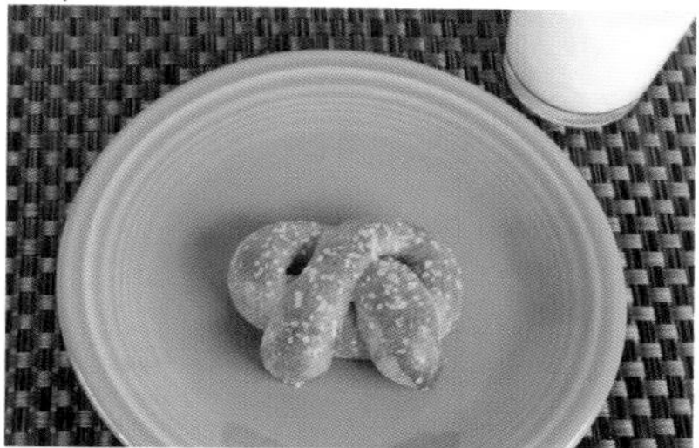
Creditable snack

Pretzel Melts

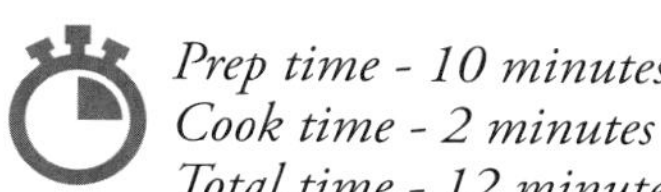
Prep time - 10 minutes
Cook time - 2 minutes
Total time - 12 minutes

Bake in oven

Yield - 12 pretzel melts

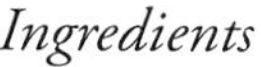
Ingredients

12 Pretzel Knots
12 1-ounce slices cheddar cheese

Directions

1. Preheat oven to 350 degrees. Line a baking sheet with foil or parchment paper, or coat with cooking spray.
2. Slice baked Pretzel Knots in half and place bottom halves on baking sheet.
3. Place a 1-ounce slice of cheese on bottom half, followed by top half of pretzel.
4. Bake pretzels until cheese melts, about 2-5 minutes.
5. Remove from oven, cool slightly and serve.

***Tip**: Make Pretzel Knots ahead of time and add the cheese just before serving.*

Pretzel Melts
provide G/B and M/MA at snack

	Toddler	Pre-School	School Age
Pretzel Melts	1/2 pretzel	1/2 pretzel	1 pretzel

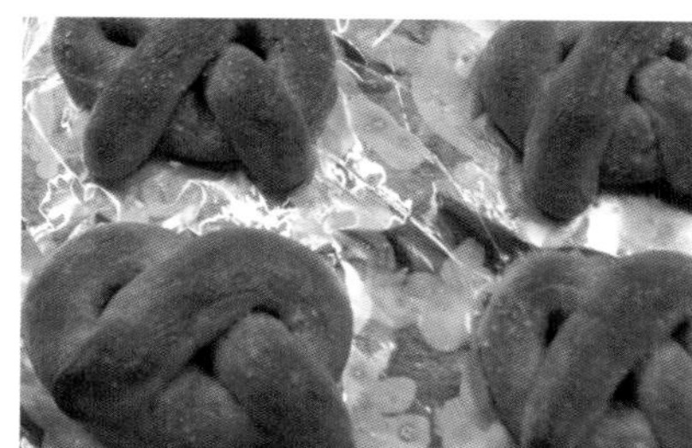
Step 4

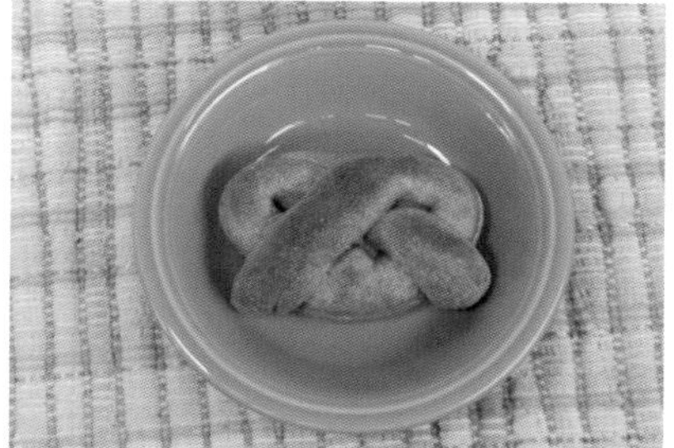
Creditable snack

Pita Nachos

Prep time - 10 minutes
Cook time - 2 minutes
Total time - 12 minutes

Bake in oven

Yield - 18 nachos

Ingredients

3 whole wheat pita bread rounds, at least 1½ ounces each
¾ cup mild salsa
¾ cup (3 ounces) shredded cheddar cheese

Directions

1. Move oven rack to about 6 inches below the broiler and preheat broiler. Line a baking sheet with foil or coat with cooking spray.
2. Top each pita round with ¼ cup salsa and ¼ cup cheese.
3. Cut each pita round into 6 triangles and place in a single layer on the baking sheet.
4. Broil until cheese has melted and edges of nachos are crisp, about 2 to 4 minutes.

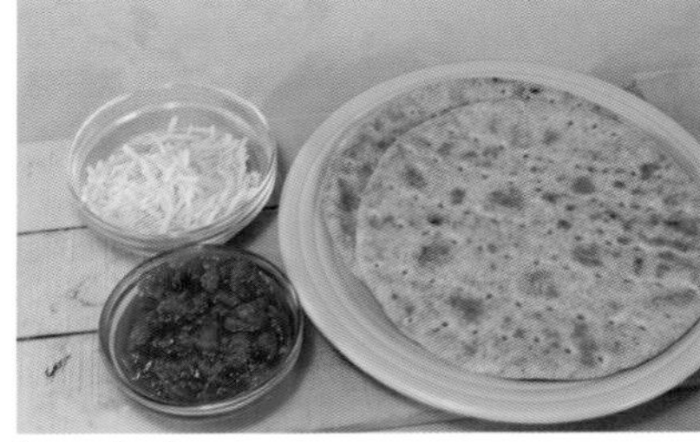
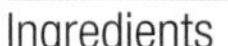
Ingredients

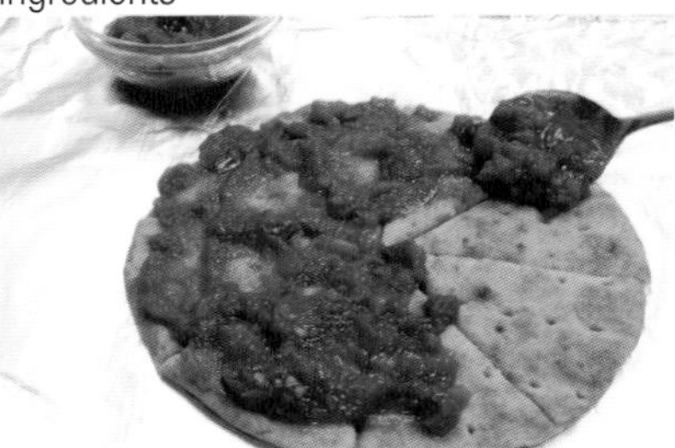
Step 2

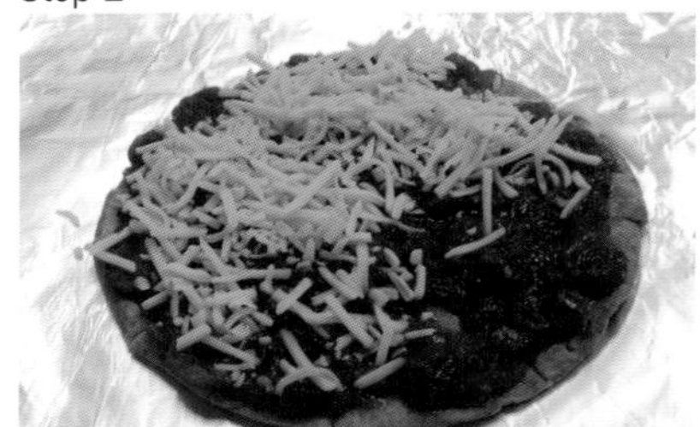
Step 3

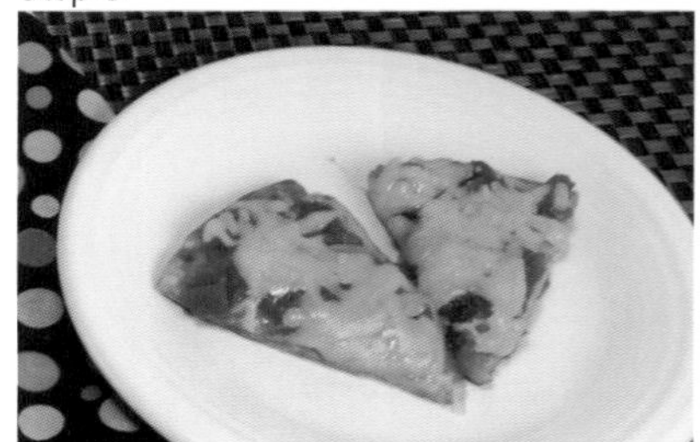
Creditable snack

Pita Nachos provide G/B and M/MA at snack			
	Toddler	Pre-School	School Age
Pita Nachos	3 triangles	3 triangles	6 triangles

Sweet Bagel Chips

Prep time - 10 minutes
Cook time - 10 minutes
Total time - 20 minutes

Bake in oven

Yield - 18 bagel chips

Ingredients

3 whole wheat bagels, at least 1½ ounces each
1 tablespoon vegetable oil
1 tablespoon sugar
1 teaspoon ground cinnamon

Directions

1. Preheat oven to 400 degrees. Line a baking sheet with foil or parchment paper, or coat with cooking spray.
2. In a small bowl, combine the sugar and cinnamon.
3. Cut each bagel into 6 slices. Brush one side of each bagel slice with oil and sprinkle with cinnamon/sugar.
4. Place bagel slices on baking sheet, cinnamon/sugar side up. Bake until crisp, about 10 minutes.

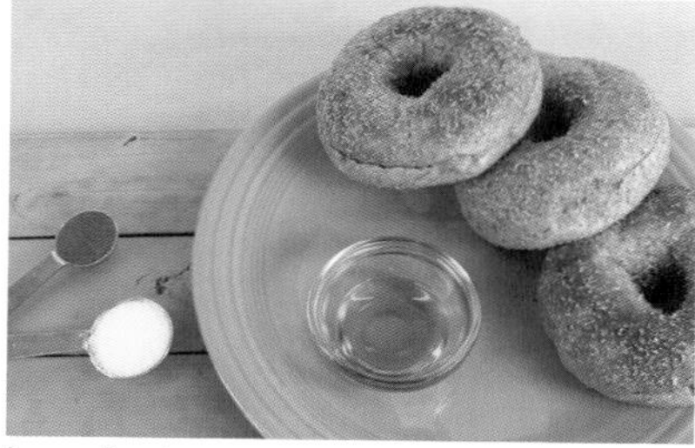
Ingredients

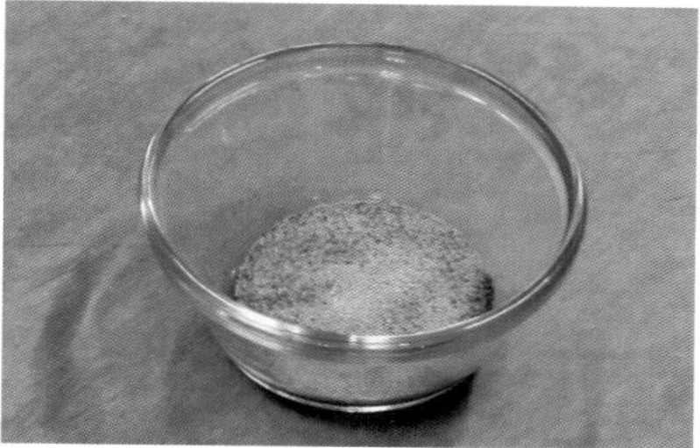
Step 2

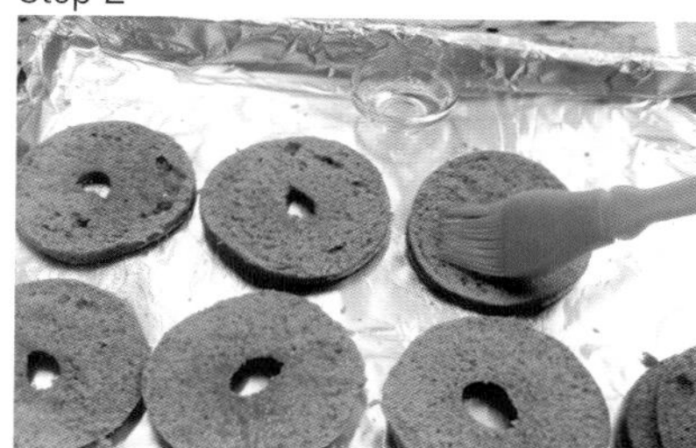
Step 3

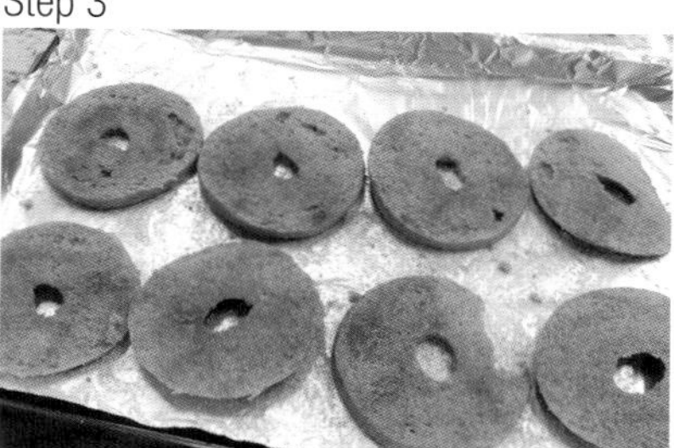
Step 4

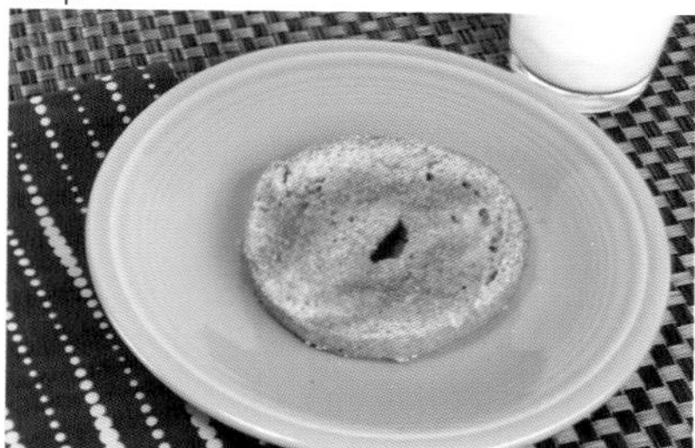
Creditable snack

Sweet Bagel Chips
provide G/B at snack

	Toddler	Pre-School	School Age
Bagel Chips	1/2 oz. or 2 chips	1/2 oz. or 2 chips	1 oz. or 4 chips
Milk	1/2 cup	1/2 cup	1 cup

Taco Cereal Trail Mix

Prep time - 10 minutes
Cook time - 5 minutes
Total time - 15 minutes

Bake in microwave

Yield - 3¾ cups

Ingredients

2 cups bite-sized square corn cereal
¾ cup bite-sized cheese crackers
¾ cup bite-sized pretzel twists
⅓ cup salted peanuts
1½ tablespoons vegetable oil
1 tablespoon water
1 tablespoon taco seasoning mix (½ packet)

Directions

1. In large microwavable bowl, mix cereal, crackers, pretzels and peanuts.
2. In small bowl, stir together oil, water and taco seasoning mix. Pour over cereal mixture, stirring until evenly coated.
3. Microwave, uncovered, on high about 5 minutes, stirring every 1½ minutes, until mixture begins to brown.
4. Spread on waxed paper or foil to cool. Store in an airtight container.

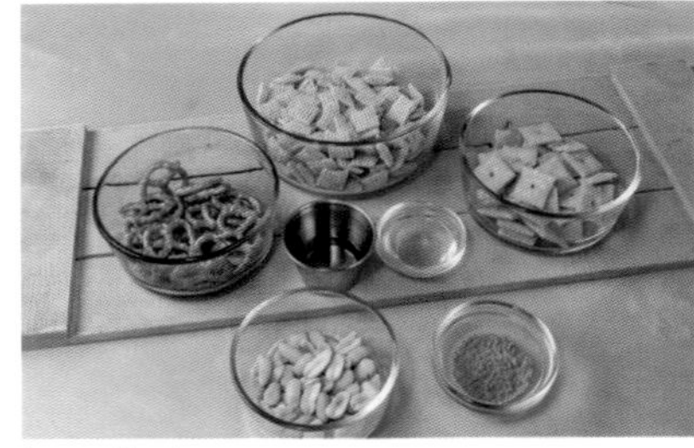

Ingredients

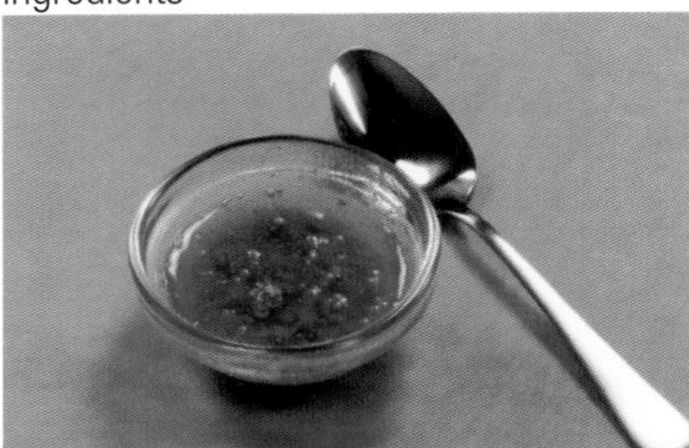

Step 2

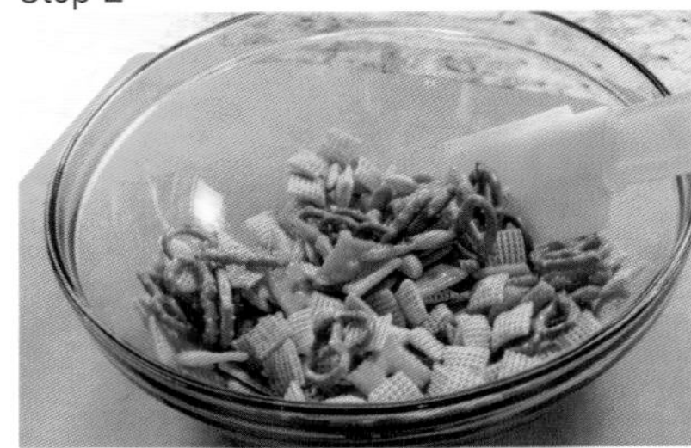

Step 3

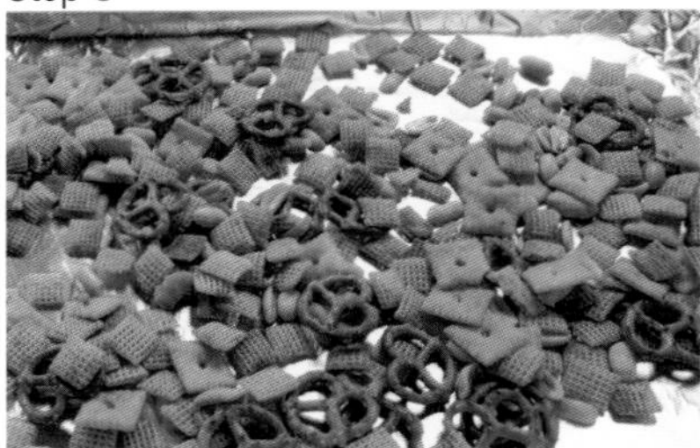

Step 4

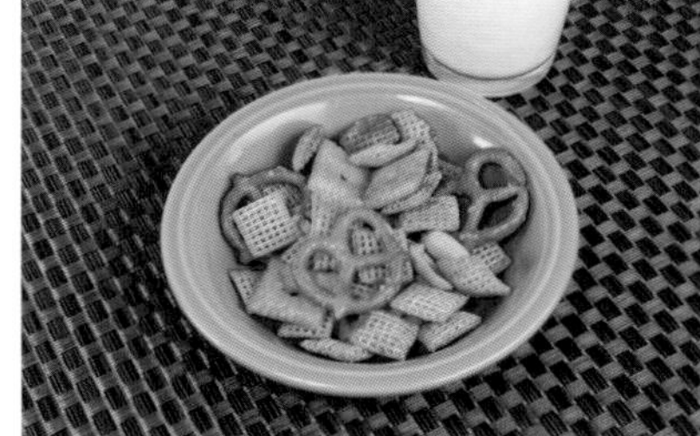

Creditable snack

Taco Cereal Trail Mix
provides G/B at snack

	Toddler	Pre-School	School Age
Taco Cereal Mix	1/2 cup	1/2 cup	1 cup
Milk	1/2 cup	1/2 cup	1 cup

Black Bean Hummus

Prep time - 15 minutes
Cook time - 0 minutes
Total time - 15 minutes

No cook, no bake

Yield - 2¼ cups

Ingredients

2¼ cups black beans, rinsed and drained
3 tablespoons water
3 tablespoons vegetable oil
2 tablespoons lime juice
1 teaspoon garlic, minced
½ teaspoon ground cumin
½ teaspoon salt

Directions

1. Using a blender or food processor, add all ingredients and process until smooth.

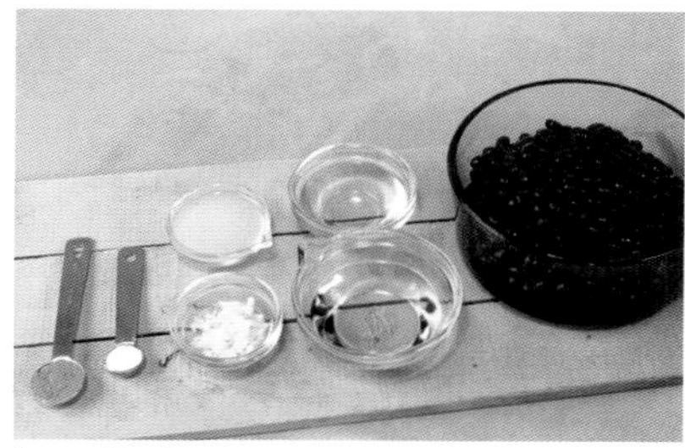

Ingredients

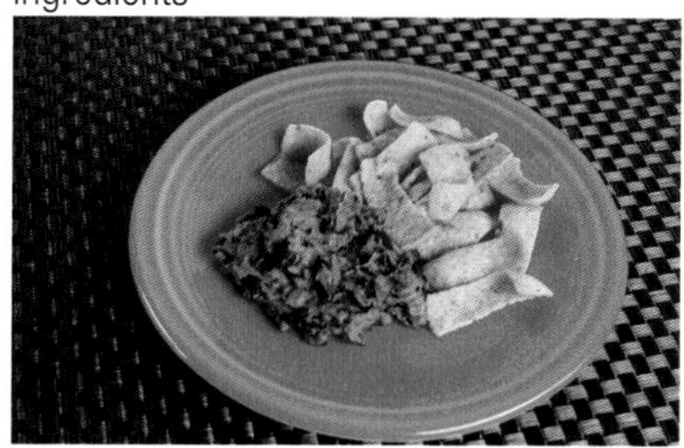

Creditable snack

Black Bean Hummus provides M/MA at snack			
	Toddler	Pre-School	School Age
Hummus	1/4 cup	1/4 cup	1/2 cup
Corn Chips	1/2 ounce	1/2 ounce	1 ounce

Caramel Yogurt Dip

Prep time - 5 minutes
Cook time - 5 minutes
Total time - 10 minutes

Cook on stovetop

Yield - 1½ cups

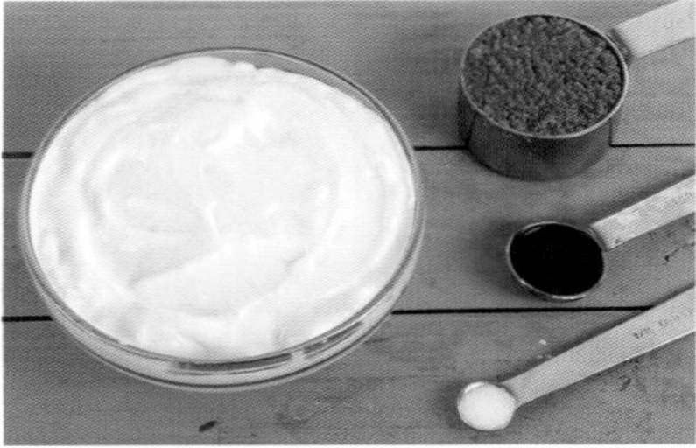
Ingredients

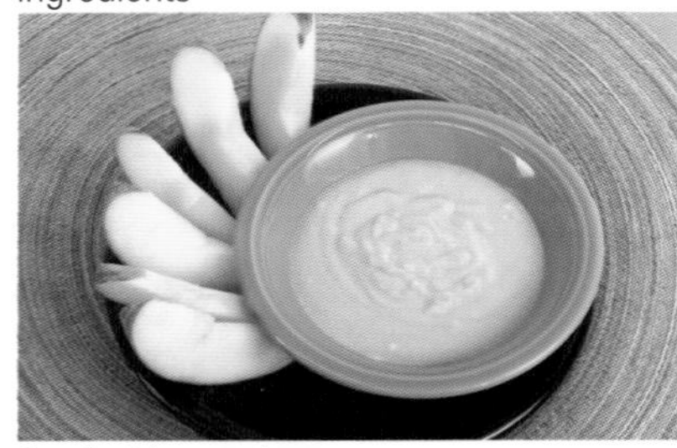
Creditable snack

Ingredients

¼ cup brown sugar
⅛ teaspoon salt
1 teaspoon pure vanilla extract
1½ cups plain yogurt

Directions

1. Combine brown sugar, salt and vanilla in a saucepan. Cook and stir constantly over medium-low heat until sugar has dissolved and the mixture has thickened, about 5-7 minutes.
2. Remove from heat and stir in yogurt until combined.
3. Transfer to a serving bowl. It will thicken more as it cools.

Caramel Yogurt Dip provides M/MA at snack

	Toddler	Pre-School	School Age
Caramel Yogurt Dip	1/4 cup	1/4 cup	1/2 cup
Apple Slices	1/2 cup	1/2 cup	3/4 cup

Cinnamon Yogurt Dip

Prep time - 5 minutes
Cook time - 0 minutes
Total time - 5 minutes

No cook, no bake

Yield - 1½ cups

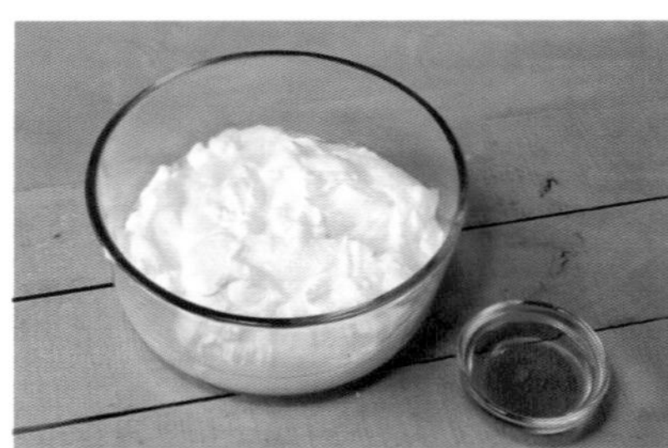
Ingredients

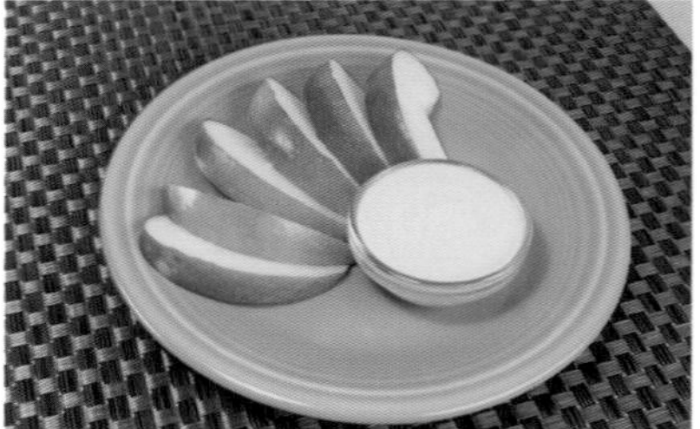
Creditable snack

Ingredients

1½ cups vanilla yogurt*
1 teaspoon ground cinnamon

Directions

1. Mix all ingredients together.

**Maximum allowable sugar in yogurt is 23 grams per 6 ounces*

Cinnamon Yogurt Dip provides M/MA at snack

	Toddler	Pre-School	School Age
Cinn. Yogurt Dip	1/4 cup	1/4 cup	1/2 cup
Apple Slices	1/2 cup	1/2 cup	3/4 cup

Carrot Dip

Prep time - 15 minutes
Cook time - 0 minutes
Total time - 15 minutes

No cook, no bake

Yield - 4 cups

Ingredients

3 cups carrots, finely shredded
1 cup plain yogurt
1 tablespoon vegetable oil
½ teaspoon salt

Directions

1. Mix all ingredients together.

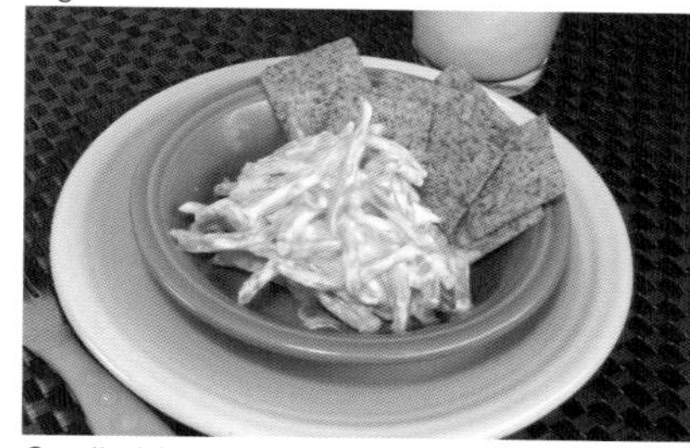

Ingredients

Creditable snack

Carrot Dip provides VEG at snack

	Toddler	Pre-School	School Age
Carrot Dip	1/2 cup	2/3 cup	1 cup
Wheat Crackers	1/2 ounce	1/2 ounce	3/4 ounce

Corn Salsa

Prep time - 10 minutes
Cook time - 0 minutes
Total time - 10 minutes

No cook, no bake

Yield - 3 cups

Ingredients

1 cup fresh tomatoes, diced
1 cup whole kernel corn, cooked and cooled
1 cup black beans, rinsed and drained
1 teaspoon taco seasoning mix

Directions

1. Mix all ingredients together.

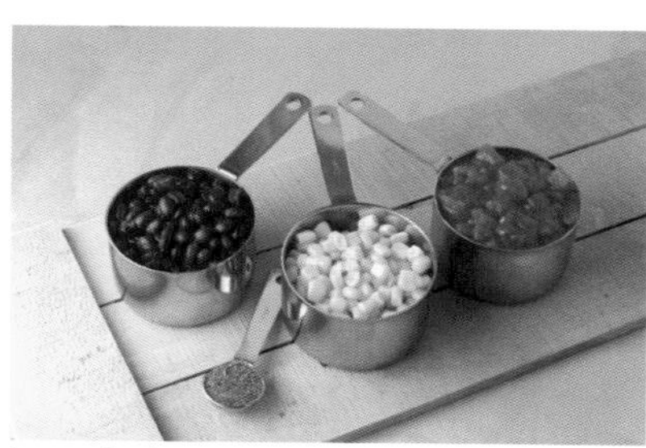

Ingredients

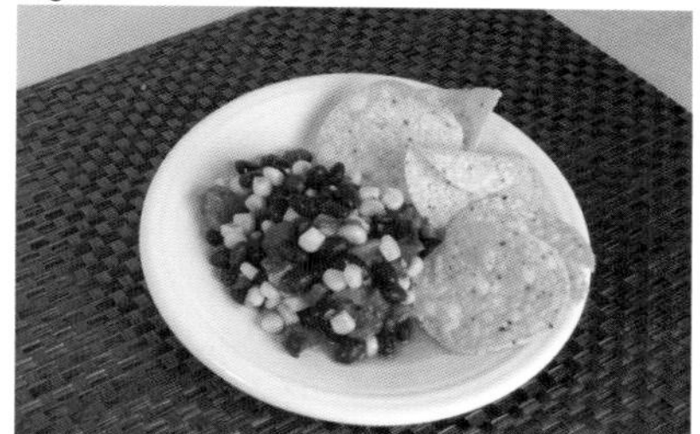

Creditable snack

Corn Salsa provides VEG at snack

	Toddler	Pre-School	School Age
Corn Salsa	1/2 cup	1/2 cup	3/4 cup
Tortilla Chips	1/2 ounce	1/2 ounce	1 ounce

Lemon Fruit Dip

Prep time - 5 minutes
Cook time - 0 minutes
Total time - 5 minutes

No cook, no bake

Yield - 1½ cups

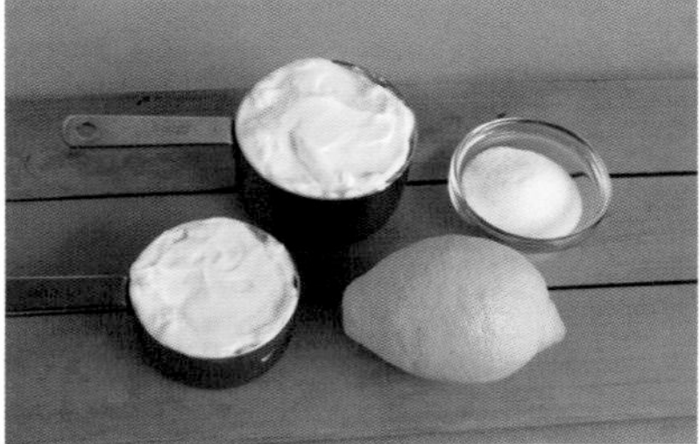
Ingredients

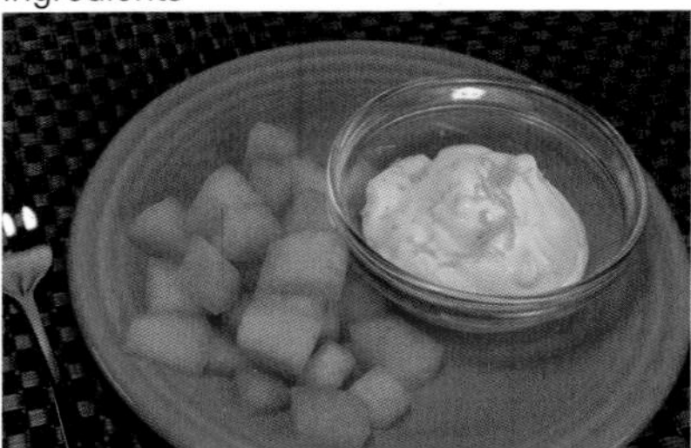
Creditable snack

Ingredients

¼ cup fresh lemon juice
1 tablespoon lemon zest
2 tablespoons sugar or to taste
1½ cups plain Greek yogurt

Directions

1. Mix all ingredients together.

Lemon Fruit Dip provides M/MA at snack			
	Toddler	Pre-School	School Age
Lemon Fruit Dip	1/4 cup	1/4 cup	1/2 cup
Melon Chunks	1/2 cup	1/2 cup	3/4 cup

Orange Bowl Dip

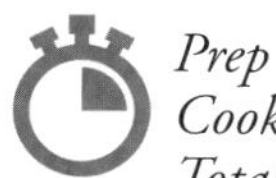

Prep time - 15 minutes
Cook time - 0 minutes
Total time - 15 minutes

No cook, no bake

Yield - 6 orange bowls

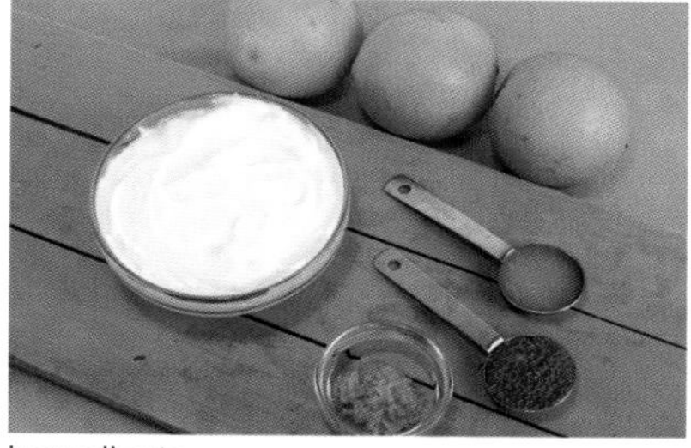

Ingredients

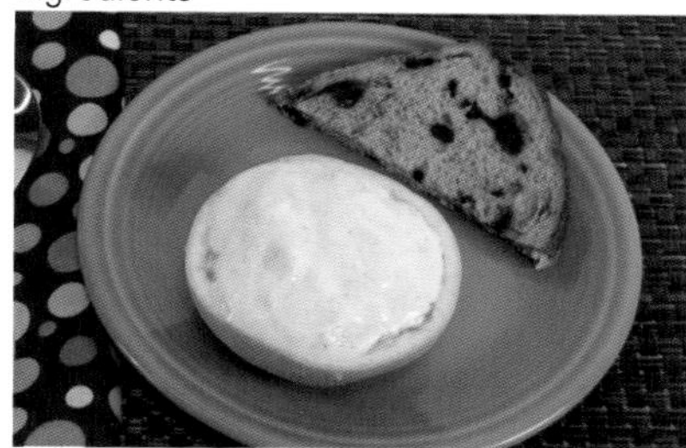

Creditable snack

Ingredients

3 whole oranges

1½ cups plain yogurt

1 tablespoon orange zest

1 tablespoon brown sugar, or to taste

1 tablespoon orange juice, squeezed from the orange pulp

Directions

1. Cut each orange in half and scoop out the pulp carefully, making 6 orange "bowls." Cut a small slice off the bottom of each "bowl" so they don't tip over.
2. Dice the orange pulp. Mix well with remaining ingredients.
3. To serve, portion the orange and yogurt mixture evenly among the six "bowls."

Orange Bowl Dip
provides M/MA at snack

	Toddler	Pre-School	School Age
Orange Bowl Dip	1/4 cup	1/4 cup	1/2 cup
Toast	1/2 oz. or 1/2 slice	1/2 oz. or 1/2 slice	1 oz. or 1 slice

Spinach Ranch Dip

Prep time - 15 minutes
Cook time - 0 minutes
Total time - 15 minutes

No cook, no bake

Yield - 2 cups

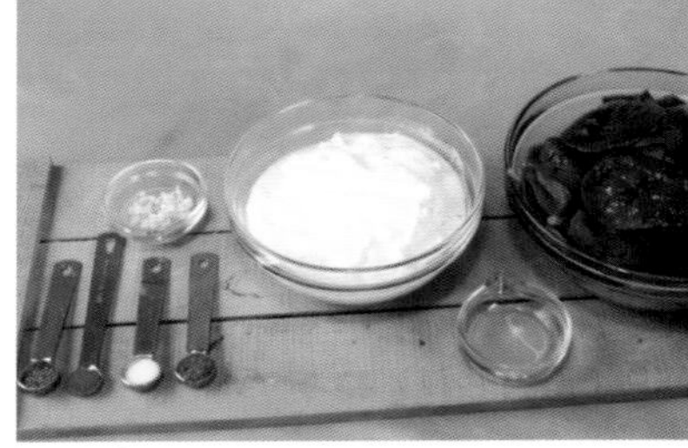
Ingredients

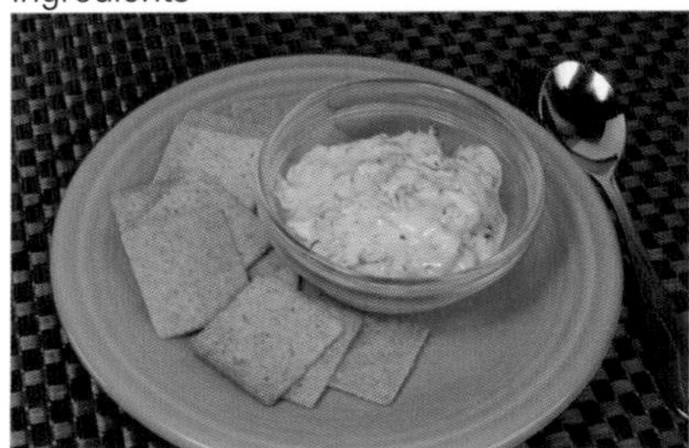
Creditable snack

Ingredients

1 cup fresh spinach, chopped
1½ cups plain Greek yogurt
¼ teaspoon fresh lemon juice
1 teaspoon fresh garlic, minced
¼ teaspoon dried dill
⅛ teaspoon paprika
⅛ teaspoon kosher salt
⅛ teaspoon black pepper

Directions

1. Thoroughly combine all ingredients.

Spinach Ranch Dip provides M/MA at snack			
	Toddler	Pre-School	School Age
Spinach Dip	1/3 cup	1/3 cup	2/3 cup
Wheat Crackers	1/2 ounce	1/2 ounce	3/4 ounce

American Flag Toast

Prep time - 15 minutes
Cook time - 5 minutes
Total time - 20 minutes

Toast in toaster or in oven

Yield - 6 slices

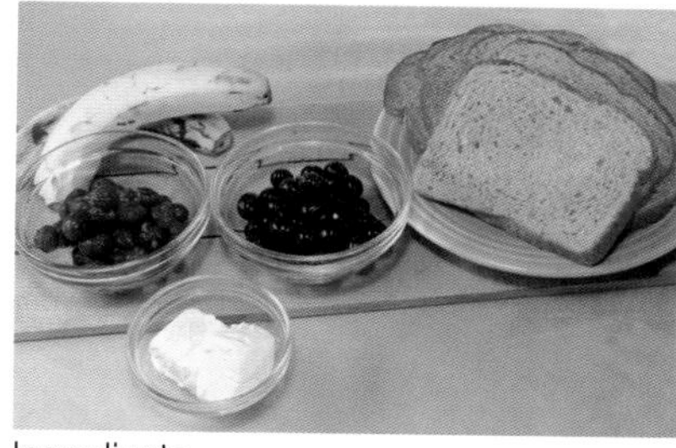
Ingredients

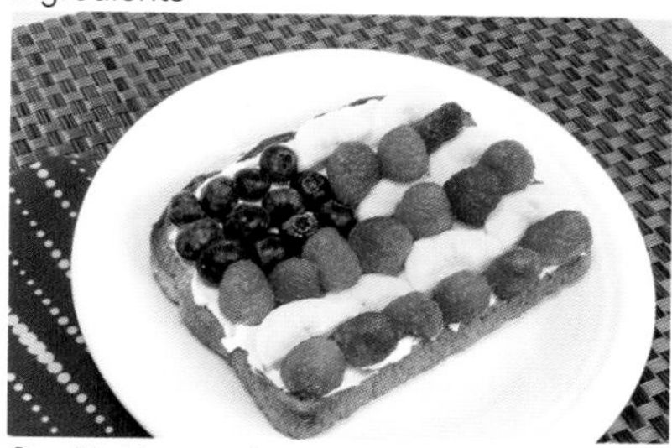
Creditable snack

Ingredients

6 slices whole grain bread, at least 1½ ounces each
⅜ cup cream cheese
¾ cup blueberries
2 medium bananas
¾ cup raspberries

Directions

1. Toast bread.
2. Slice bananas into half circles.
3. Spread a thin layer of cream cheese on toast.
4. Place blueberries in the upper left corner to represent the "stars."
5. Alternate rows of raspberries and banana slices to represent the "stripes" on the United States flag.

American Flag Toast
provides G/B and FR at snack

	Toddler	Pre-School	School Age
Flag Toast	1 slice	1 slice	2 slices

Baked Apple Pretzel Boats

Prep time - 15 minutes
Cook time - 35 minutes
Total time - 50 minutes

Bake in oven

Yield - 6 apple halves

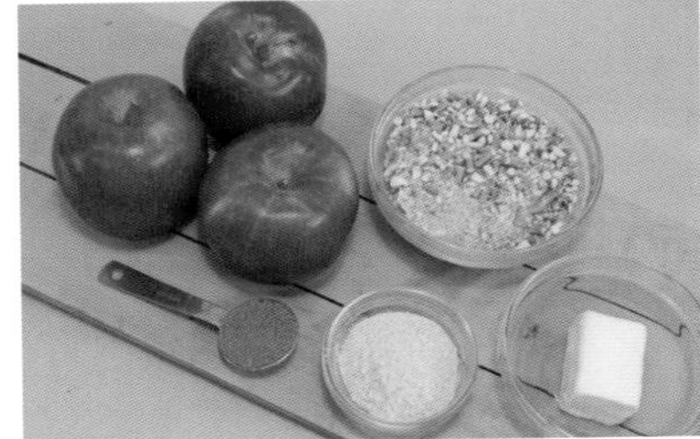

Ingredients

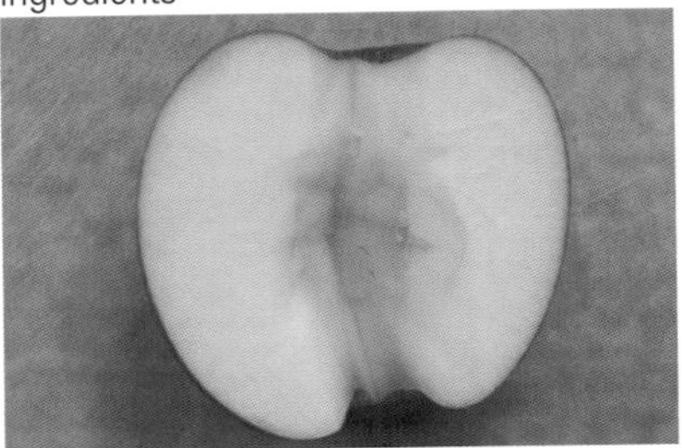

Step 2

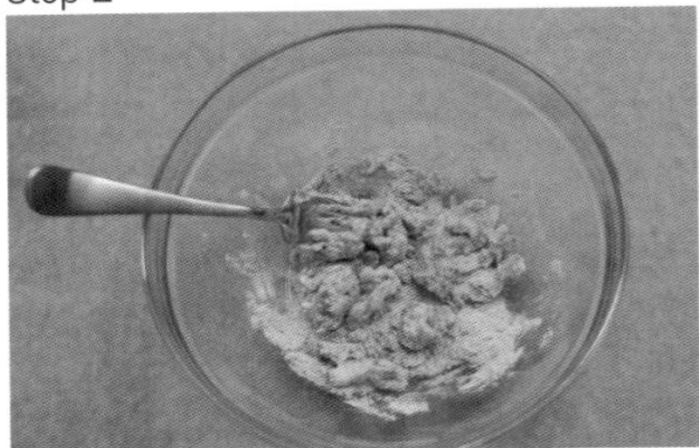

Step 3

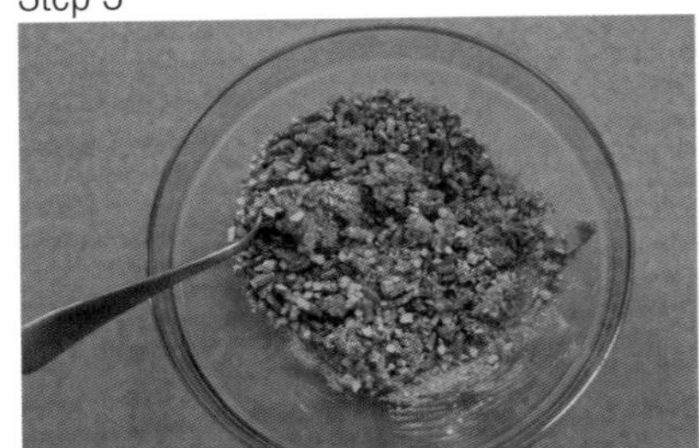

Step 4

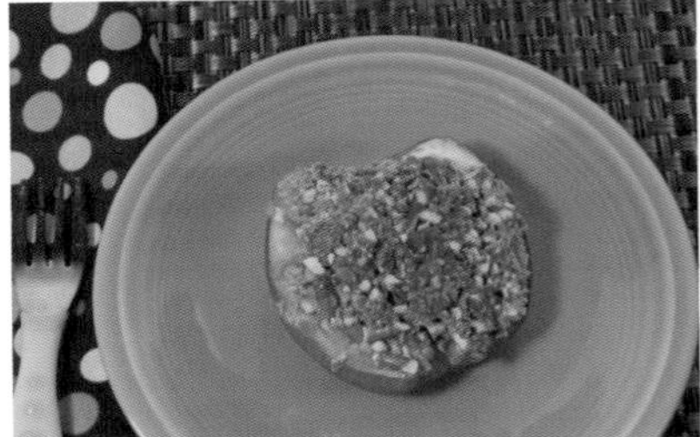

Creditable snack

Ingredients

3 tablespoons unsalted butter, softened
3 tablespoons whole wheat flour
1 tablespoon brown sugar
3 ounces pretzels, crushed
3 apples, halved and cored

Directions

1. Preheat oven to 375 degrees. Line a baking sheet with foil or parchment paper, or coat with cooking spray.
2. Thoroughly combine butter, flour and brown sugar.
3. Mix in pretzels.
4. Portion mixture on top of each apple half.
5. Bake until apples are soft and topping is crisp, about 35 to 40 minutes.

Baked Apple Pretzel Boats provide FR at snack			
	Toddler	Pre-School	School Age
Apple Pretzel Boats	1/2 apple	1/2 apple	1 apple

Creamy Dreamy Whipped Fruit

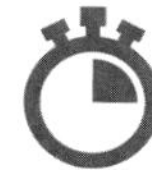

Prep time - 10 minutes
Cook time - 0 minutes
Total time - 10 minutes

No cook, no bake

Yield - 3 cups

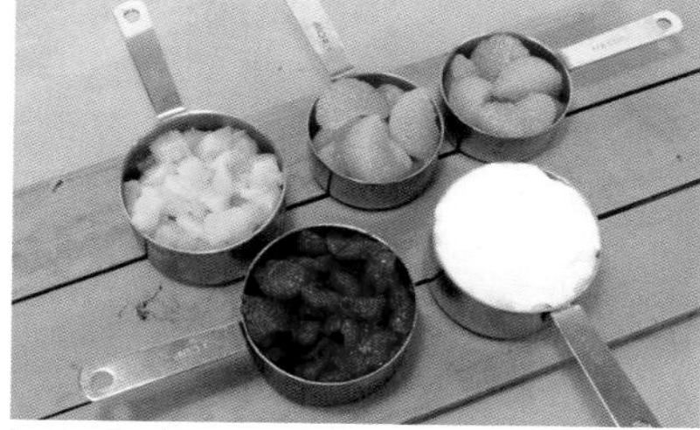
Ingredients

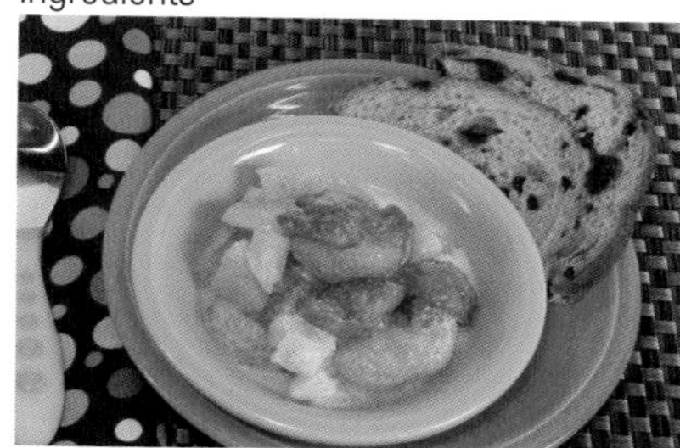
Creditable snack

Ingredients

1 cup whipped topping
1 cup mandarin oranges, drained
1 cup pineapple tidbits, drained
1 cup strawberries, sliced
—if frozen, thawed and drained

Directions

1. In large bowl, gently mix all ingredients together.

Creamy Dreamy Whipped Fruit provides FR at snack			
	Toddler	Pre-School	School Age
Whipped Fruit	1/2 cup	1/2 cup	3/4 cup
Toast	1/2 oz. or 1/2 slice	1/2 oz. or 1/2 slice	1 oz. or 1 slice

Fresh Fruit Cone

Prep time - 15 minutes
Cook time - 0 minutes
Total time - 15 minutes

No cook, no bake

Yield - 6 cones

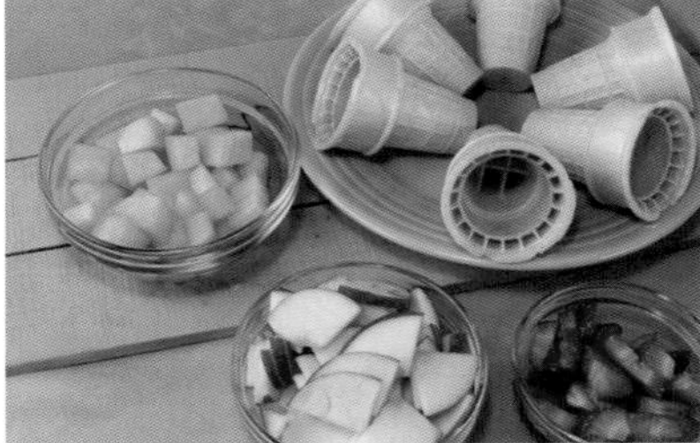
Ingredients

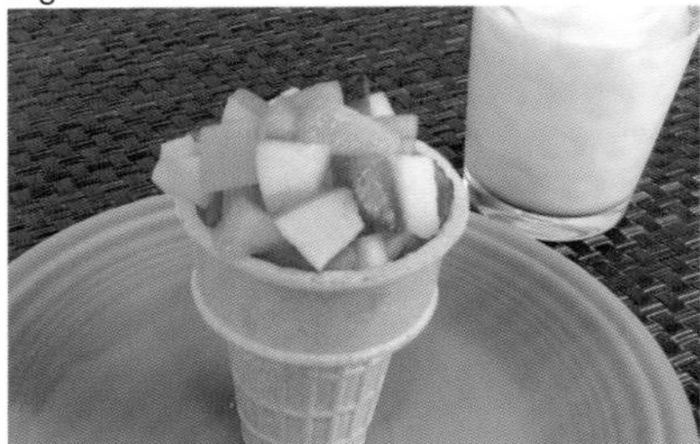
Creditable snack

Ingredients

1 cup cantaloupe, finely diced
½ cup strawberries, finely diced
1½ cups apples, finely diced
6 ice cream cones

Directions

1. In a bowl, combine the fruit.
2. Place ½ cup of fruit in each cone.

Fresh Fruit Cone provides FR at snack			
	Toddler	Pre-School	School Age
Fresh Fruit Cone	1 cone	1 cone	2 cones
Milk	1/2 cup	1/2 cup	1 cup

Fruity Dippers

Prep time - 10 minutes
Cook time - 0 minutes
Total time - 10 minutes

No cook, no bake

Yield - 1½ cups dip

Ingredients

1½ cups plain yogurt
2 tablespoons unsweetened cocoa
1 cup bananas, sliced
1 cup strawberries, sliced
1 cup pears, sliced

Directions

1. Mix the yogurt and cocoa together.
2. Serve with fruit "dippers."

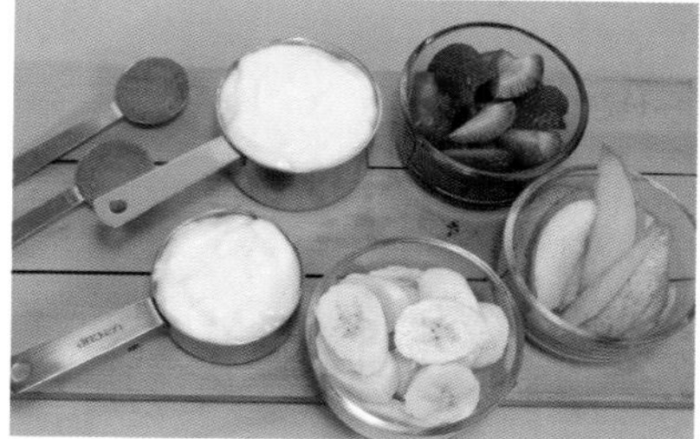

Ingredients

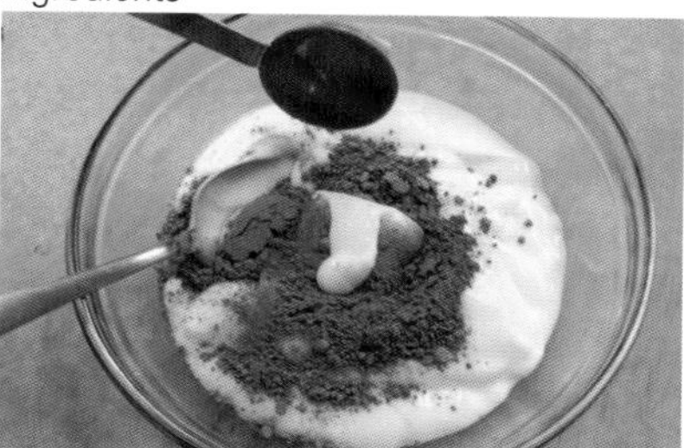

Step 2

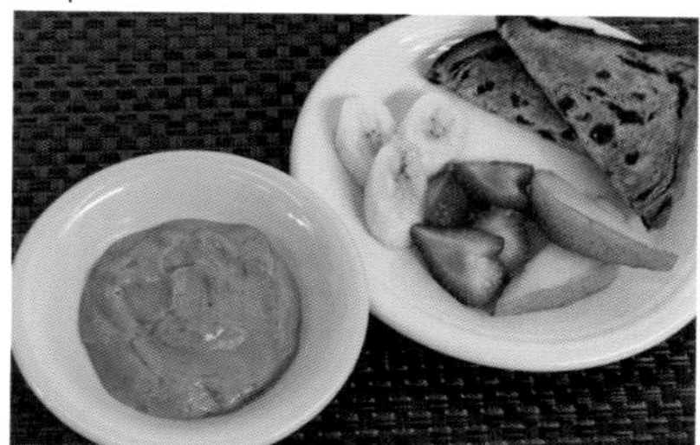

Creditable snack

Fruity Dippers provide M/MA and FR at snack			
	Toddler	Pre-School	School Age
Yogurt	1/4 cup	1/4 cup	1/2 cup
Fruit	1/2 cup	1/2 cup	3/4 cup
Raisin Toast	1/2 oz. or 1/2 slice	1/2 oz. or 1/2 slice	1 oz. or 1 slice

Mini Fruit Pizza

Prep time - 15 minutes
Cook time - 0 minutes
Total time - 15 minutes

No cook, no bake

Yield - 6 fruit pizzas

Ingredients

3 whole wheat English muffins, at least 1½ ounces each, split
2 cups frozen mixed berries, thawed and drained
1 cup peaches, drained and chopped
⅜ cup vanilla yogurt

Directions

1. Lay out muffin halves on a work surface.
2. In a bowl, mix the berries and peaches.
3. Spread 1 tablespoon of yogurt on each muffin half. Top with ¼ cup fruit and serve remaining fruit on the side.

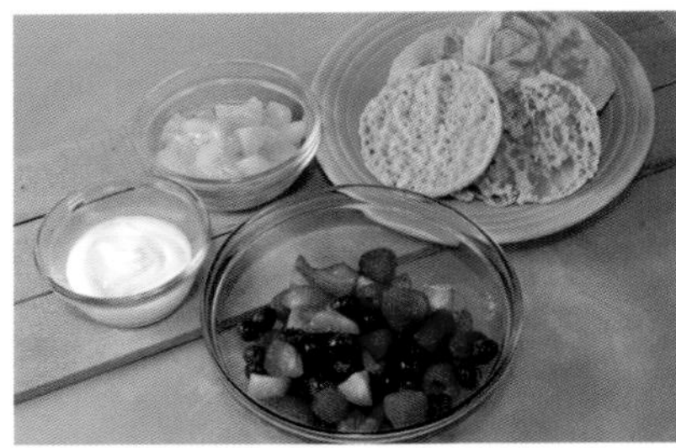

Ingredients

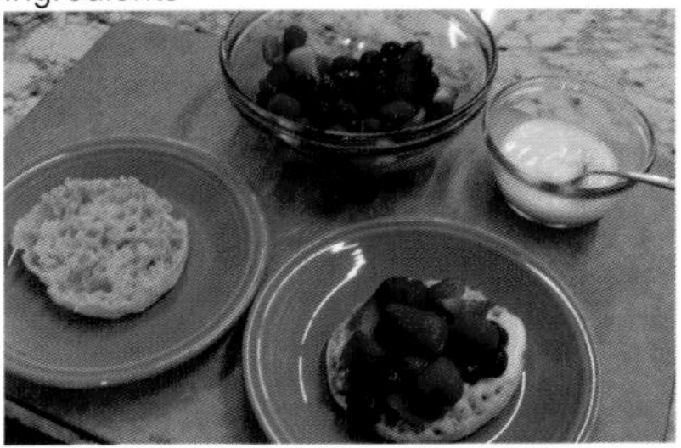

Step 3

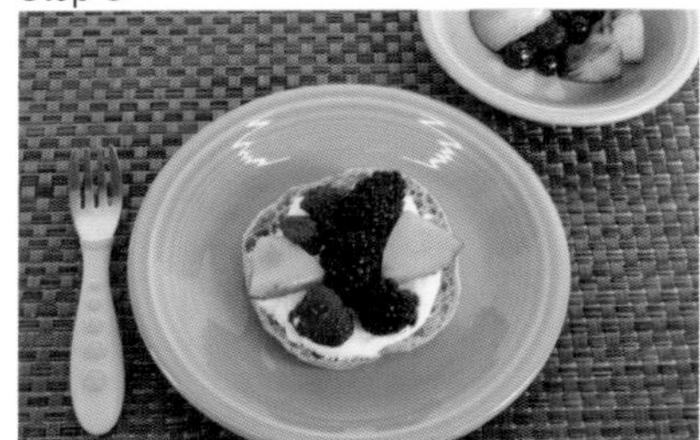

Creditable snack

Mini Fruit Pizza provides G/B and FR at snack			
	Toddler	Pre-School	School Age
Mini Fruit Pizza	1 round	1 round	2 rounds
Extra Fruit	1/4 cup	1/4 cup	3/8 cup

Broccoli-Cheese Quesadillas

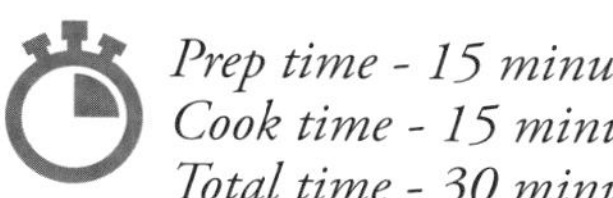

Prep time - 15 minutes
Cook time - 15 minutes
Total time - 30 minutes

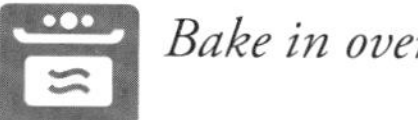

Bake in oven

Yield - 3 quesadillas

Ingredients

2 tablespoons butter
4 cups broccoli, finely chopped
6 6-inch whole wheat tortillas
1½ tablespoons vegetable oil
¾ cup (3 ounces) shredded mozzarella cheese
¾ cup salsa

Directions

1. Preheat oven to 400 degrees. Line baking sheet with foil or parchment paper, or coat with cooking spray.
2. Add butter to skillet and melt over medium heat. Add broccoli and cook until tender, about 7 minutes.
3. Brush one side of each tortilla with the oil and place, oiled side down, on baking sheet.
4. Spread the broccoli evenly over each tortilla, followed by ¼ cup of cheese. Top each with another tortillas, oiled side up, and place on the baking sheet.
5. Bake until cheese melts, about 8 minutes. Rotate pan halfway through baking.
6. Serve with two tablespoons of salsa.

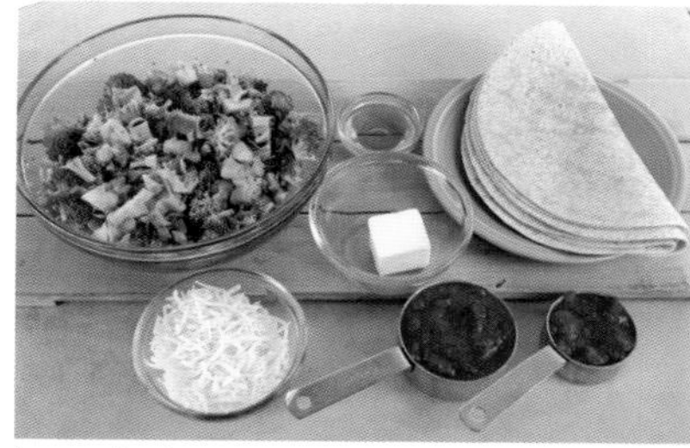

Ingredients

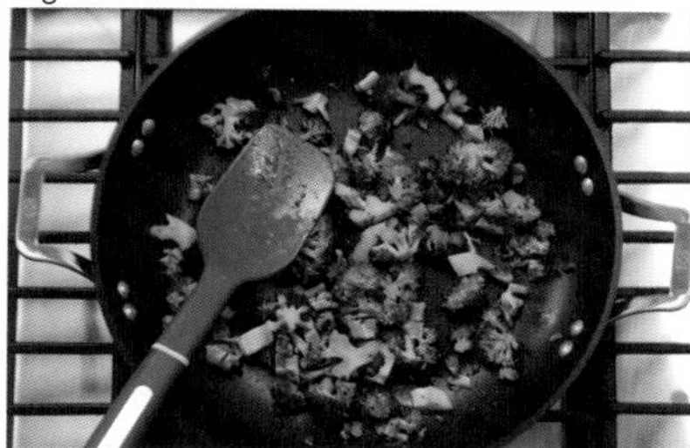

Step 2

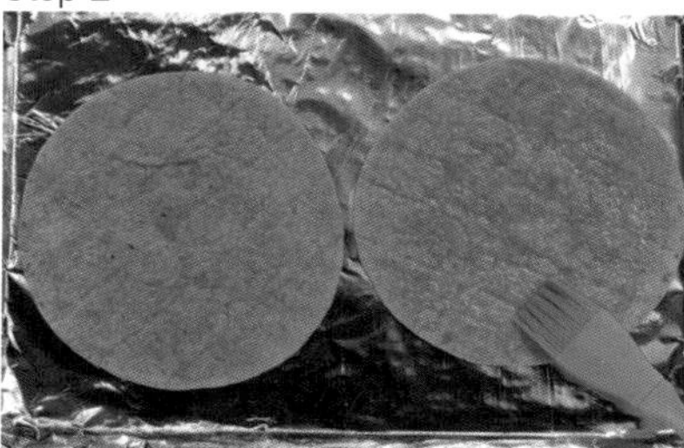

Step 3

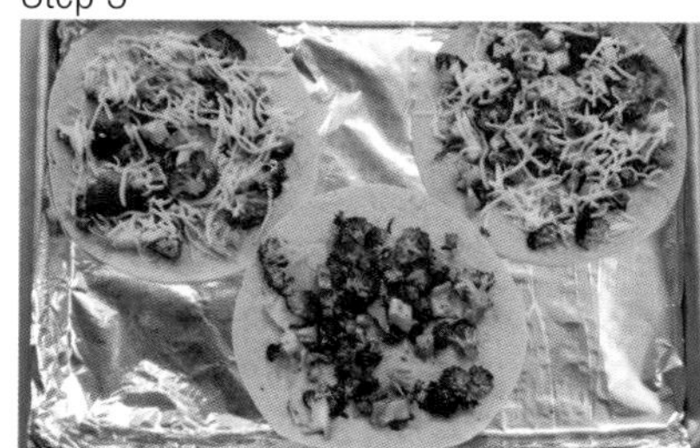

Step 4

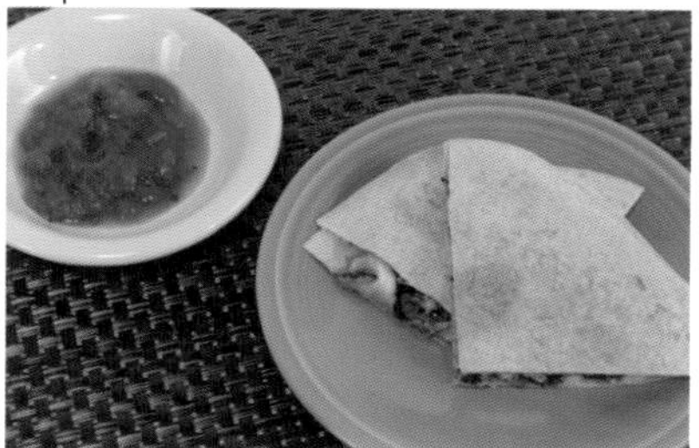

Creditable snack

Broccoli-Cheese Quesadillas
provide G/B, M/MA and VEG at snack

	Toddler	Pre-School	School Age
Quesadillas	1/2 quesadilla	1/2 quesadilla	1 quesadilla

Cheesy Baked Broccoli Bites

Prep time - 15 minutes
Cook time - 20 minutes
Total time - 35 minutes

Bake in oven

Yield - 4 cups

Ingredients

4 cups frozen broccoli florets
1 cup (4 ounces) shredded cheddar cheese
1 egg
2 tablespoons water
½ cup plain bread crumbs

Directions

1. Preheat oven to 350 degrees. Line baking sheet with foil or parchment paper, or coat with cooking spray.
2. Cook broccoli according to package directions, about 10 minutes.
3. Once cool to the touch, place broccoli in a colander lined with paper towels and squeeze out the excess moisture.
4. In a bowl, whisk the egg and water. Mix the bread crumbs and cheese in a separate bowl.
5. Dip the broccoli in the egg wash and then into the bread crumb mixture and place on the baking sheet.
6. Bake until golden brown, about 10-15 minutes.

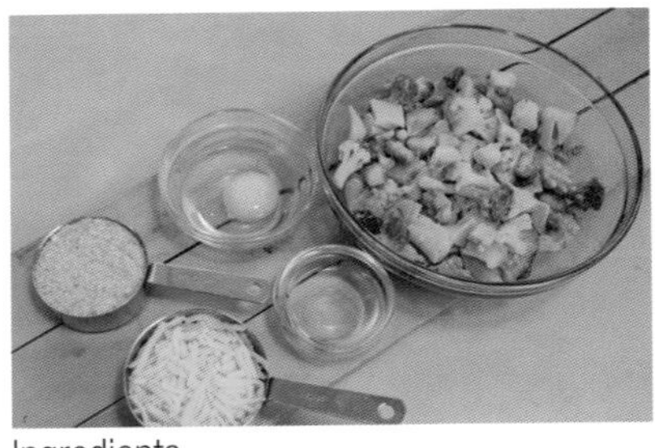

Ingredients

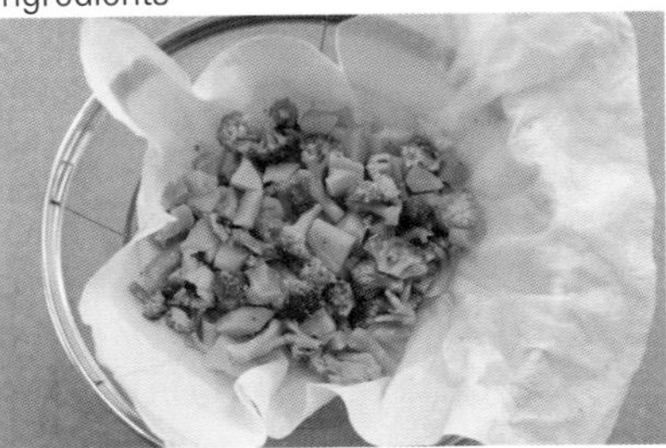

Step 3

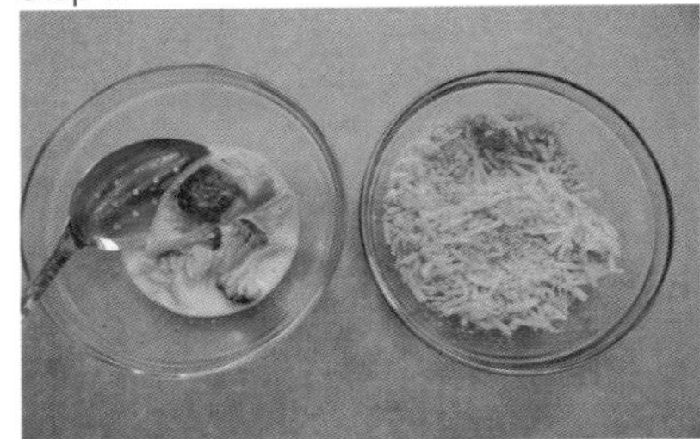

Step 5

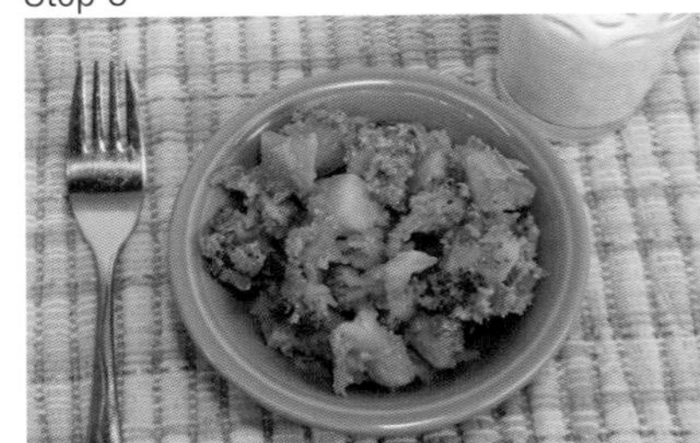

Creditable snack

Cheesy Baked Broccoli Bites provide M/MA and VEG at snack			
	Toddler	Pre-School	School Age
Broccoli Bites	2/3 cup	2/3 cup	1 cup

Cheesy Zucchini Sticks

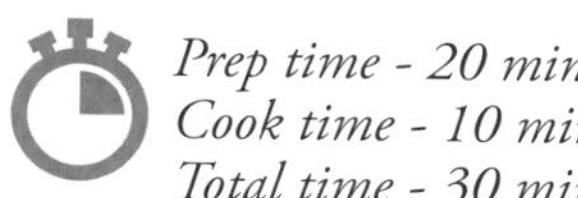
Prep time - 20 minutes
Cook time - 10 minutes
Total time - 30 minutes

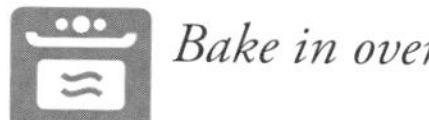
Bake in oven

Yield - 6 zucchini sticks

Ingredients

2 medium zucchini
6 1-ounce sticks string cheese
½ cup seasoned bread crumbs
2 eggs
1 tablespoon water
1 tablespoon vegetable oil

Directions

1. Preheat oven to 400 degrees. Line a baking sheet with foil or parchment paper, or coat with cooking spray.
2. With a vegetable peeler or mandolin, slice zucchini lengthwise into thin ribbons.
3. Wrap each cheese stick with zucchini ribbons and secure with toothpicks.
4. In a small bowl, beat eggs and water together. Place bread crumbs in a separate bowl.
5. Dip each zucchini-wrapped cheese stick in the egg mixture and then coat completely with the bread crumbs.
6. Place on baking sheet and brush with the oil.
7. Bake until golden and the cheese begins to melt, about 10 minutes.
8. Remove toothpicks before serving.
9. Serve with warmed marinara sauce.

Cheesy Zucchini Sticks
provide M/MA at snack

	Toddler	Pre-School	School Age
Zucchini Sticks	1 stick	1 stick	2 sticks
Marinara Sauce	2 tablespoons	2 tablespoons	4 tablespoons
Milk	1/2 cup	1/2 cup	1 cup

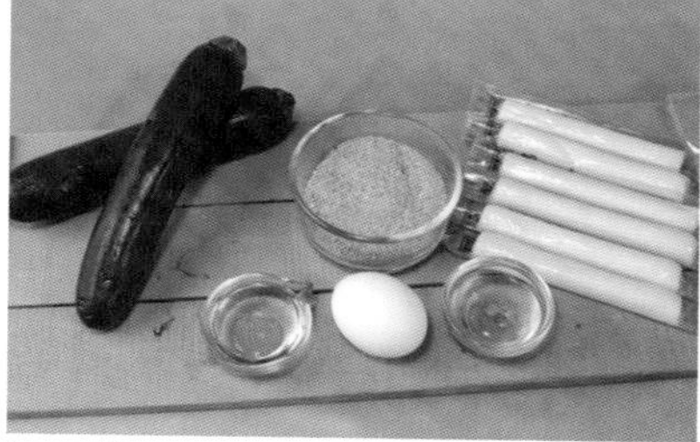
Ingredients

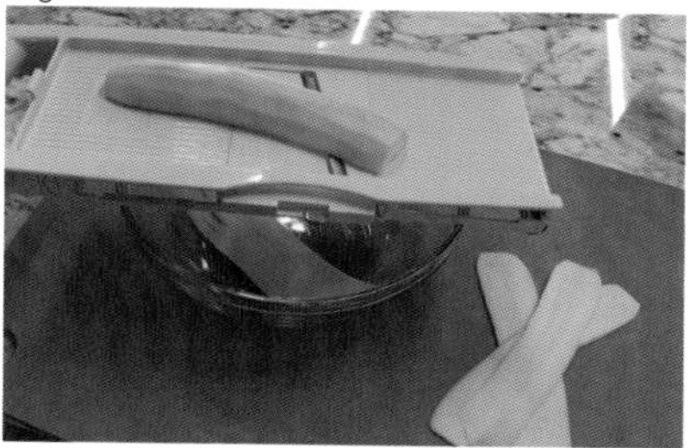
Step 2

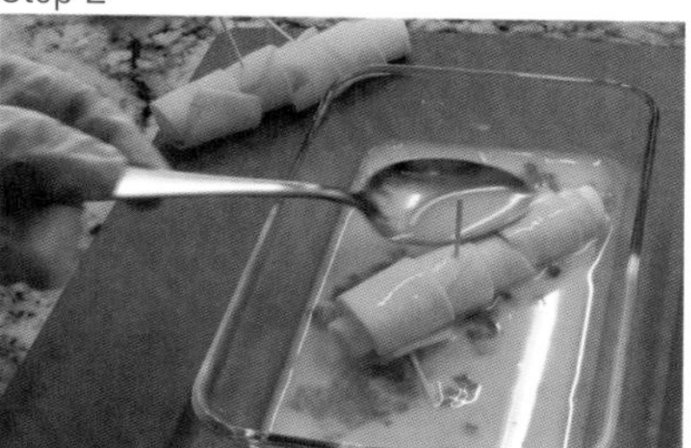
Step 5a

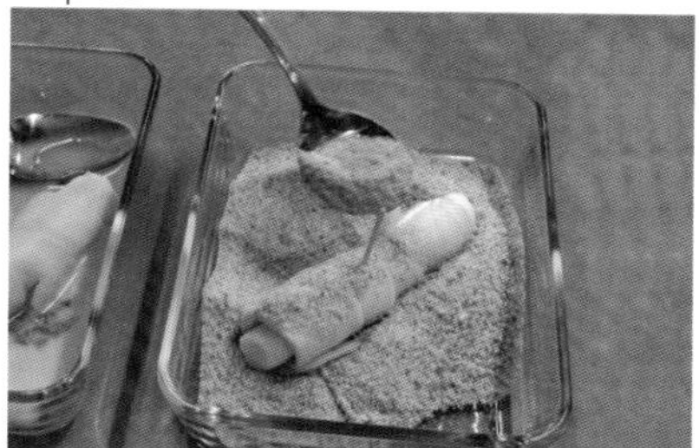
Step 5b

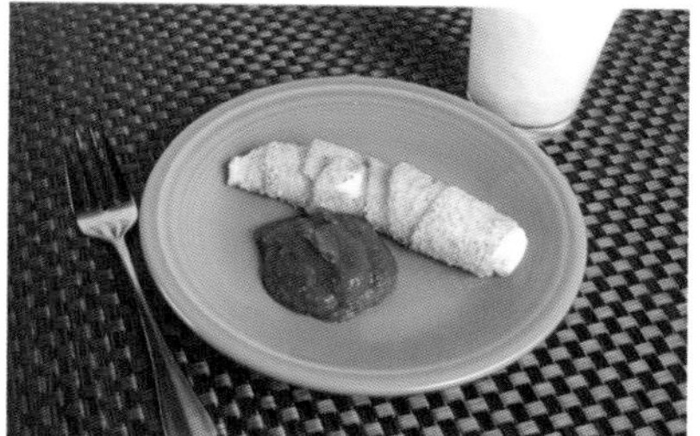
Creditable snack

Potato Nachos

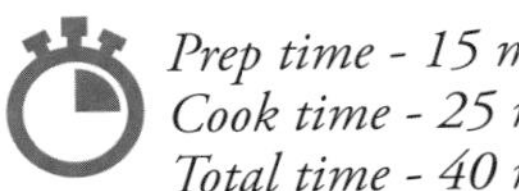

Prep time - 15 minutes
Cook time - 25 minutes.
Total time - 40 minutes

Bake in oven

Yield - 18 wedges

Ingredients

3 8-ounce russet potatoes, each cut into 6 thick wedges
1½ tablespoons vegetable oil
½ teaspoon taco seasoning
½ teaspoon garlic salt
½ cup black beans, rinsed and drained
¼ cup tomatoes, diced
¼ cup green onions, sliced
1 cup (4 ounces) shredded cheddar cheese

Directions

1. Preheat oven to 425 degrees. Line a baking sheet with foil or parchment paper, or coat with cooking spray.
2. In a small bowl, stir together the oil, taco seasoning and garlic salt.
3. Place the potato wedges in a large bowl and brush with the seasoned oil to coat completely.
4. Spread potatoes in a single layer on baking sheet and bake, turning occasionally, until potatoes are golden brown and crispy, about 25 to 30 minutes.
5. Shortly before potatoes are done, heat the black beans until warmed through.
6. Transfer potato wedges from baking sheet to a large plate. Top with the black beans, diced tomatoes, green onions and cheese.

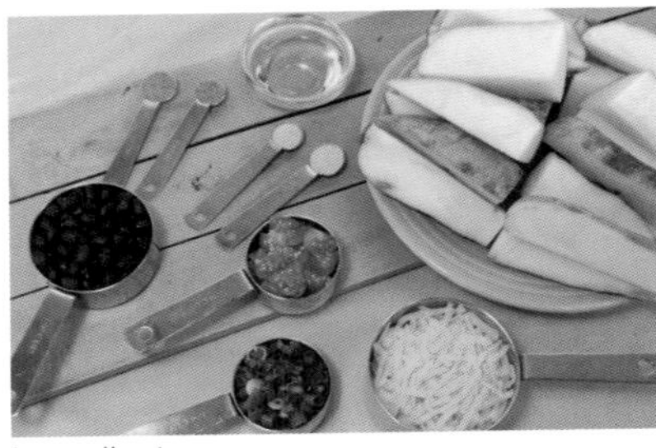

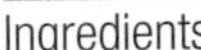

Ingredients

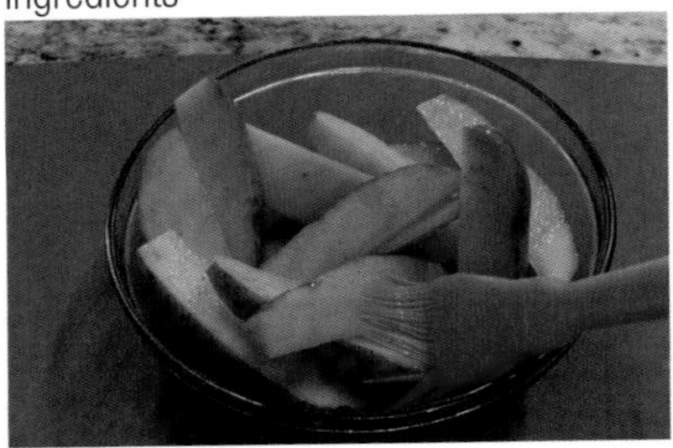

Step 3

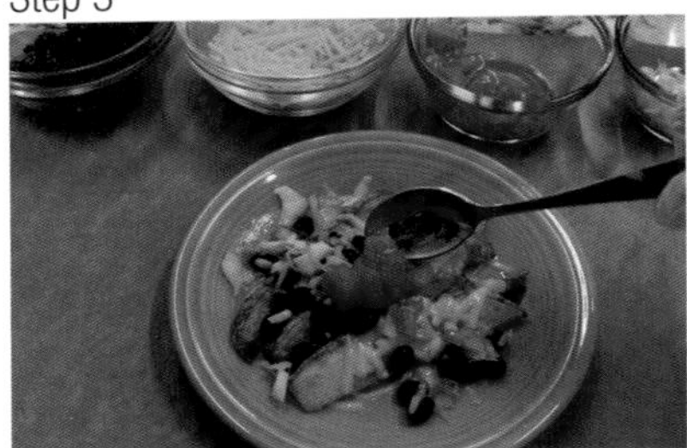

Step 6

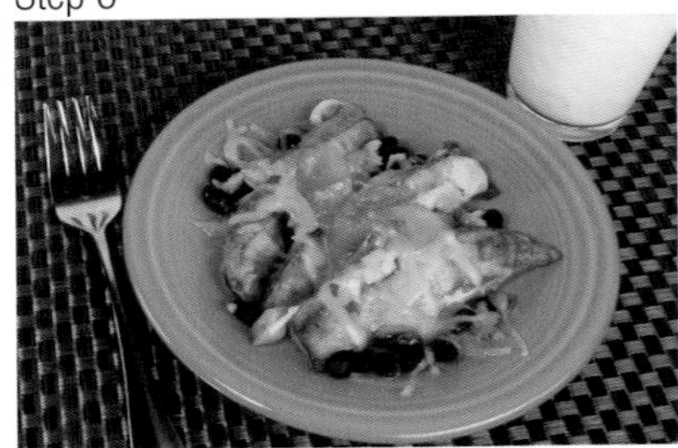

Creditable snack

Potato Nachos provide M/MA and VEG at snack			
	Toddler	Pre-School	School Age
Potato Nachos	3 wedges	3 wedges	5 wedges

Veggie Kebabs

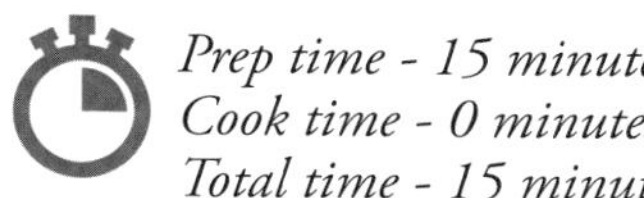

Prep time - 15 minutes
Cook time - 0 minutes
Total time - 15 minutes

No cook, no bake

Yield - 6 kebabs

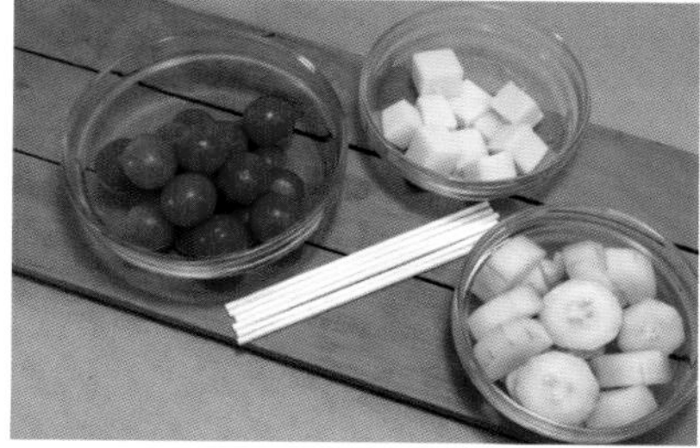
Ingredients

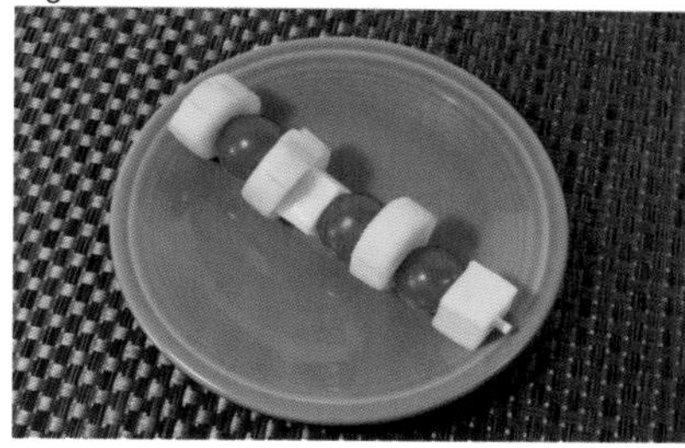
Creditable snack

Ingredients

3 ounces chunk mozzarella cheese, cut into 12 ½-inch cubes
1½ cups cherry tomatoes
1½ cups cucumbers, peeled and cubed
6 child-safe sticks

Directions

1. Using child-safe lollipop sticks or thin drinking straws, thread a cherry tomato, cucumber cube and cheese cube and repeat. Each kabob should have ½ ounce of cheese (2 cubes) and ½ cup of vegetables.

Veggie Kebabs provide M/MA and VEG at snack			
	Toddler	Pre-School	School Age
Veggie Kebabs	1 kebab	1 kebab	2 kebabs

Veggie Pita Pizza

Prep time - 15 minutes
Cook time - 15 minutes
Total time - 30 minutes

Bake in oven

Yield - 6 pizza rounds

Ingredients

3 whole wheat pita bread rounds, at least 1½ ounces each
3 tablespoons grated Parmesan cheese
1½ cups (6 ounces) shredded mozzarella cheese
1 teaspoon Italian seasoning
1 cup fresh roma tomatoes, seeded and diced
½ cup chopped spinach,
—if frozen, thawed and moisture squeezed out

Directions

1. Preheat oven to 425 degrees. Line two baking sheets with foil or parchment paper or coat with cooking spray.
2. With a knife, cut the pita bread in half crosswise to make 6 rounds.
3. In a bowl, combine the cheeses with the Italian seasoning.
4. In a separate bowl, combine tomatoes and spinach.
5. Place pita rounds on baking sheet and top each with ¼ cup of the tomato/spinach mix. Sprinkle each round with ¼ cup cheese.
6. Bake for 15 minutes or until cheese is melted and pita is crispy.

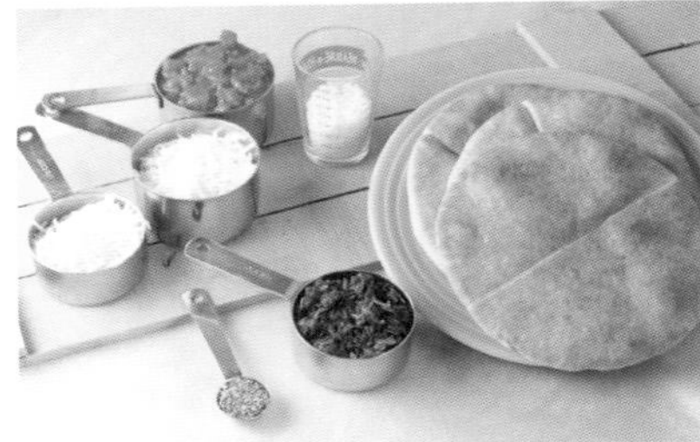

Ingredients

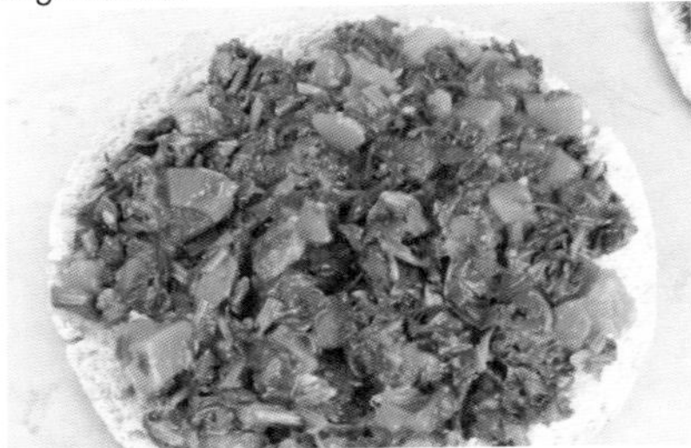

Step 5

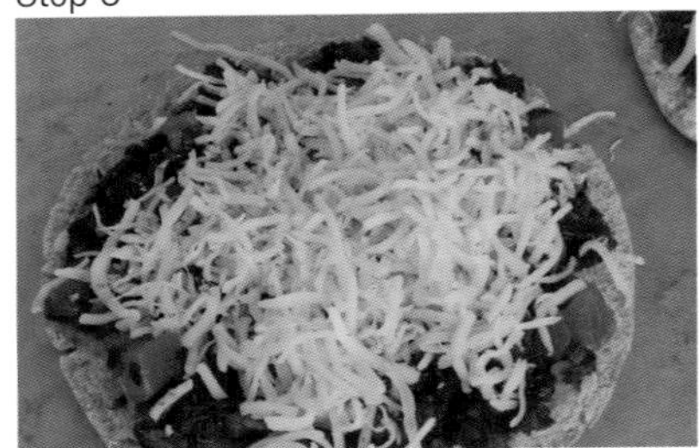

Step 6

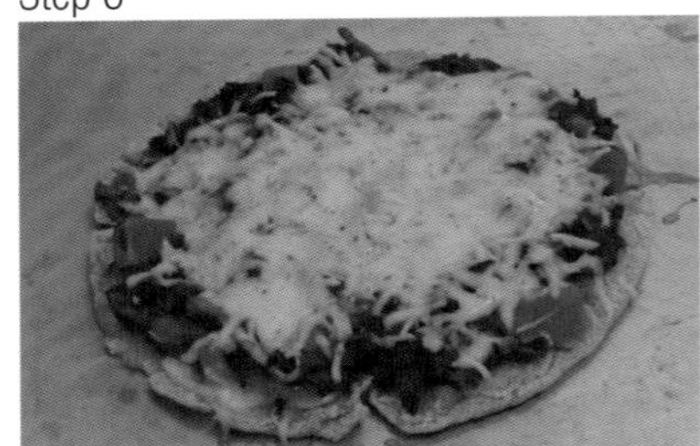

Step 7

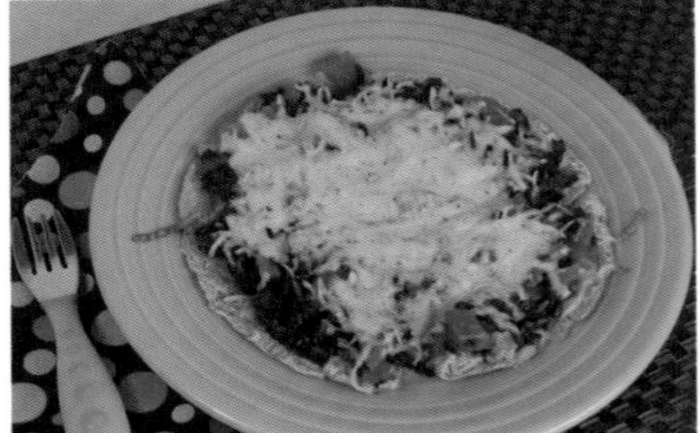

Creditable snack

Veggie Pita Pizza
provides G/B and M/MA at snack

	Toddler	Pre-School	School Age
Veggie Pita Pizza	1 round	1 round	2 rounds

Carrot Swirl Bites

Prep time - 10 minutes
Cook time - 0 minutes
Total time - 15 minutes

No cook, no bake

Yield - 12 swirl bites

Ingredients

3 8-inch whole wheat tortillas
6 tablespoons plain cream cheese
2¼ cups carrots, shredded
¾ cup raisins

Directions

1. Lay tortillas on work surface and spread 2 tablespoons cream cheese on each.
2. Sprinkle ¾ cup grated carrots and ¼ cup raisins on each tortilla and roll up.
3. Slice each tortilla into 4 bites. Serve with cut side up.

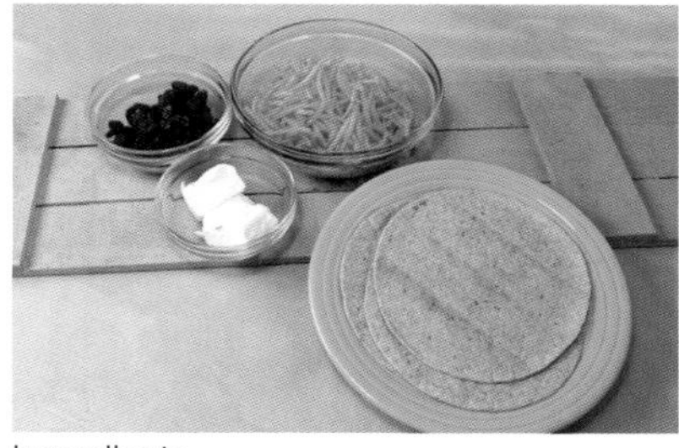

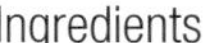

Ingredients

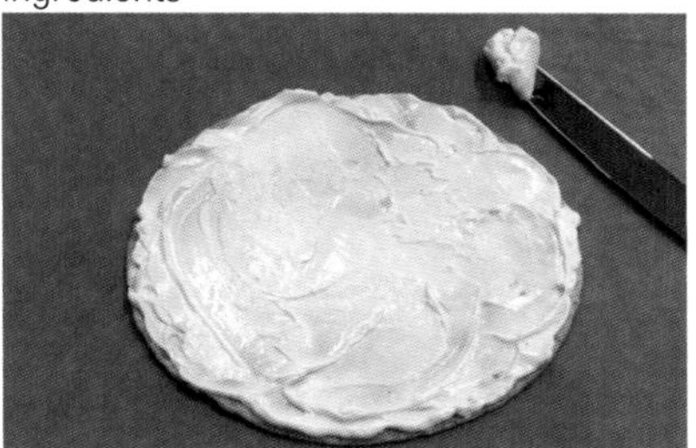

Step 1

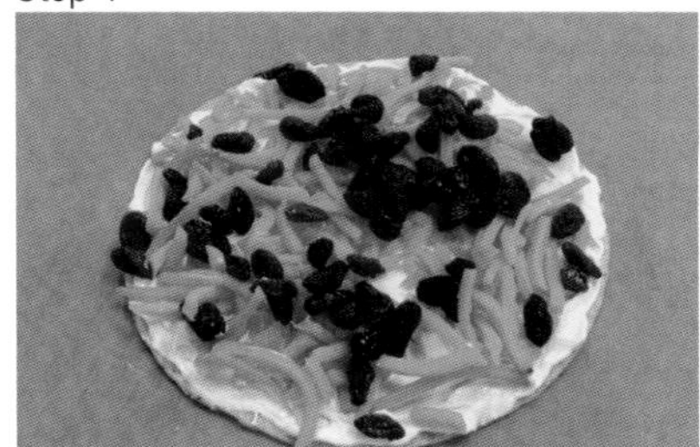

Step 2

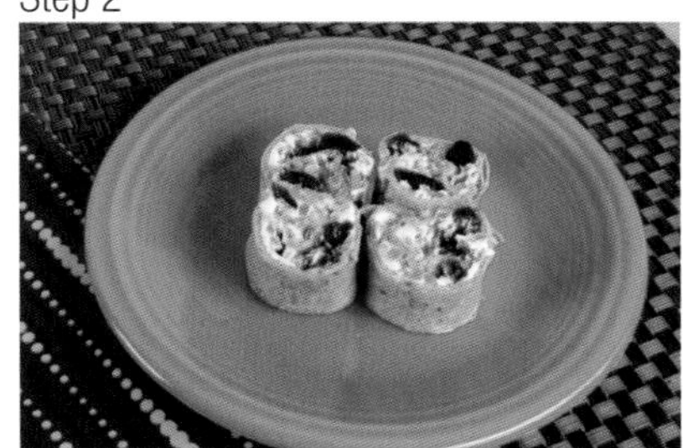

Creditable snack

Carrot Swirl Bites provide G/B and VEG at snack			
	Toddler	Pre-School	School Age
Swirl Bites	2 bites	2 bites	3 bites

Crackerwiches

Prep time - 10 minutes
Cook time - 0 minutes
Total time - 10 minutes

No cook, no bake

Yield - 12 crackerwiches

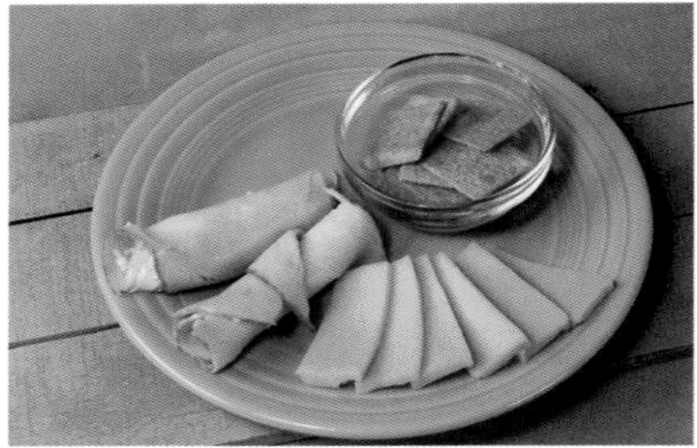
Ingredients

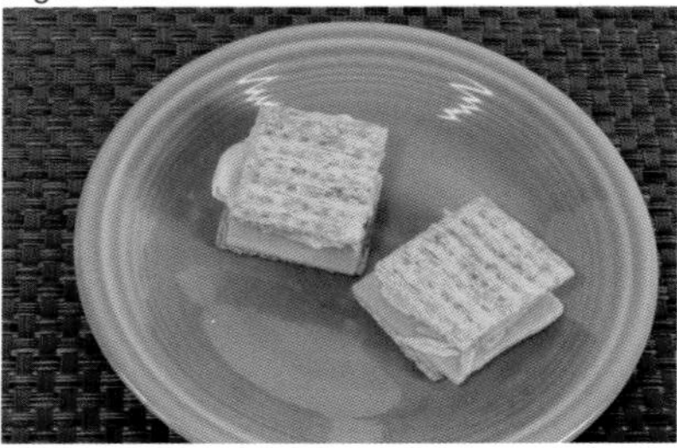
Creditable snack

Ingredients

3 1-ounce slices cheddar cheese
3 ounces turkey, thinly sliced
24 whole wheat crackers, at least 6 ounces total

Directions

1. Cut each slice of cheese into 4 squares.
2. Cut each slice of turkey into squares of the same size.
3. Assemble ingredients as follows: 1 cracker, 1 square cheese (¼ ounce), 1 square turkey (¼ ounce), 1 cracker.

Crackerwiches provide G/B and M/MA at snack			
	Toddler	Pre-School	School Age
Crackerwiches	2	2	4

Ham Pinwheels

Prep time - 15 minutes
Cook time - 2 minutes
Total time - 17 minutes

Bake in oven

Yield - 12 pinwheels

Ingredients

3 8-inch whole wheat tortillas
2½ ounces turkey ham, sliced into strips
⅜ cup (1½ ounces) shredded cheddar cheese

Directions

1. Preheat oven to 400 degrees. Line a baking sheet with foil or parchment paper, or coat with cooking spray.
2. Lay tortillas on baking sheet. Sprinkle ¾ ounce turkey ham and ½ ounce (2 tablespoons) of cheese on each tortilla.
3. Warm in oven just until cheese melts, about 2 minutes.
4. Roll up and slice each tortilla into four pieces.

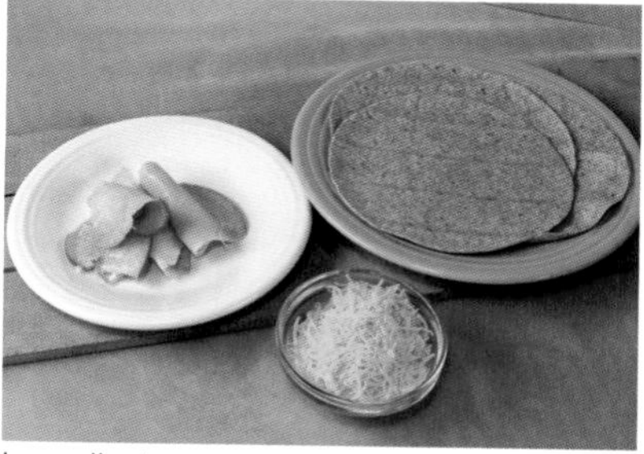

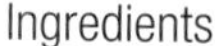

Ingredients

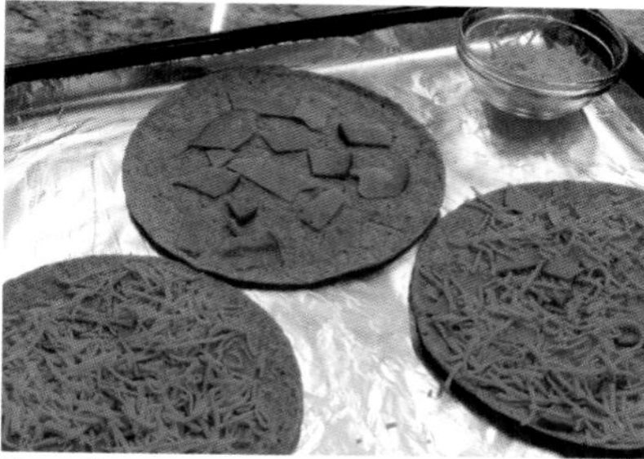

Step 2

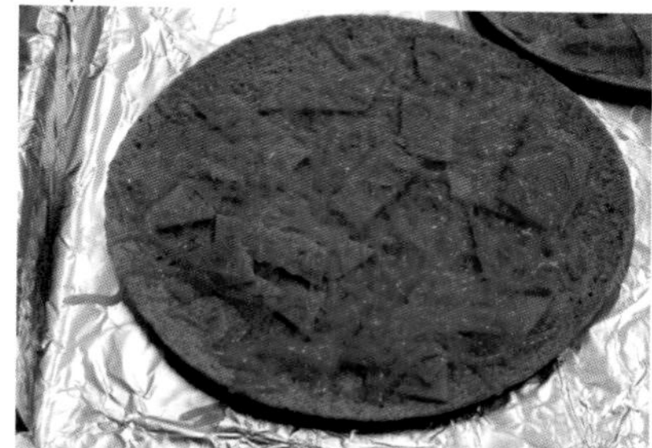

Step 3

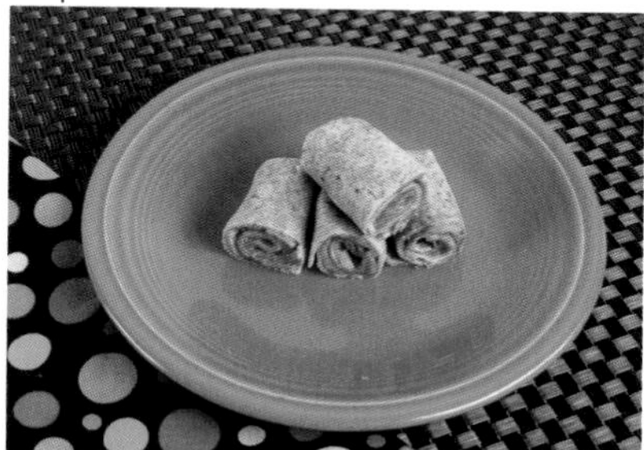

Creditable snack

Ham Pinwheels provide G/B and M/MA at snack			
	Toddler	Pre-School	School Age
Ham Pinwheels	2 pinwheels	2 pinwheels	4 pinwheels

Mini Bagel Cucumber Sandwiches

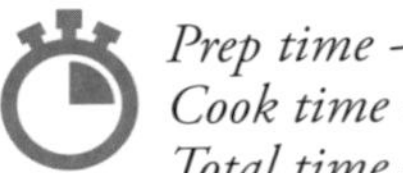

Prep time - 10 minutes
Cook time - 0 minutes
Total time - 10 minutes

No cook, no bake

Yield - 6 sandwiches

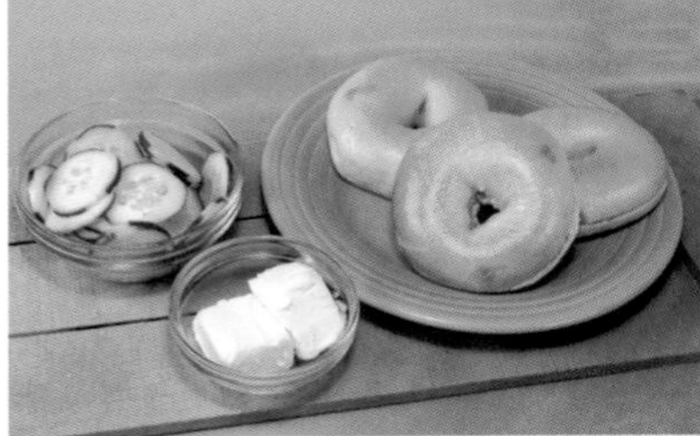
Ingredients

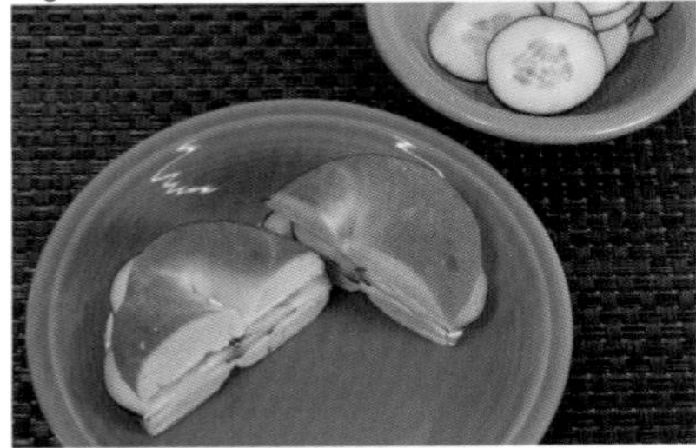
Creditable snack

Ingredients

6 whole wheat mini bagels, at least 1 ounce each
6 tablespoons plain or veggie-flavored cream cheese
3 cups cucumbers, thinly sliced
Salt and pepper to taste

Directions

1. Cut each bagel in half and spread with 1 tablespoon cream cheese.
2. Top with ¼ cup of cucumber slices, salt and pepper, and top with remaining bagel half. Serve remaining cucumbers on the side.

Mini Bagel Cucumber Sandwiches provide G/B and VEG at snack			
	Toddler	Pre-School	School Age
Bagel Sandwich	1 sandwich	1 sandwich	2 sandwiches
Extra Cucumbers	-	-	1/4 cup

Tuna Stackers

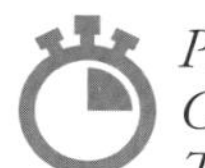

Prep time - 15 minutes
Cook time - 0 minutes
Total time - 15 minutes

No cook, no bake

Yield - 12 stackers

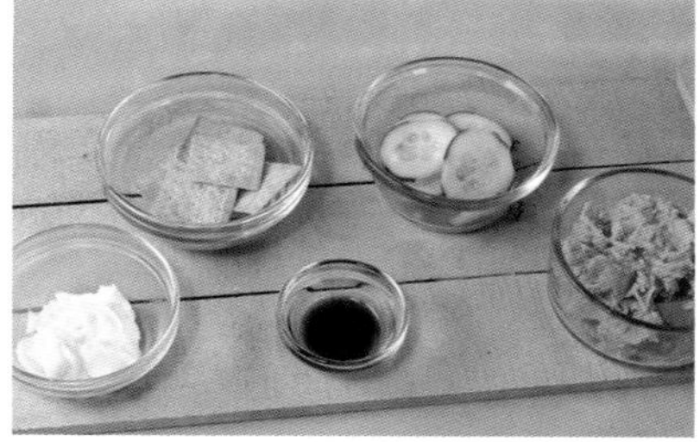

Ingredients

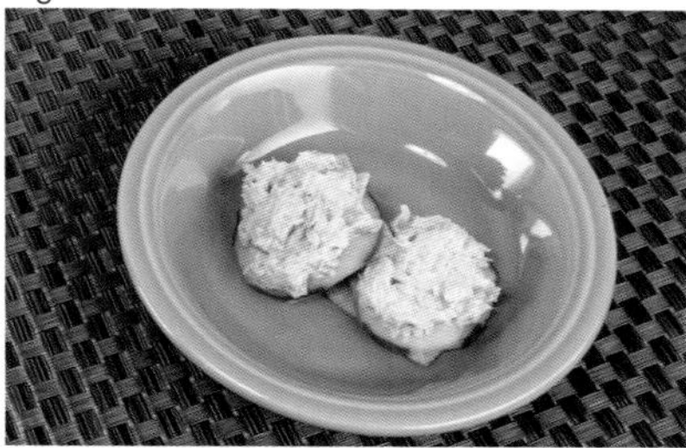

Creditable snack

Ingredients

3 ounces water-packed tuna, drained
3 tablespoons mayonnaise
½ teaspoon soy sauce
12 wheat crackers, at least 3 ounces total
¼ cup cucumbers, sliced

Directions

1. In a bowl, combine the tuna, mayonnaise and soy sauce. Mix well.
2. Top each cracker with a cucumber slice and then with a portion of the tuna salad.

Tuna Stackers provide G/B and M/MA at snack			
	Toddler	Pre-School	School Age
Tuna Stackers	2 stackers	2 stackers	4 stackers

Apple-Cinnamon Yogurt

Prep time - 5 minutes
Cook time - 0 minutes
Total time - 5 minutes

No cook, no bake

Yield - 2½ cups

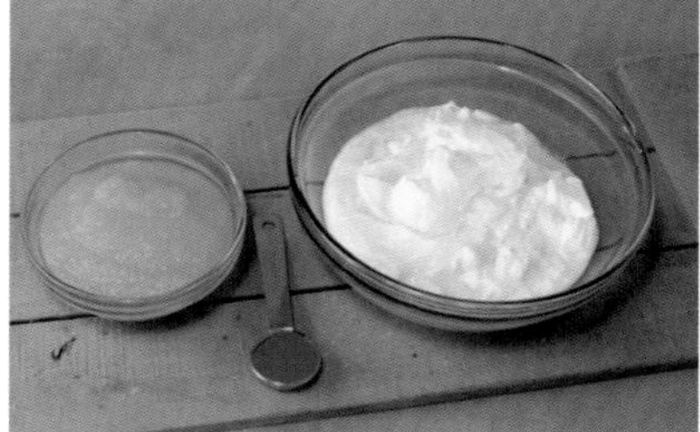
Ingredients

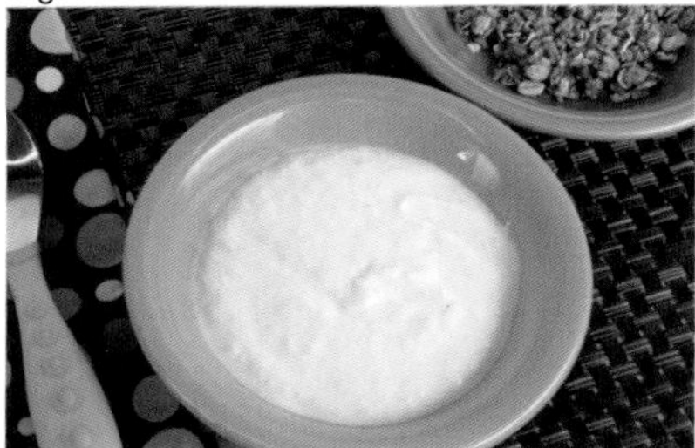
Creditable snack

Ingredients

1½ cups plain yogurt
1 cup unsweetened applesauce
1 teaspoon ground cinnamon

Directions

1. Mix all ingredients together. Spoon into dishes and serve.

Apple-Cinnamon Yogurt provides M/MA at snack			
	Toddler	Pre-School	School Age
Yogurt	1/4 cup	1/4 cup	1/2 cup
Granola	1/8 cup	1/8 cup	1/4 cup

Cream Cheese Bagel Butterflies

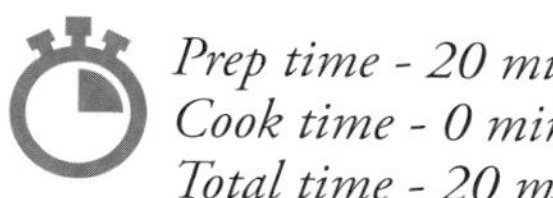

Prep time - 20 minutes
Cook time - 0 minutes
Total time - 20 minutes

No cook, no bake

Yield - 6 bagel halves

Ingredients

3 whole wheat bagels, at least 1½ ounces each
3 cups strawberries, sliced and divided
6 tablespoons plain cream cheese

Directions

1. Cut each bagel in half.
1. Reserve 1½ cups strawberries for side serving. Also, set aside 24 strawberry slices to make the "butterflies."
2. Place the remaining strawberries and the cream cheese into a food processor or blender. Pulse just a few times to make strawberry cream cheese.
3. Spread 1 tablespoon of cream cheese on each bagel half. Then arrange slices of strawberries to look like a butterfly.
4. Serve the remaining sliced strawberries on the side.

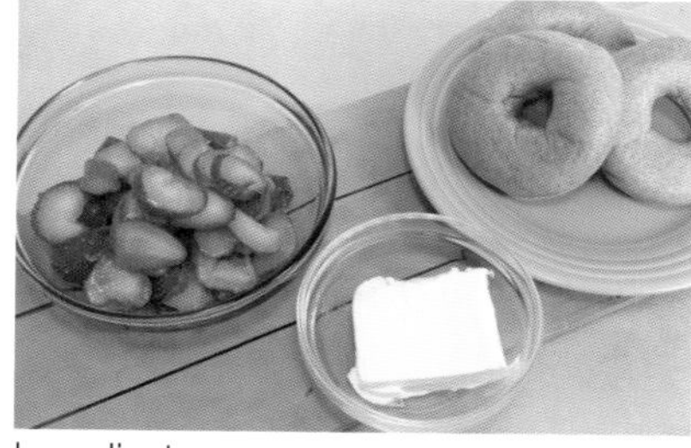

Ingredients

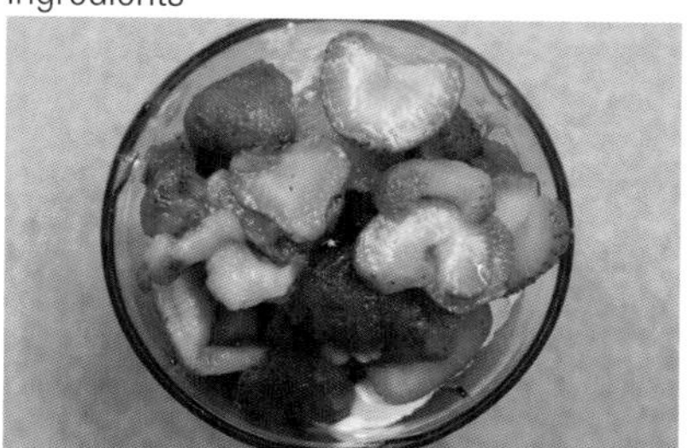

Step 2

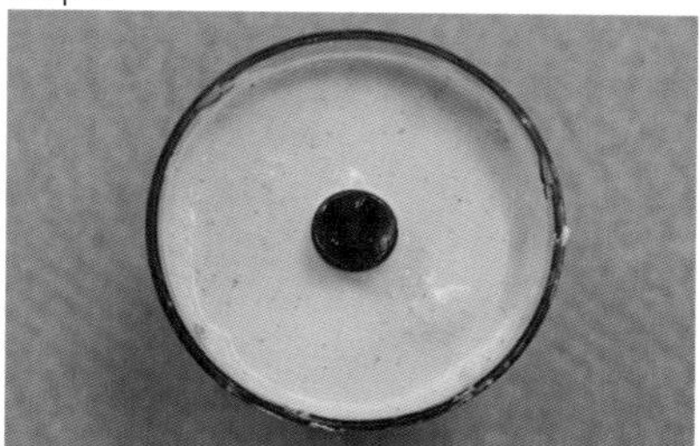

Step 3

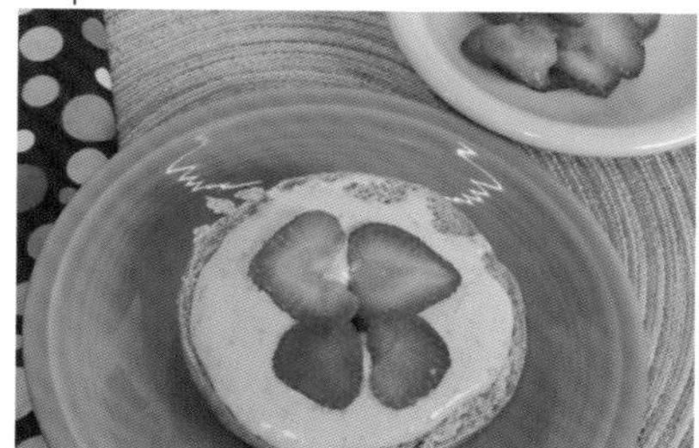

Creditable snack

Cream Cheese Bagel Butterflies provide G/B and FR at snack			
	Toddler	Pre-School	School Age
Bagel Butterflies	1/2 bagel	1/2 bagel	1 bagel
Extra Strawberries	1/4 cup	1/4 cup	3/8 cup

Fruity Toast Snacks

Prep time - 15 minutes
Cook time - 5 minutes
Total time - 20 minutes

Toast in toaster or in oven

Yield - 6 snacks

Ingredients

3 slices whole grain bread, at least 1½ ounces each
¾ cups cottage cheese
1 cup bananas, sliced
1 cup strawberries, sliced
1 cup kiwi fruit, peeled and sliced

Directions

1. Toast bread.
1. Spread ¼ cup cottage cheese on each slice of bread, then top with ¼ cup fruit slices. Cut in half.
2. Serve the remaining ¼ cup of fruit on the side.

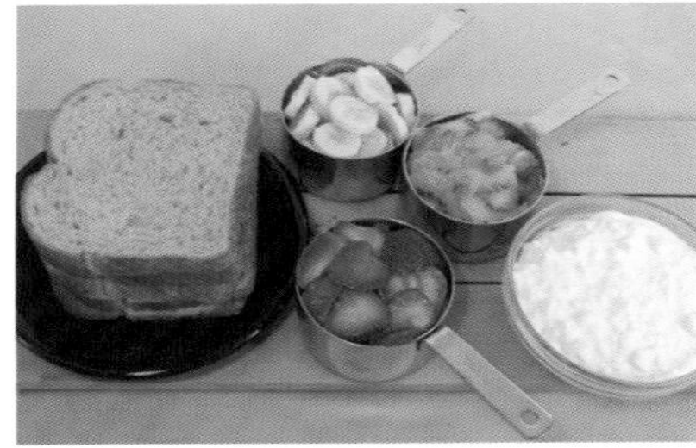

Ingredients

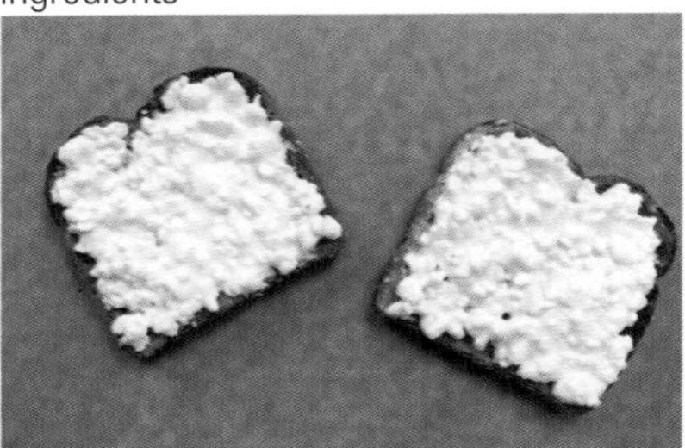

Ingredients

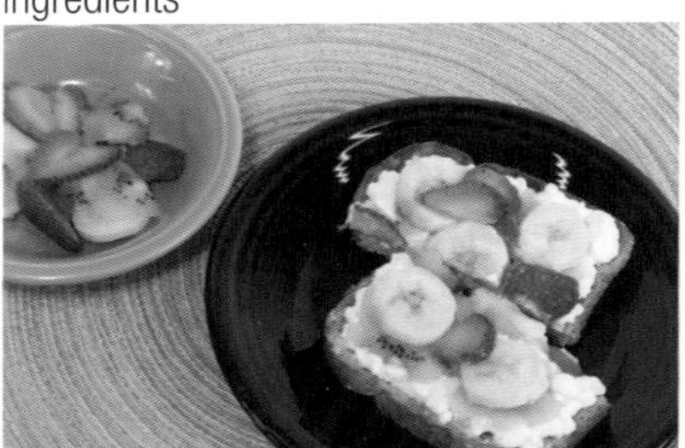

Creditable snack

Fruity Toast Snacks provide G/B and FR at snack			
	Toddler	Pre-School	School Age
Fruity Toast Snacks	1/2 slice	1/2 slice	1 slice
Extra Fruit	1/4 cup	1/4 cup	3/8 cup

Oatmeal Biscuits

Prep time - 15 minutes
Cook time - 10 minutes
Total time - 25 minutes

Bake in oven

Yield - 15 biscuits

Ingredients

1 cup instant oats
¾ cup whole wheat flour
⅓ cup brown sugar
1½ teaspoons baking powder
⅛ teaspoon salt
2 tablespoons butter, softened
1 large egg
1 teaspoon vanilla extract

Directions

1. Preheat to 325 degrees. Line a baking sheet with foil or parchment paper, or coat with cooking spray.
2. In a large bowl, combine oats, flour, baking powder and salt.
3. In another bowl, cream the butter and brown sugar until smooth and fluffy. Add the egg and vanilla. Mix well.
4. Add the dry ingredients to the wet ingredients and mix until dry ingredients are just incorporated. Don't over-mix.
5. Using a 2-ounce scoop, drop batter onto the baking sheet and flatten with a spatula.
6. Bake for 10-12 minutes until semi-firm. Don't overcook. Allow to cool on wire rack.

Variation

Add raisins or chopped nuts.

Oatmeal Biscuits provide G/B at snack			
	Toddler	Pre-School	School Age
Oatmeal Biscuits	1 biscuit	1 biscuit	2 biscuits
Milk	1/2 cup	1/2 cup	1 cup

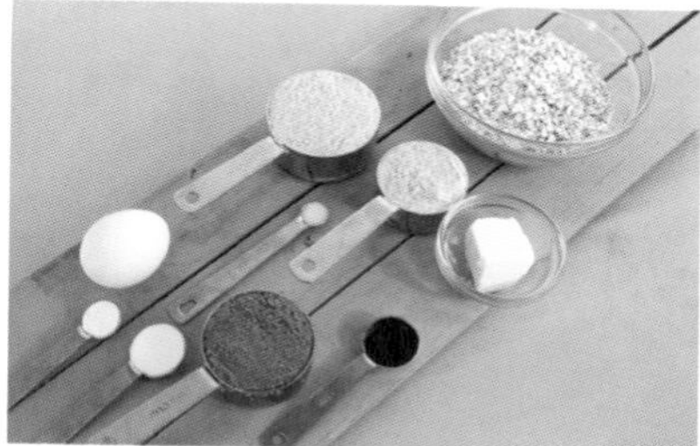

Ingredients

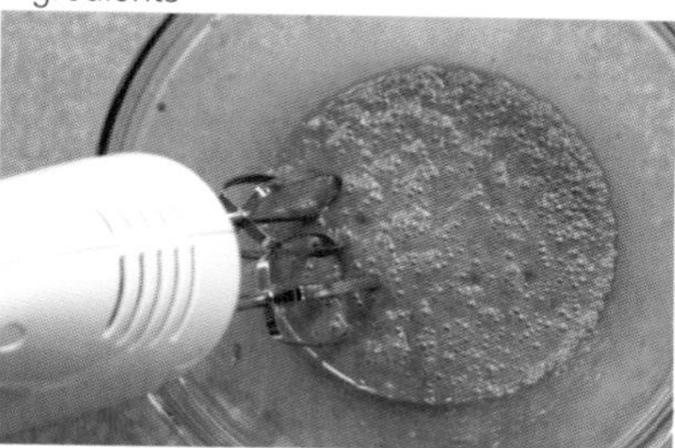

Step 2

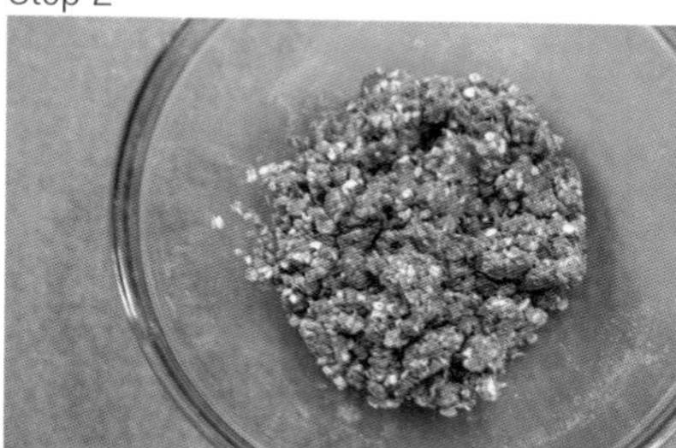

Step 3

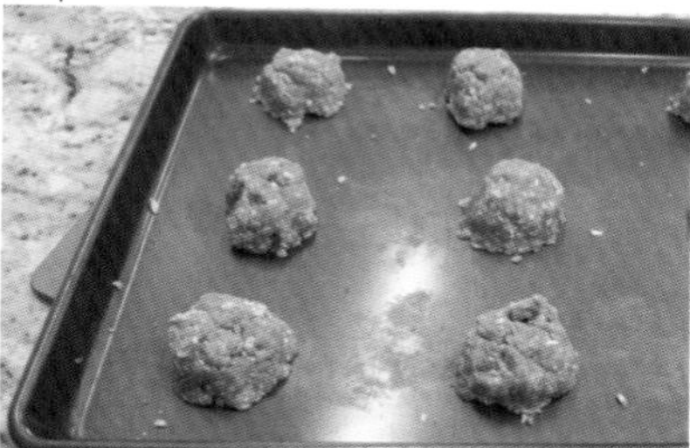

Step 5

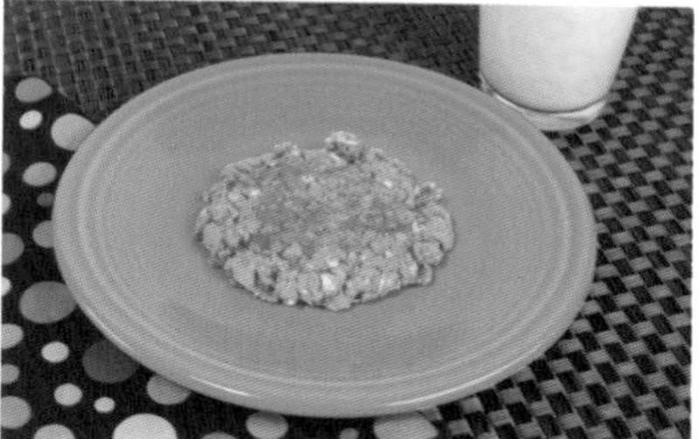

Creditable snack

Raisin Energy Snacks

Prep time - 15 minutes
Cook time - 30 minutes
Total time - 45 minutes

Bake in oven

Yield - 24 snacks

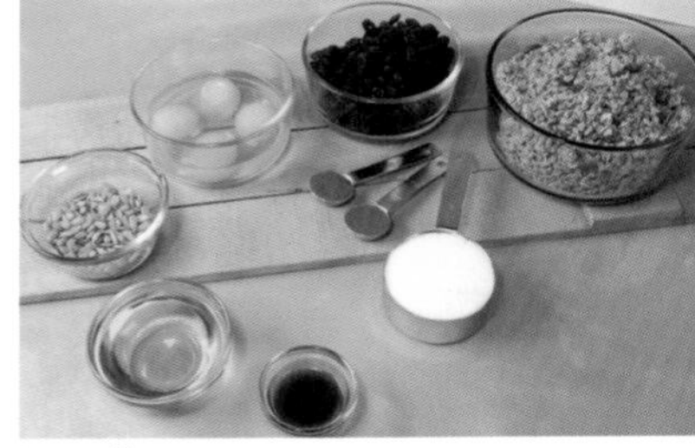
Ingredients

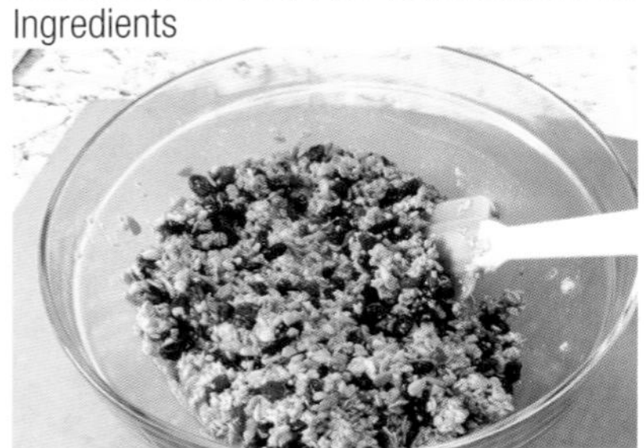
Step 4

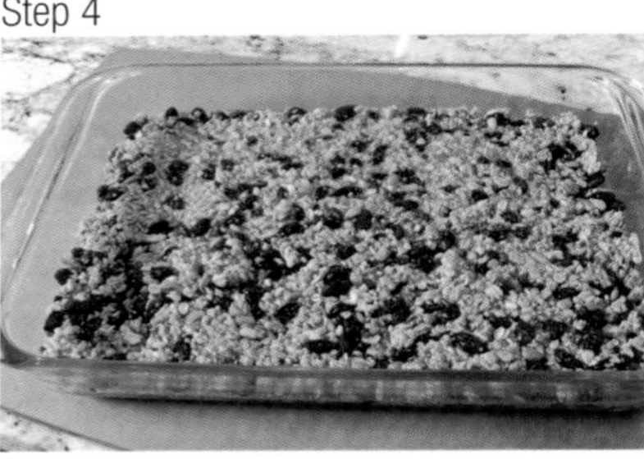
Step 5

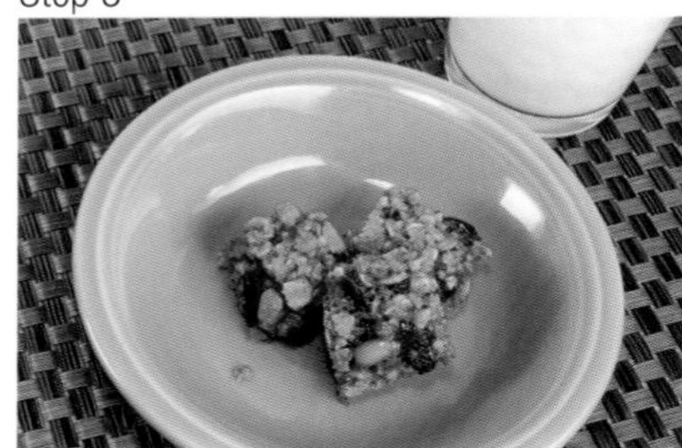
Creditable snack

Ingredients

4 eggs
½ cup sugar
3 tablespoons vegetable oil
2 teaspoons ground cinnamon
1½ teaspoons vanilla extract
3⅓ cups plain granola
2 cups raisins
⅜ cup raw sunflower kernels

Directions

1. Preheat oven to 300 degrees. Grease 9x13-inch baking pan or coat with cooking spray.
2. In a large bowl, beat eggs and sugar with whisk until smooth.
3. Beat in oil, cinnamon and vanilla.
4. Stir in remaining ingredients; mix well.
5. Turn mixture into baking pan and spread evenly.
6. Bake until golden brown, about 30 minutes.
7. Cool 5 minutes in pan. Loosen edges with spatula and invert onto wire rack to cool completely.
8. Cut into 24 squares.

Raisin Energy Snacks provide G/B at snack			
	Toddler	Pre-School	School Age
Energy Snacks	1 square	1 square	2 squares
Milk	1/2 cup	1/2 cup	1 cup

LOOK & COOK

A step-by-step guide to healthy meals in family child care homes

By Partners in Nutrition and
the Chef Marshall O'Brien Group

About the Authors

Partners in Nutrition

Partners in Nutrition's mission is to increase access to nutritious food for children attending early care and education programs, with specific emphasis on children from low-income households and communities of color.

Our primary lever is increasing participation in the USDA Child and Adult Care Food Program (CACFP) among eligible programs. The CACFP is a federal food support program that provides funds to eligible early care and education programs for serving meals and snacks that meet the meal pattern requirements. Partners in Nutrition engages in outreach to eligible programs and provides culturally-specific training and technical assistance to support participation.

We also provide training to program owners, directors and teachers, including training required for licensing, national accreditation programs and Quality Rating and Improvement Systems. We have several publications that support early care and education providers and also provide consulting services to support general center operations, including compliance checks for licensing requirements and paperwork audits.

In addition to programmatic work, we also work on policies and systems change. Specifically, we participate in local, regional, statewide and national coalitions that have missions aligned with our own. We also actively seek to identify barriers to healthy food access in early care and education programs, and lead community-driven solutions to remove those barriers, including through policy change and administrative rule making.

Chef Marshall O'Brien Group

The Chef Marshall O'Brien Group's mission is to help children and families eat more nutritious food, that will allow them to lead happier, healthier lives. We strive to teach people that nourishing is different from eating. When we eat nourishing food, we perform better in everything we do.

The Group is made up of chefs, dietitians, researchers, writers and videographers. The role of the researchers and dietitians is to understand current best nutrition practices and translate these practices into the right foods that produce the desired results. Since people will only eat the right foods if they taste good, our chefs use the recommended foods to create recipes that taste great. We call this "Putting Delicious in Nutritious."

The Chef Marshall O'Brien Group works with home-based early care providers and centers, schools, the YMCA, fire, police and public works departments, cities and corporations on staff wellness and nutrition strategies that help people perform better. We love early care providers, centers and schools because children are the future of this country. When children are provided the right nutrition, they develop to their full potential, both physically and mentally, and learn lessons that will help them throughout their lives.

In producing this book, we hope to provide a tool for home providers and centers that makes it easier for them to do the wonderful work they do in nourishing our children. We are proud to join with Partners in Nutrition on this project.

Index